Mad Cows and Mother's Milk

Mad Cows and Mother's Milk

The Perils of Poor Risk Communication

WILLIAM LEISS AND

DOUGLAS POWELL

Second Edition

McGill-Queen's University Press
Montreal & Kingston • London • Ithaca

© McGill-Queen's University Press 2004
ISBN 0-7735-2817-2

Legal deposit fourth quarter 2004
Bibliothèque nationale du Québec

First edition 1997
Printed in Canada on acid-free paper

McGill-Queen's University Press acknowledges the
support of the Canada Council for the Arts for our
publishing program. We also acknowledge the financial
support of the Government of Canada through the Book
Publishing Industry Development Program (BPIDP)
for our publishing activities.

Library and Archives Canada Cataloguing in Publication

Leiss, William, 1939–
Mad cows and mother's milk : the perils of poor risk
communication / William Leiss and Douglas Powell. –
2nd ed.
Order of authors reversed on previous ed.
Includes bibliographical references and index.
ISBN 0-7735-2817-2
1. Health risk communication. 2. Health risk assessment.
I. Powell, Douglas A. (Douglas Alan), 1962–
II. Title.
T10.68.L44 2004   363.1′072   C2004-903654-8

Typeset in New Baskerville 10/12
by Caractéra inc., Quebec City.

Magnus and Marco, Great Danes, this is their book, conceived during the sorrow after the passing of Magnus (1987–96), companion dog, beribboned master of the show ring, and diligent supervisor of projects in study and barnyard; and completed in the darkest bitterness and regret in January 1997 following the sudden death at ten months of age of Marco, whose guileless charm had ensnared all who knew him.

William Leiss

This book is dedicated to my wife, Wendy, and our children, Madelynn, Jaucelynn, Braunwynn, and Courtlynn, who have once again shared in both the work and the accomplishment.

Douglas Powell

Contents

Preface to the First Edition   ix

Preface to the Second Edition   xiii

PART ONE   WAITING FOR THE SCIENCE

1 Mad Cows or Crazy Communications?   3

2 A Diagnostic for Risk Communication Failures   26

3 Dioxins, or Chemical Stigmata   41

4 Hamburger Hell   77

5 Silicone Breasts   99

PART TWO   WAITING FOR THE REGULATORS

6 Lost in Regulatory Space: rBST   123

7 Gene Escape   153

8 Mother's Milk   182

9 Ten Lessons   210

PART THREE   NEW PERILS FOR RISK
MANAGERS

10   Two Stinking Cows: The Mismanagement of BSE Risk
     in North America   229

11   A Night at the Climate Casino: Canada and the Kyoto
     Quagmire   262

12   Life in the Fast Lane: An Introduction to Genomics
     Risks   296

     Appendix   341

     Notes   351

     Bibliography   413

     Index   443

Preface to the First Edition

The work of risk communication occurs within the great divide that often separates two evaluations of risks: those of scientific experts on the one hand, and those of members of the public on the other. Good risk communication practice seeks to bridge that divide by ensuring that the meaning of scientific risk assessments is presented in understandable terms to the public – and, equally, by ensuring that the nature of the public's concerns is known to and respected by risk managers. All too frequently no decent effort is made on either account, and a risk information vacuum interposes itself between experts and the public, blocking the exchanges that ought to be occurring regularly. Trapped in the resulting solitudes, experts bemoan the public's irrationality while being repaid with the public's contempt for their indifference and arrogance.

These solitudes represent risk communication failures. The seven case studies in this book show how and why they happen and how costly they can be, in monetary terms as well as in needless anxieties and the stalemating of effective risk management decision making. In the concluding chapter we draw some lessons from these cases that, if learned and applied to others both present and emerging, might reduce the failure rate and its attendant costs.

Many hands were involved in this book, but one person – Jackie Botterill, a graduate student in the School of Communication, Simon Fraser University – coordinated all those efforts and compiled the text, endnotes, and bibliography. The fact that we were able to pull all of this together in a relatively short time is due almost entirely to her skill and dedication. In addition to the collaborators noted below, we had able help from a number of graduate students who served as research associates: Anne-Marie Nicol, Epidemiology and Health Care, University of British Columbia; Eric Smith, Communications, Simon Fraser University; and Melanie Power, Policy Studies, Queen's University. During the period 1993–95, graduate students in the School of Communication at SFU did much of the primary research for chapter 3 (Pascal Milly and Tim Southam) and some early work on biotechnology regulation (Christine Massey).

Douglas Powell is the senior author for chapters 1, 4, and 6; William Leiss is senior author for chapters 2, 3, and 9; we have joint responsibility for the remainder. At the head of the various chapters we have sought to recognize others who helped us with specific case studies; in three of them (chapters 5, 7, and 8) our collaborators also did the initial draft of the case study report and are therefore entitled to join us in the authorship credit. However, the two of us are responsible for the entire text of this book in its final form.

Our collaborators are listed here in order of appearance: Amanda Whitfield (chapter 1) is a graduate student in the Department of Food Science, University of Guelph. Steve E. Hrudey (chapter 3) is Eco-Research chair in Environmental Risk Management and professor, Department of Public Health Sciences, University of Alberta. Linda Harris (chapter 4) is assistant professor of Food Science at the University of California, Davis. Conrad G. Brunk (chapter 5) is professor of Philosophy, Conrad Grebel College, University of Waterloo. Angela Griffiths (chapter 7) holds a PHD in Resource Management and Environmental Studies from UBC and is an associate at the Macleod Institute for Environmental Analysis, Calgary; Katherine Barrett is a doctoral student in the Department of Botany, UBC. Pascal Milly (chapter 8) is a postdoctoral fellow at the Centre interuniversitaire de recherche sur la science et la technologie, Université du Québec à Montréal.

Financial support for the research came from the following grants to William Leiss: Social Sciences and Humanities Research Council (SSHRC), Strategic Grants in Science and Technology Policy, "The Flow of Science into Public Policy," 1991–95 (initial research for chapters 3, 7, and 8), Simon Fraser University; SSHRC Research Grant, "Case Studies in Risk Communication," 1994–97; Tri-Council Secretariat and Imperial Oil Ltd., Eco-Research Chair in Environmental Policy, Queen's University, 1994–99. Some of the research by Douglas Powell undertaken during his graduate program at the University of Guelph was supported by the Natural Sciences and Engineering

Research Council, Agriculture and Agri-Food Canada, Ontario Ministry of Agriculture, Food and Rural Affairs, Ontario University
Research Incentive Fund, and Monsanto Canada. Later support was
provided by the Science and Society Project at the universities of
Guelph and Waterloo.

Douglas Powell is most grateful to colleagues at the University of
Guelph who helped to shape the original ideas for several chapters
herein while he was completing his doctoral thesis research, especially
Mansel Griffiths, Trevor Watts, Linda Harris, and Gord Surgeoner. He
also thanks Bill Leiss, who helped to fit parts of the thesis into the
book project, provided encouragement along the way, and came up
with the snappy book title; Ken Murray, an accomplished and passion-
ate individual who financed the Science and Society Project and who
has provided continuous personal support; and the many friends and
family who have shared what they know about agriculture and food.

Both authors appreciate greatly the encouragement and support
received from two of the finest gentlemen and scholars in the risk
studies field, Paul Slovic and Howard Kunreuther.

William Leiss is most grateful to Holly Mitchell, administrative assistant for the Environmental Policy Unit (EPU), School of Policy Studies, Queen's University, for concealing that fact that she, and not he,
actually runs the research chair program there. To Keith Banting,
director of the school, for securing the chair program for the school
in the face of stiff competition and for his tolerance of the fourth-
floor unorthodoxies that almost certainly were not a part of his original design. To Queen's University, for providing such an extraordinarily supportive platform for conducting public policy research and
dissemination. To the EPU's postdoctoral fellows Michael Mehta,
Debora VanNijnatten, and Éric Darier (now at the University of Lan-
caster), for scholarly collaboration and for their interest in farm life.
To the very accommodating and accomplished staff of McGill-Queen's
University Press. To Maureen Garvie, for expert copy-editing. To
Philip Cercone, executive director of the press, for being Italian and
thus reinforcing my sentimental attachment to (almost) all things
originating there – and incidentally for agreeing to publish so many
of my books. And to Marilyn Lawrence, who has somehow endured
ten of these projects over a period that is now alarmingly close to
thirty years, who joins me in the dedication and who thinks that our
Great Danes, Yoko and Theo, and our Belgian mares, Molly, Tosca,
and Tess, deserve a good deal of the credit.

D.P.   W.L.
Guelph, Ontario   Digging Dog Farm, Selby, Ontario

Preface to the Second Edition

Three brand-new, extensive case studies have been added for this edition – on BSE (mad-cow disease) in North America, climate change and the Kyoto Protocol, and genomics. The format for these new studies follows that developed for the seven originally published in the first edition, which may be summarized as follows. Risk management issues that come to public attention are predominantly those touching on human health concerns, environmental concerns, or some combination of both. In this context, risk can be described as the chance that something bad or undesirable might happen, either to the population as a whole or to some specific individuals or groups.

At the core of all such risk issues is a highly technical characterization of what the nature and scope of the risk is thought to be by specialists in the relevant fields, who may be physicists, biologists, chemists, engineers, climate modellers, or medical researchers. Then additional precision is provided by the work of statisticians, who try to assign a more specific probability to the chance of occurrence: Are we talking about a one-in-a-hundred risk, or a one-in-a-million chance? They also seek to determine what important uncertainties lie behind the apparent precision of the "risk number." And immediately, from the standpoint of ordinary citizens, who worry about health risks but are inexpert in the technical aspects of their description, this is where the trouble starts.

The trouble arises first with science. There is a widespread belief that the findings reported in peer-reviewed and published scientific papers have a kind of authoritative status as "facts," which stand far above the careless ruminations found in the ordinary discourses of mortals – for example, in remarks by politicians. To be sure, this popular belief has a substantial basis, namely, the strong, shared commitment of scientists to a formal methodology for the conduct of research. Although shoddy or even fraudulent work periodically slips through the peer-review process, these are rare events indeed, and they are not the source of the popular misunderstanding of science. Rather, it is to be found in the failure to understand that scientific results are, like every other product of the human imagination, an *interpretation* of some body of evidence, not "facts" as such; that all such interpretations are of necessity limited by the existing overall state of knowledge; and that nature is subtle and does not yield its secrets easily.

Above all, the popular misunderstanding often overlooks the reality that science is cumulative, tentative, always incomplete, and never-ending. The best advice to be given to any concerned citizen who expresses alarm over media reports of apparently frightening revelations of a new scientific study is: wait for the next study before taking any action (to be sure, there are exceptions to this rule).

This advice is doubly sound where risks are concerned. As mentioned, the purely scientific aspects of a risk characterization are themselves an interpretation of a certain limited body of evidence (for example, what happened to the rats when they were dosed with a certain chemical?). But when all of the other relevant considerations are added, in order to figure out whether this study's findings are something anyone should worry about ("If it happened to the rats, will it do the same to humans?"), the situation gets messier and messier. The risk assessor might say: "Well, based on this study, it's possible that there might be two additional cases of cancer in the population at similar levels of exposure." At which point the issue is off and running. Rarely does the dialogue continue right on the spot, as it should – for example, with the question, addressed to the risk assessor: "How sure are you of that?" Which could elicit the following reply: "Of course, I assume you know that we're talking about the 95 per cent confidence level here." And the rejoinder: "What does that mean?" And the reply: "Well, we're 95 per cent certain that there wouldn't be more than two additional cases, but, as I'm sure you realize, it's quite possible that there will be fewer than two additional cancers, and possibly none at all."

The discipline of risk communication arises with the realization that most of us, listening to such a dialogue, need a lot of help – and rarely get what we need. We need help in understanding what scientists are talking about, especially since their work appears to be advancing at a blistering pace, with something fresh and momentous coming out each week. We need a great deal of help in coming to terms with probabilities, which form the essential language of risk: "What do you mean, there's a 10 per cent probability this might occur: Is it or isn't it going to happen?" "You tell me that 10 per cent of the exposed population might get sick under these circumstances, but what I want to know is, will it happen to me or my kids?" And we require some help in figuring out just what bad outcomes can or cannot be prevented or lessened, and how this can be done, by some combination of creative scientific research, sound risk assessments, enlightened government policy – and good (responsible) behaviour on the part of citizens.

There are some reasons for optimism on this score, despite the prevailing view in some expert circles that the public is hopeless when it comes to risk. The technical language of risk is used more frequently in media reporting, as a way of framing the explanation of events, and over time this contributes to increased risk literacy among the public. Both the print and electronic media report regularly on new scientific studies of general interest, in part because leading journals, especially *Science* and *Nature*, take steps to provide journalists with news about forthcoming studies. For someone like me, a lifelong, dedicated reader of daily newspapers, what has happened in the last decade is nothing short of astonishing: at least once or twice every week, prominent (often front-page) coverage is given to a new scientific study, complete with an extensive summary, quotations from the study authors and other scientists, and references to other relevant work. Many of these articles are about revisions to previously reported interpretations; for example (quite recently), a re-analysis of data about the usefulness of mammography screening for breast-cancer risk strongly criticized the earlier work, which had received enormous media publicity. At least for the declining segment of the population that still reads newspapers, the resources currently available for tracking scientific studies relevant to popular health concerns have never been better.

Then there is the Internet. In well-connected countries like Canada, surfing the world-wide web for information has become a daily routine. Self-directed investigations of health and environmental issues are conducted by many individuals. It is safe to say that no other previous resource, including public libraries, could have ever dreamed about putting an equivalent amount of information at the fingertips of the ordinary citizen. This previously undreamed-of opportunity is simultaneously a cautionary tale. The Internet offers no peer review, and advocacy is everywhere, as one should expect. Risk issues do not lose any of their complexity just because a lot of technical information is suddenly accessible in one's home study. To take only one example, some public health officials are quite concerned about the Internet-based campaigns, launched by individuals and groups, advising parents to avoid having their children vaccinated for common infectious diseases, because of alleged collateral risks, such as autism. As we know from the world of advertising, arguments can be persuasive without necessarily being informative or balanced. Parents can make serious mistakes with their children's health by deciding to trust some sources over others. More generally, the proliferation of spam e-mails offering alternative sources for health remedies offers a clue to the level of interest among the public in playing around with self-diagnosis and self-medication.

This new context for health risk communication has inspired me and a group of like-minded colleagues to launch an experimental, web-based public information resource, using a single risk issue as a test case (http://www.emcom.ca). "Emcom" is an acronym for "endocrine modulator communication," although the issue is better-known under the heading "endocrine disruptors." The risk refers to the possibility that very small concentrations of certain chemicals, industrially produced in some cases and naturally occurring in others, could cause a wide range of serious, adverse health impacts for both children (developmental effects) and adults. Some of the risk factors are well described for other animals – the endocrine system is common in all mammals – and can appear to be quite frightening. The problem is, no one yet knows whether most people should worry very much about these particular risks. At the same time, enough news is circulating about them to create a need for reliable and understandable expositions of the relevant scientific research. This is what the "emcom" website seeks to provide. The site is managed by a group of university-based researchers who have staked their professional reputations on the claim that the site's contents will be found to be accurate, complete, up-to-date, readily understandable by a non-expert member of the public, and interactive. It is also free of any advocacy for or against a course of action with respect to the issues, and it includes a number of innovations in information presentation, including animated graphics and "layered" documentation (very short papers supplemented by longer and more technical expositions).

The "emcom" site design and strategy were conceived as a template that could address any health or environmental issue of significant public interest. The web-based strategy has tremendous advantages over conventional print publication, including ease of updating and revision, interactive responsiveness, ready addition of new sources and references, linkages with complementary sites, and the ability to use colour graphics to aid comprehension of technical data. (All of which presuppose the availability of a high-speed Internet connection, of course.) In a way, then, the "emcom" website represents a fourth current case study, in addition to the three reported in this new edition. To be sure, the public's grasp of the risk issues reviewed in those three chapters – BSE in North America, climate change, genomics – could benefit enormously from the availability of similarly targeted web-based resources, which do not now exist, although the interested reader can find a good deal of supplementary insight by following the many web-links contained in the endnotes to each chapter. (For one of the studies, that on climate change and the Kyoto Protocol, a number of helpful graphics will be found among the PowerPoint presentations on my website: http://www.leiss.ca/presentations/.)

Chapter 10 (BSE) is a solo effort. The senior author for chapter 11 (climate change) is Stephen Hill, Assistant Professor, Environmental and Resource Studies, Trent University, who holds a BSC. in chemical engineering from Queen's and a PhD in environmental science from the Faculty of Environmental Design, University of Calgary. For chapter 12 (genomics) the senior author is Michael Tyshenko, who has both a doctorate in molecular biology and a master's in public administration from Queen's University, and is currently a postdoctoral fellow at the McLaughlin Centre for Population Health Risk Assessment, University of Ottawa.

The remaining chapters are unchanged from the first edition.

W. L.
Ottawa
April 2004

PART ONE

Waiting for the Science

1 Mad Cows or Crazy Communications?

WITH AMANDA WHITFIELD

BSE has caused the biggest crisis in the history of the European Union.
Franz Fischler, European Union's agricultural commissioner[1]

On 20 March 1996, British Health Secretary Stephen Dorrell rose in the House to inform colleagues that scientists had discovered a new variant of Creutzfeldt-Jakob disease (CJD) in ten victims, and that they could not rule out a link with consumption of beef from cattle with bovine spongiform encephalopathy (BSE), also known as mad cow disease.[2]

Overnight, the British beef market collapsed, and politicians learned how to enunciate the names of the diseases. Within days, the European Union banned exports of British beef; consumption of beef fell throughout Europe, especially in France and Germany, and in Japan, where suspicion of foreign food runs high. The unsettling dialogue among uncertain science, risk, and politics was played out in media headlines, where it continues to this day. Beef consumption across the European Union dropped 11 per cent in 1996, and the BSE crisis cost the E.U. U.S.$5 billion in subsidies to the beef industry.[3] In February 1997 junior Agriculture Minister Angela Browning told the House of Commons that compensation payments to farmers for destroyed cattle to the end of 1996 amounted to £553 million and payments to abattoirs totalled £162 million in that same period. The culling and slaughtering of cattle goes on.[4]

The minister's announcement of 20 March 1996 was the culmination of fifteen years of mismanagement, political bravado, and a gross underestimation of the public's capacity to deal with risk. Of all the lessons to be drawn from the BSE fiasco, the most important is this: there is a terrible risk in seeking to comfort the public with "no-risk" messages. For almost a decade the British government and its leading scientific advisors insisted there was no risk – or that the risk was so infinitesimally small that it could be said there was no risk – of BSE leading to a similar malady in humans, CJD, even in the face of contradictory evidence. The no-risk message contributed to devastating economic and social effects for Britons, a nation of beef-eaters, to the mass slaughter of British cattle, and to a decrease in global consumption of beef, all at a cost of billions of dollars.

BACKGROUND: AN ANIMAL HOLOCAUST

BSE is a slowly progressing, fatal nervous disorder of adult cattle that causes a characteristic staggering gait and is similar to a handful of rare, neurological diseases that affect humans and other animals. The most common of these diseases is scrapie, which causes sheep compulsively to scratch themselves on fence posts or whatever is available. The human equivalent of scrapie is called Creutzfeldt-Jakob disease, which normally occurs in about one person per million every year throughout the world. All of these ailments have long incubation times, from two to seven years in cattle and up to thirty years in humans, but once symptoms appear, the victim rapidly degenerates. There is no known treatment.

Besides the characteristic "spongy" brain (literally, holes in the victims' nerve cells) and the deposition of a fibrous scrapie protein in the brain, these ailments also share the way they are transmitted: by direct contact with the brain (or products derived from the brain) of an infected person or animal. CJD is similar to another human disease, kuru, a fatal infection that was common among Papua New Guinean tribes who handled and ate the brains of their dead during mourning rites. Cases of CJD have been linked to the use of dura mater (a tough lining that surrounds the brain and is used as repair material in neurosurgery) from an infected cadaver. Unsterile instruments or electrodes used during brain surgery have been identified as the source in several cases. At least one case has been linked to corneal transplants. And ten people in the U.K. have died of CJD after receiving injections of human growth hormone prepared from the pituitary glands of human cadavers unknowingly infected with CJD. A 1993 inquest was told that the 1,900 Britons who were given growth hormone as children from 1959 to 1985 (because their bodies did not make enough naturally) were all potentially at risk of developing CJD. The use of cadaver-derived growth hormone was suspended in Britain and North America in 1985 after a genetically engineered version became available.

The epidemic of BSE that emerged in British cattle in the late 1980s seems related to several factors, including the large proportion of sheep to cattle compared with other countries; the high incidence of scrapie in sheep and, until recently, the absence of a scrapie control program; and changes in the methods of rendering ruminant offal that were implemented in the early 1980s. When animals such as cows or sheep are sent for slaughter, meat is processed for human consumption, but the remaining portions, such as entrails, hooves, and whatever else cannot be used, form what is called offal. This offal is then rendered using temperatures in excess of 100°C, yielding a meat and bone meal that has many uses. One such use is as an inexpensive source of high-quality protein in animal feed. The leading theory – although still just a theory – is that diseases like scrapie and BSE are spread when an infected sheep or cow is slaughtered and its by-products fed to other animals.

BSE was first discovered among Britain's cattle in 1986. (Examination of cattle brains held in archive from 1980–86 has not turned up any cases of BSE.[5]) In June 1988 the British government made BSE a reportable disease and by July had instituted a ban on ruminant offal in cattle feed. In August the government decided to slaughter and incinerate all cows suspected of having BSE and to provide compensation to farmers at 50 per cent of the animal's estimated worth. By December 1988 the milk from any suspect cows was also destroyed. Although the rate of increase of new cases has dropped dramatically since the ban was imposed (taking into account the long incubation period), 166,380 cases of BSE at more than 32,400 British farms had been reported by 15 November 1996.[6]

But while the process of infection has been tentatively identified, the cause of BSE, scrapie, and CJD remains a mystery that challenges the basic tenets of biology. In 1982 Stanley Prusiner, a neurologist at the University of California, San Francisco, building on the work of others, first provided evidence that scrapie in sheep was caused by an agent that contained no nucleic acid, something he dubbed a "prion" or infectious protein.[7] Prusiner's suggestion was greeted with ridicule. Bacteria, viruses, and every living organism contain either deoxyribonucleic acid (DNA) or in some instances only ribonucleic acid (RNA), which encodes the proteins required for life. Surely, his critics argued, there must be nucleic acid: it just hadn't been found yet. Nevertheless, after more than a decade of research, the idea of prions is holding up and winning respectability.

Prusiner first identified the infectious protein by removing the brains of sheep infected with scrapie, literally blending them in a high-tech blender, and injecting portions of the resulting solution into healthy sheep, which then went on to develop scrapie. The infectious agent Prusiner identified retained its ability to cause scrapie on its own in the face of any and all techniques that normally destroy nucleic acids and viruses.

In 1985 the gene encoding the scrapie-inducing protein was cloned by Charles Weissmann at the University of Zurich, and it was discovered to produce a protein normally occurring in the brains of healthy sheep. The equivalent human gene was soon found, and specific changes or mutations in the prion gene structure were linked to the 10 per cent of CJD cases that are deemed to be hereditary, that is, to exist in certain families and be passed on from generation to generation. When the defective human prion gene was injected into experimental mice, they too developed the symptoms of CJD.

Current thinking is that the normal prion protein is required for some type of cell-to-cell communication in nerve cells in the brain, but that when the disease-causing form of the protein is present, it somehow interacts with the normal prion protein, making it difficult for the latter to be broken down. Experimental evidence is accumulating to support such a model.[8] Further, whatever is causing mad cow disease and related ailments is able to survive temperatures in excess of 100°C. This mutant form of the protein accumulates and, over time, leads to diseases like CJD, scrapie, and BSE.

At the crux of the BSE crisis is the question of whether humans can develop CJD after eating beef from cattle infected with BSE. In other words, can the infectious agent jump the species barrier?

"THERE IS NO RISK"

United Kingdom newspapers reported the new malady in the mid-1980s, although it was not until 1990 that North American newspaper coverage began. Throughout this time, British government sources were adamant that meat and other products from cattle infected with BSE posed no risk to humans. The 1990 coverage was prompted by the discovery that the infectious prion did in fact appear to be crossing the species barrier – to cats.

Several cases of English cats developing feline spongiform encephalopathy were discovered and thought to be due to the use of rendered ruminant protein in cat food. The news about BSE appearing in cats initiated the first crisis of confidence in British beef, and consumption plummeted. David Maclean, Britain's Food minister at the time, was quoted in the *New York Times* on 24 January 1990 as saying "the cow disease does not pose a health risk to humans. We are not in the business of subjecting our people to unsafe food." Nevertheless, a scientific committee set up by the U.K. Ministry of Agriculture Fisheries and Food – the Tyrell committee – said in the same article that "it was not known whether people could contract the disease."[9] By 20 May 1990 Maclean had shifted his position slightly, stating that BSE posed "a very remote risk to human health."[10] In response to the first European threats of a ban on British beef – initially by France – David Curry, Britain's junior minister of Agriculture, was quoted as saying "our meat presents no health hazards." The ban is "a question of agricultural protectionism."[11] Then Agriculture Minister John Gummer sought to reassure the public that all was well by urging his four-year-old daughter, Cordelia, to eat a hamburger with him for the benefit of the television cameras. *The Economist* described events more succinctly, stating already in May 1990 that the widely reported death of the first cat "proved beyond scientific doubt that nobody trusts MAFF any more."[12]

While consumption eventually did recover, questions continued to be raised by the scientific community, the British public, and trading partners. The United States banned British beef imports in 1989, and Canada followed in 1990. All the while the British government insisted that humans were not at risk. In the summer of 1995, questions about the causes, risks, and controls of BSE began to appear more frequently in the European press. On 12 July 1995 a U.K. consumer group called for a new inquiry into BSE, after it became clear some cattle were still being fed the recycled organs of other cows, despite the 1988 ban – and a number of other prohibitions on the use of specified bovine offals, introduced in the early 1990s – demonstrating that good rules need great enforcement. In short, actions have to match words, a recurring theme in the case of BSE and several other studies presented in later chapters.

On 15 August 1995 Granada Television's *World in Action* broadcast a documentary about a nineteen-year-old boy who had died from CJD in May.[13] He was the first known British teenage victim killed by the rare brain disease, which normally attacks the elderly. The disease is so uncommon in teenagers that there had only been three other reported cases in the world. Also mentioned was a seventeen-year-old girl in Wales who was in a deep coma and also believed to be suffering from CJD. Her relatives blamed her illness on eating hamburgers contaminated with beef from cattle with BSE. The story also quoted prominent scientists who said anything unusual – like two teenagers dying from CJD – was cause for concern. In response, the government said there would be no inquiry into the death of the boy and insisted, "We continue to believe there's no evidence that BSE can cause CJD in humans."[14]

By October 1995 these random stories began to pique the interests of journalists, who did their job and started investigating other cases. On 24 October 1995 the *Daily Post* newspaper in Liverpool revealed it had discovered two more cases of CJD: one was a sixty-four-year-old farmer's wife who had died three weeks earlier, the other a forty-two-year-old Liverpool businessman.[15] The story recounted how three farmers had already died from CJD and a fourth was seriously ill. Two days later a paper was published in the medical journal the *Lancet* recounting the cases of the two teenage Britons who were the rare, young victims of CJD. The report also said the cases were not linked to BSE.[16]

On the industry side, representatives of slaughterhouse owners were summoned to a meeting with Agriculture Minister Douglas Hogg on 9 November 1995, following the release of evidence that some carcasses were leaving abattoirs without all the offal removed. They were told to smarten up or be prosecuted. Again, the rules drafted within the bureacracy of MAFF were not being enforced on the slaughterhouse floor.[17]

By the middle of November 1995 media coverage began to increase. BBC Television reported that nearly a quarter of Britons had either stopped eating beef or were eating less, fearing BSE could infect people.[18] Another television program claimed that up to six hundred BSE-infected cattle were being consumed in Britain every week.[19] And by 17 November 1995 the first report of a school banning beef from its cafeterias surfaced. The chief cook wrote to parents: "I am a farmer's daughter myself and while I don't want to see farmers put out of work I don't feel the Ministry of Agriculture is doing enough to reassure the public."[20] In response, a Meat and Livestock Commission spokeswoman said: "There is no scientific basis for banning beef – there's a lot of misinformation going around."[21] These conflicting perspectives typified the words frequently cited in the media coverage, where the debate bounced back and forth, with industry and government saying there was no scientific evidence that BSE could cross the species barrier into humans, and the public saying, in effect, "we don't believe you."

On 23 November 1995 the government, patting itself on the back, stated that mad cow disease would soon be eradicated in Britain: "We shall be seeing an end of it in not too long," said Lord Lucas of Crudwell.[22] He also joined other peers in urging the public to start eating British-produced, "welfare-friendly" veal, rather than foreign imports that might have used the veal crate system. Of course some of those other countries, notably Germany and France, called for bans of British beef imports because of BSE. As with the use of growth promoters in beef, one country's scientific standard is another's non-tariff trade barrier. (North American beef has been banned in the E.U. since 1988 on the grounds that it is produced using growth promoters, which are prohibited in the E.U. – this despite clearance from the E.U.'s own veterinary experts that such growth promoters are scientifically safe.[23])

A scientific debate about the possibility of BSE causing CJD surfaced in British academic journals. In a series of letters to the *British Medical Journal* that appeared on 24 November 1995, American and European doctors called for extensive new research into whether people actually could catch CJD by eating beef from cattle infected with BSE. Sheila Gore of the Biostatistics Unit of the Medical Research Council said that by April 1995 BSE had been confirmed in more than 53 per cent of dairy herds in Britain and that the new cases of CJD in humans were worrying. In a statement that was widely quoted elsewhere, she said: "Taken together, cases of Creutzfeldt-Jakob disease in farmers and young adults are more than happenstance."[24] Two days later Dr Stephen Dealler, writing in the *British Food Journal*, claimed that most adult British meat-eaters would, by the year 2001, have ingested a potentially fatal dose of meat infected with BSE. He also said that the medical and dietary professions should question the present policy of "waiting passively" to see if the incidence of CJD rises in the United Kingdom.[25]

It was in this climate of public discussion that, on 30 November 1995, Professor Sir Bernard Tomlinson, one of the U.K.'s leading brain disease experts, told BBC Radio 4's *You and Yours* consumer program that he no longer ate meat pies or beef liver and "at the moment" would not eat a hamburger "under any circumstances." He said there was growing evidence (although he offered none in his remarks on that program) that CJD could be caught from infected beef products.

Although there had been occasional trade publication coverage in North America, the first general report surfaced in Canada in the *Vancouver Sun* on 4 December 1995, reporting that one of Britain's leading physiologists, Professor Colin Blakemore of Oxford, had joined the list of scientists warning that mad cow disease could pass to humans. "There is growing evidence of a transmission to humans, and I believe there is a strong chance we are going to suffer the most frightening epidemic," he said.[26]

On 4 December 1995 the British government fought back, when Health Secretary Stephen Dorrell insisted there was "no conceivable risk" of people becoming infected with CJD from eating beef.[27] Dorrell said that he was still prepared to eat beef himself and to give it to his own children, echoing the 1991 testimony of John Gummer. On

6 December 1995 the British caterers association said school caterers should consider using more chicken, turkey, and pork until the controversy over mad cow disease had been resolved. And what was the government's response? In Wales, Agriculture Minister Gwilym Jones told the Commons the public should not overreact to concerns about BSE, insisting there was no scientific evidence linking BSE and CJD, and declaring, "I am more than content to go on eating beef on a regular basis." He went on to say, "We must not overreact to this issue."[28]

Even British Prime Minister John Major became embroiled in the debate, telling Parliament, "There is currently no scientific evidence that BSE can be transmitted to humans or that eating beef causes CJD."[29] In response, more schools banned beef. Sue Dibb, co-director of the independent watchdog Food Commission, responded that "nobody is trusting what is coming out of Government any more. The Government seems to be more interested in propping up the beef industry rather than admitting that there may be a risk, however small it may be. I think what is happening is that every time a minister gets up and says beef is safe, there is absolutely no danger, there is absolutely no risk, a whole lot more people stop buying beef because they don't trust the Government."[30]

Another week went by and reports about the public's concerns continued unabated. Hence on 14 December 1995 Agriculture Minister Douglas Hogg, along with a clutch of government experts, spent two hours with a group of journalists, reviewing the scientific evidence, which, in the minister's interpretation, meant that the latest BSE scare was unfounded. Within hours of the meeting two hundred more schools had banned beef. On 18 December 1995 the Meat and Livestock Commission confirmed that beef sales had dropped 15 per cent.[31] A *Sunday Times* opinion poll found that one in five said they had stopped eating beef.[32]

The newspapers discovered a couple of more people thought to be suffering from CJD. On 9 January 1996 the BSE story finally garnered wide distribution in North America, with front-page coverage in the *New York Times* and a wire story that was reprinted in many papers.[33] British beef companies were starting to show the effects, reporting lower sales and earnings. Then, on 17 January 1996, two months after the situation had assumed crisis proportions, Britain's meat industry and leading supermarkets announced they were launching an unprecedented joint campaign to allay customers' fears over beef. Full page advertisements were placed in national newspapers assuring consumers that they could serve British beef with confidence. "Your favourite supermarkets are usually in hot competition. On one thing, though, they're in total agreement. British beef. Just as they have always sold it with the utmost confidence, so they continue to do so. Roasts, steaks, stews, mince, burgers, pies or sausages, whatever takes your fancy, you can share their confidence." A Meat and Livestock Commission spokesman denied the campaign reflected growing concern over the safety of beef.[34]

Rudimentary risk communication theory would suggest that such an advertisement would fail, simply because it sought to deny the existence of concern. Research has suggested that efforts to convince the public about the safety and benefits of new or existing technologies – or in this case the safety of the food supply – rather than enhancing public confidence, may actually amplify anxieties and mistrust by denying the legitimacy of fundamental social concerns.[35] The public carries a much broader notion of risk, one incorporating, among other things, accountability, economics, values, and trust. During the preceding years the risk messages from industry and government had never included timely references to the latest scientific developments, and they had also consistently failed to acknowledge both the content and context of the evolving public concerns about BSE risks. Moreover, the announced actions for controlling the spread of BSE in cattle had been poorly enforced.

To summarize, although for almost ten years the British government and industry had been trumpeting a no-risk message, in the run-up to Christmas 1995 beef consumption in the United Kingdom had fallen 20 per cent, and 1.4 million British households had stopped buying beef. Thousands of schools had taken beef off the menu. And several prominent scientists had predicted a medical catastrophe if a link between BSE and CJD eventually were to be proved. All this occurred months before the 20 March 1996 announcement of a putative link between BSE and CJD. When evidence of a link (albeit of a tentative sort) was reported to the government, there was no choice but to release it, for otherwise it would have leaked out. So, while the 20 March statement by Health Secretary Dorrell was a spectacular news event with all the more sensational aspects of a risk story – uncertainty, dread, catastrophe, the possible involvement of children – the announcement also was made in a climate of extreme mistrust of the U.K. Ministry of Agriculture Fisheries and Food. It shattered any remnants of credibility enjoyed by the British government.

"MAYBE THERE IS A RISK"

During 1994 and 1995 ten victims displaying an unrecognized and consistent pattern of CJD were identified by the U.K. CJD Surveillance

Unit. The victims were much younger than in previous cases, with the oldest being forty-two and the average age twenty-seven-and-a-half, whereas in the experience of the medical profession until that time, people usually did not contract CJD until after the age of sixty-three. The illness also lasted longer than usual, an average of thirteen months compared with the normal six. Some of the outward characteristics of the patients differed from traditional CJD, but most importantly, the pattern of neurological damage in brain tissue was unique. Specifically, there were much larger aggregates of prions in the brains in cases of what came to be called new variant-CJD (nvCJD) than had been seen in previous cases. Scientists found no evidence of genetic or medical factors common to the ten victims and consistent with acquiring CJD.[36] This led the U.K. Spongiform Encephalopathy Advisory Committee (SEAC) to state in March 1996 that, in the absence of any other available explanation at the time, the cases were "most likely" to have been caused by exposure to BSE-infected cattle brain or spinal cord before 1989.

Thus on 20 March 1996 Stephen Dorrell also announced that he was following through on a series of new recommendations from SEAC, including:

- requiring the carcasses of cattle aged over thirty months to be deboned in licenced plants supervised by the Meat Hygiene Service with trimmings from those animals to be classified as offal containing a health risk;
- imposing a ban on the use of mammalian meat and bonemeal in feed for all farm animals;
- urging public health watchdogs, in consultation with SEAC, to review their advice in light of the new findings; and,
- requesting SEAC to consider what further research was necessary.[37]

The British and international media immediately gave front-page status to this story. Thus all the more prominence was bestowed on the accompanying statement by Health Secretary Dorrell, who, in a classic case of Orwellian doublespeak, insisted in response to reporters' questions that the government had always followed the advice of senior medical staff: "The Government has consistently taken the advice of scientists on this subject," he said. "It's not true the Government has said there's no link. The Government has said there's no evidence of a link ... What has happened today is that SEAC has revised its advice both on the possibility of a link between BSE and CJD and the action we should take."[38] As we have seen, the "no evidence" assertion was not a fair representation of the developing scientific understanding. The minister's desperate equivocations and hair-splitting reached the public at the same time as did Professor Richard Lacey's widely cited prediction of a rapid rise in the incidence of CJD, with somewhere between five thousand and 500,000 Britons possibly stricken by the year 2000, and Dr Stephen Dealler's estimate that by 2010 as many as ten million Britons might have CJD, assuming high infectivity.[39]

Scapegoats were needed and were found everywhere. Junior Scottish minister the Earl of Lindsay conceded that the government may have "unwittingly" tempted farmers not to destroy infected animals by failing to offer full compensation to them between 1986 and 1990.[40] Tim Lang, professor of food policy at Thames Valley University and chairman of the National School Meals Campaign, blamed intensive farming for the "tragedy" of BSE and called for modern farming techniques to be fundamentally changed. "We are in a mass experiment which is killing us. Never before have diseased ruminants (sheep) been fed to other ruminants (cows) and then fed to humans," he said. "We have interfered with the whole process of nature and what is now happening is one of our worst nightmares."[41] Months later Richard Packer, MAFF's permanent secretary, told the European Parliament's committee of inquiry into BSE that the mad cow crisis was "an act of God." Packer did make a small concession: "Some of the things we have done we might with the benefit of hindsight have done differently. To that extent the U.K. government accepts responsibility – but that is not very much of the responsibility."[42]

Within days the E.U. banned all British beef exports and government supporters began blaming the media. Tory Lord Soulsby of Swaffham Prior, a veterinarian, said the crisis had its origins in "media hyperbole" and pressed the government for "positive steps" to generate public confidence by more "aggressive" information. "The British public will believe the science of the situation if it was put to them in a more effective way," he said.[43] By the end of April it was revealed that hygiene inspectors had found that one in twenty slaughterhouses and plants dealing with beef offal were failing to meet new controls to combat the threat of BSE.[44]

Far removed from the hyperbole and the negotiations between the U.K. and the E.U. over banned British beef products, science began to shore up the initially tenuous link between BSE and CJD. In April 1996 researchers at Oxford University and a government lab reported in *Nature* a new analysis of the genetic sequences of prion proteins in cattle, sheep and humans. While the overall DNA sequences of cattle and sheep are more similar to each other than to humans, two crucial changes that affected the three-dimensional structure of the prion protein – and remember that protein conformation is crucial to the onset of prion diseases – were found to be much more similar in cattle and humans than in sheep.[45]

By August new research at MAFF revealed that cattle infected with BSE could pass the disease on to their offspring.[46] A seven-year project begun in 1989 at the government's Central Veterinary Laboratory in Weybridge, Surrey, set out to compare the rates of BSE in calves born to infected and BSE-free cattle. Unfortunately, many calves were fed with potentially infected feed early in the experiment, which complicated subsequent analysis. According to a news story in *Nature*,[47] of 333 calves born to mothers with BSE, 273 had died by 14 July. Initial histological examination showed that forty-two suffered from BSE. An equivalent group was the offspring of BSE-free cattle; thirteen of these animals had developed the disease. The implications for child-bearing women were widely speculated upon in the British press.

In a comprehensive statistical analysis of BSE in British cattle, Anderson *et al.* reported that the epidemic may disappear almost entirely by as early as 2001 without the need for culling (although the uncertainties are large).[48] This study immediately prompted the British government to reneg on a deal with the E.U. to carry out a selective cull of another 147,000 or so animals (in addition to the slaughter of all cattle over thirty months old) deemed to be at high risk for developing BSE – creating more political drama.[49]

In September, two provisional tests for CJD were reported in scientific journals, following a June 1996 publication about a live test for scrapie developed by Dutch researchers.[50] Inga Zerr and colleagues of Georg-August-Universitaet in Gottingen wrote in the 27 September 1996 issue of the *Lancet* that they had developed a test using the cerebrospinal fluid of suspected CJD victims and that the test was 80 per cent accurate. The previous day Hsich *et al.*[51] had reported a similar test, although both currently will work only if a patient has already developed the outward symptoms of the disease. This again sparked outrage in the British press, when an accompanying editorial in the *Lancet* asked: "Why were laboratory tests for spongiform encephalopathies developed in the USA and in Germany, countries that have worldwide average incidences of CJD ... and no BSE? Why did it take a report of 10 cases of new variant CJD to force the U.K. Ministry of Agriculture Fisheries and Food to pay serious attention to BSE research, doubling its research investment for 1996/97 to 10.4 million pounds from 5.4 million pounds the previous year?"[52] During this time there were also widespread allegations of secrecy and witholding of data at MAFF, but such stories are difficult to confirm.[53]

A panel of scientists chaired by Charles Weissmann of the Institute of Molecular Biology in Zurich told the E.U. Commission in October 1996 that predictions about the eradication of the disease are based on assumptions that might not "hold true," and it warned the commission that the risk of the disease becoming endemic cannot be discounted.[54]

The most convincing evidence of transmissability to date appeared on 24 October 1996, when a team headed by John Collinge, of Imperial College School of Medicine at St Mary's Hospital in London, reported in *Nature* that the biochemical characteristics of nvCJD are closer to those of BSE than those of classical CJD.[55] Each of the different forms or causes of CJD produces a slightly different neurological pattern as well as a traceable molecular marker when passed through experimental mice. Collinge *et al.* extracted the disease-causing agent from cases of CJD – attributed to inheritance, human growth hormone, no known cause (spontaneous), and nvCJD – and passed it through experimental mice. They then compared the molecular patterns of the agent and found that of the four strains, nvCJD was different from the other three CJD strains and much more similar to BSE. Not proof, but further evidence that BSE and nvCJD were in fact linked.

Again there were front-page headlines. The E.U. warned there could be no relaxation of the ban on British beef products and said there was now no excuse for further delay by the government in carrying out the selective cull of 147,000 cattle. European Commission Agriculture Commissioner Franz Fischler was quoted as saying the research "shows that the risk of transmission to humans is a fact – it is not the proof, but it is one more proof." British Prime Minister John Major retorted: "There's no new, fresh public health concern. People can eat beef as safely today as they could yesterday, and I think it is perfectly safe." He did, however, admit that there "might" be a link between eating infected beef and developing CJD – although one can only wonder at the juxtaposition of these two statements, after all that had happened up to that point. The U.K. National Farmers' Union insisted there was no reason for consumers to be "alarmed." And the Meat and Livestock Commission pressed ahead with its Festival of British Beef in London, determined to get across its message that the meat was safe.[56] By December Britain had relented and agreed to go ahead with the selective slaughter demanded by the E.U.[57]

A report in the *Lancet* predicted that the death toll from nvCJD would be in the hundreds within seven years; this was greeted by some as good news because it was not the doomsday scenario of hundreds of thousands.[58] By the end of 1996 thirteen people had died from nvCJD in the United Kingdom and one in France (an additional two victims had been diagnosed by cerebral biopsy in the U.K. but are still alive). The latest was nineteen-year-old Victoria Lowther, who died in a hospice in Carlisle, Cumbria, four months after first showing signs of nvCJD.[59] The chairman of the school Victoria had attended was quoted as saying: "She had her whole life in front of her and was one of those girls who had it all. She had good looks. She was a stunning girl – bright, clever, very popular. It all happened so quickly. In a matter of six months she slid downhill rapidly."

"THERE IS A RISK": THE NORTH AMERICAN RESPONSE

The events from March 1996 to the present do not exist in a vacuum; rather, they are the latest in a series of public controversies in Britain related, in this case, to the public perception or confidence of the food supply and the U.K. Ministry of Agriculture Fisheries and Food, involving listeria, botulism, salmonella, and BSE. More importantly, though, media coverage originating in Britain raised several questions peripheral to the BSE issue that forced a reconsideration of agricultural practices in Canada and the United States, such as the use of rendered sheep and cattle offal as a protein-rich feed supplement for cattle. The issue was succinctly described in media accounts as turning herbivores into carnivores, or, feeding dead animals to animals that only ate plants.

How the United States and Canada reacted to the 20 March 1996 news offers additional insights into differing interpretations of effective risk management and communication. Media coverage in both countries was extensive. Richard Lacy and other U.K. critics became instantly credible, widely quoted in North American coverage, predicting CJD deaths at between five thousand and 500,000 by the year 2000.[60] The Humane Society of the United States issued a press release on 21 March 1996 stating that "some scientists speculate that this disease could become an epidemic as deadly as AIDS" and noting the availability of a former cattle-rancher turned vegan-activist, Howard Lyman, who was called an expert on "mad-cow" disease.[61]

Immediately following the U.K. announcement, the U.S. Department of Agriculture (USDA) and the U.S. Food and Drug Administration (FDA) announced stricter inspection of live cattle imported from Great Britain prior to 1989 and an expansion of current "antemortem" inspection of BSE.[62] The USDA statement also noted the agency's BSE surveillance program had examined over 2,660 specimens from forty-three states and no BSE had ever been detected in cattle from the United States. And the USDA said it was working with state and public health counterparts, scientists and industry representatives to review current policies and regulations concerning BSE. These were all concrete actions, issued in a timely manner and subsequently widely reported. On 22 March 1996, USDA's Animal and Plant Health Inspection Service (APHIS) hosted a six-hour meeting of about seventy government and private animal health experts to review the BSE-CJD link. Again, this was widely reported. In most stories USDA officials were quoted as saying the risk of BSE developing in the United States was small, and then outlined why that was and stressed the control measures in place.

This did not happen in Canada. Agriculture and Agri-food Canada (AAFC) issued no public statement[63] but choose instead to respond to individual media inquiries. This is a tedious task and increases the chance of inconsistent messages entering the public domain.

The Canadian minister of Agriculture was quite adamant there was no risk of BSE developing in Canada. The actions of the ministry in handling the 1993 discovery of an Albertan cow with BSE – it had been imported from the U.K., and AAFC quickly ordered the destruction of 363 cattle still in Canada that had originated in the U.K., as well as the entire herd of the infected animal – were widely lauded and used as evidence that regulators knew what they were doing. Heidi Grogan, manager of public affairs for the Canadian Cattlemen's Association in Calgary, was quoted as saying that "the main thing in 93–94 was taking measures that would assure human health was the No. 1 priority, because we didn't know enough about the research. We thought the measures were warranted, and clearly they were."[64]

Officials repeatedly said that Canada had a BSE surveillance program in place. Yet journalists never asked, or if they did they failed to report, the details of this surveillance program. During a 23 October 1996 telephone conversation, an Agriculture Canada official said the surveillance program amounted to between 250 and 400 animals per year[65] – certainly sufficient to ensure confidence, but no journalist had ever asked. In fact, the official was just pulling the numbers together in October 1996, seven months after the 20 March 1996 announcement, and seven months after the United States revealed, without being asked, the number of animals checked for BSE.

In both countries questions were immediately raised about the practice of feeding herbivores ruminant protein. A cursory examination of letters to the editor shows widespread consumer outrage at the practice. Jeremy Rifkin announced March 28 that his Washington-based Foundation for Economic Trends would sue the FDA to try to ban the feeding of rendered animal parts to cattle.[66] Other groups launched similar suits.[67] The FDA again responded in a timely manner, saying on the same day that it would consider banning ruminant protein in cattle and sheep feed and make a decision within ten to fourteen days. By 29 March 1996, USDA and FSIS announced they were expediting regulations prohibiting ruminant protein in ruminant feeds, boosting surveillance, and expanding research.[68] The same day, the National Cattlemen's Beef Association, the American Sheep Industry Association, the National Milk Producers Federation, the American Veterinary Medical Association, the American Association of Bovine Practitioners, and the American Association of Veterinary Medical Colleges issued a statement supporting the moves and instituting a voluntary ban on ruminant protein in ruminant feed.[69] Chandler Keyes, vice president for congressional relations at the U.S. National Cattlemen's Beef Association (NCBA), described the association's decision to back a voluntary ban on the feeding of ruminant proteins to ruminants in the following words: "When there is a rocket coming down toward you, you can't wait to act. Sometimes you have to pull the trigger and move."[70]

Different again in Canada, where an Agriculture and Agri-Food Canada official was quoted as saying they were consulting with industry groups and that an announcement was expected that day.[71] It never came, at least not publicly. Even after a 3 April statement by the World Health Organization calling for a global ban on the use of ruminant tissue in ruminant feed – by a committee chaired by a Canadian – Agriculture and Agri-Food Canada remained silent, occasionally being quoted that government officials were trying to broker a consensus between packers, producers, renderers, and feed mills.[72] As far as any Canadian consumer knows, they're still trying. However, as the FDA move to legislate a ban on ruminant protein in ruminant feed neared completion in late 1996, Canadian agriculture officials began publicly to state that Canada would have to follow suit or face trade sanctions.

On 8 April 1996, the U.S. Centers for Disease Control and Prevention (CDC) announced it would add CJD to its four-state sentinel program, and twenty-one states began ordering the slaughter of 113 British cattle known to be in the United States. In a widely reported bulletin on 8 August 1996, CDC reiterated its advice to physicians to be on the lookout for CJD.[73]

But even good management can sometimes fail to be communicated. During the Oprah Winfrey show of 16 April 1996, the host announced in dramatic fashion that she would stop eating hamburgers because of fears over BSE and expressed shock after a guest said meat and bone meal made from cattle was routinely fed to other cattle to boost their meat and milk production. The camera showed members of the studio audience gasping as Howard Lyman explained how cattle parts were rendered and fed to other cattle. Even though the National Cattlemen's Beef Association had supported a voluntary ban on ruminant protein in ruminant feed, chief scientist Gary Weber appeared dumbfounded by Lyman's claims and never explained the risk management procedures undertaken by the industry. Instead, Weber was reduced to arguing that "cows weren't vegetarians because they drank milk" while the cameras showed audience members rolling their eyes in disbelief. News of the popular show's content swept through the Chicago cattle futures markets, contributing to major declines in all the beef contracts as traders feared it would turn Americans away from beef.[74]

The Canadian Cattlemen's Association began circulating an information memo on 27 March 1996 to grocery officials across Canada to inform consumers that "BSE is a British issue and does not affect the Canadian consumer. Canadian consumers can continue to be confident in the safety and wholesomeness of our product."[75] But consumers have a much broader notion of risk. To say BSE was only a British issue was to ignore the numerous stories in Canadian media outlets criticizing the practice of using ruminant protein in feed – in Canada. Again, the message denied the legitimacy of a consumer concern, which usually makes things worse.

COWS DON'T EAT COWS; COWS EAT GRASS

As the British saga unfolded during the rest of 1996, the key issue for North American regulators and the cattle industry was the use of rendered ruminant protein in ruminant feed, although the issue was largely confined to discussion in trade publications. Even here, regulators in the two countries differed significantly in their approach to the issue. American regulators often talked about scientific uncertainties and the need to reduce or minimize risk, while Canadian officials openly questioned the validity of the scientific link between ruminant protein in ruminant feed and the development of transmissible spongiform encephalopathies (TSEs, as the family of diseases are known), stating instead that the science "wasn't there" and that the decisions were being driven more by public perception and trade considerations than science. Such a stance shows a flagrant disregard for the British experience with TSEs.

The FDA was always clear about its intent for a ban on ruminant-protein in ruminant feed. In May, spokesperson Lawrence Bachorik was quoted as saying, "There is no Bovine Spongiform Encephalopathy

(BSE) in this country. Any measure we take would simply add an extra layer of protection."[76] The rendering industry, along with the NCBA, however, saw the proposed rule as an unnecessary infringement. These groups, instead, proposed an alternative, Hazard Analysis & Critical Control Point (HACCP) risk analysis approach to prevent the introduction of BSE in the United States.[77,78] When the FDA appeared cool to the idea, the renderers continued to argue that "government efforts to deal with the issue of BSE are motivated more by fear and politics than by science."[79] In the same story, Dr Don Franco, director of scientific services at the U.S. National Renderers Association, told the group's annual meeting that American efforts to deal with BSE were "self flagellation" because there has been literally no incidence of the disease here.

No matter: on 2 January 1997, the U.S. Food and Drug Administration proposed a ban on ruminant protein in ruminant feed. Said the FDA statement: "Because of concerns that BSE could in the future be identified scientifically as the cause of a new TSE in humans, FDA and USDA officials said the protection of public health depends on the development of a strategy to control possible routes of TSE expansion in food animals."

Donna E. Shalala, U.S. secretary of Health and Human Services, was quoted as saying, "This is a precautionary measure – there have been no reported cases of BSE in this county. It will add another level of safeguards to protect the U.S. against the potential risk from these diseases." FDA Commissioner David A. Kessler added, "In essence, this proposal would build a protective barrier against the spread of BSE."[80] Even NCBA, which had supported the HACCP route, said in a statement that the FDA proposed rule was "an appropriate next step to prevent Bovine Spongiform Encephalopathy (BSE) from ever occurring in the U.S." NCBA also noted that while they had in the past supported the HACCP approach, they would expect the final regulation, if passed as is, to have little effect on the cost of producing beef and milk because, even before beef and dairy producers voluntarily removed ruminant derived protein by-products from their feed in April, they used only 15 per cent of the available by-products.[81] Lawrence Altman wrote in front-page coverage in the New York Times that the FDA's "precautionary step is being proposed because of strong evidence that the disease can be spread through animal feed contaminated with rogue proteins known as prions."[82] Altman also quoted Kessler as saying that the proposed ban "reflected new scientific information that a team headed by Dr John Collinge, a British expert on Creutzfeldt-Jakob disease, reported in the journal Nature in October."

That "strong evidence," based on the British experience and Collinge *et al.* was apparently not enough for Canadian regulators. Whereas American regulators, at least in the public domain, emphasized controls to prevent the occurrence of BSE and moved forward with legislation, Canadian regulators insisted there was "no risk." Appropriately, the Canadian Feed Industry Association exploited the fallacy of the no-risk argument. If, as the Canadian minister of Agriculture stated, there was no risk of BSE developing in Canada, then why impose a ban?[83] Graham Clarke, chief red meat inspector with the feeds division of Agriculture and Agri-food Canada, responded in the same story that even though there was no risk in Canada, and no conclusive science to support the WHO recommendation, there was a concern over public perceptions and the possibility of the issue becoming a non-tariff trade barrier.

Even one of Canada's better-known science journalists, Stephen Strauss of the *Globe and Mail,* argued the mad cow crisis was more perception that science, writing in his year-end roundup that "After years of suggestive evidence, it was all but confirmed that the brain-rotting condition could be transmitted from cow to cow-eating human ... Was the risk of a rare disease so great that every Bossy in the British Isles would have to be killed? Scientific arguments foundered on the shoals of human irrationality. People are not reasoning machines, they are fearing machines and, when there's a scare, politicians and scientists better tremble."[84]

Those differences in the approach to BSE risk – is it science, as the FDA says, or is it perception, as AAFC says? – became increasingly clear over the summer of 1996. In July Clarke was quoted as saying that even though the FDA was moving toward a legislated ban on ruminant protein in ruminant feed, it did not mean that legislation was imminent in Canada. "Our concern is that we get a lot of co-operation, because we can't make it work without that," he stated; Ag Canada was reluctant to "penalize an industry on the basis of not very good science. We're not going to be pushed into making rash decisions."[85]

The sniping at the science by Canadian regulators continued in July 1996, when Dr Norman Willis, director general of Animal and Plant Health, Agriculture and Agri-food Canada, told the Canadian Veterinary Medical Association's annual convention in Charlottetown on 6 July 1996 that "actions were taken out of sheer paranoia, with people significantly hyped by the media. We took actions that went way beyond ones that were scientifically justified." Willis added, "We wouldn't have political interference. We wouldn't have non-science factors influence the actions we took. BSE blew that all away ... Canada and other trading countries couldn't hold with science-based decisions. There was just too much at stake by way of trade."[86]

The Canadian Cattlemen's Association also began to hedge its bets, arguing that the HACCP approach to mitigating BSE risk was more appropriate than a ban on ruminant protein in ruminant feed. Dave Andrews, a rancher from Brooks, Alberta, and the CCA president, was quoted as saying, "It seems they are going in a much more reasonable direction than they were planning." He added that Agriculture and Agri-Food Canada "has been leaning on the CCA to be the catalyst to get the stakeholders involved in this at the table to discuss what we are going to do." Note that the FDA apparently did not have similar problems. Andrews also admitted that little progress had been made so far in Canada and that Canadian beef industry leaders were meeting with the National Cattlemen's Beef Association at its mid-year meeting in Tennessee.[87]

After the Tennessee meeting, CCA, to its credit, changed its tune. Andrews was quoted as saying that CCA must be proactive on the issue, and that, "We've come to realize that we can't ignore this issue as an industry." Canada must follow the proposed ban in the United States, said Andrews, or be subject to trade sanctions.[88] By this time the Canadian government was "waiting to see where the U.S. goes before it puts its own rules on feeding animal byproducts to mammals into place."[89]

Even with the January 1997 announcement of the proposed FDA ban, there was silence from the Canadian government – and there still is only silence – beyond blanket assurances of the type issued for ten years by the British government. Leadership by abdication may be the Canadian way, but given both the public discussion of BSE to date and the newest scientific findings, such a strategy must be regarded as irresponsible and archaic.

DORRELL BSE STATEMENT — FULL TEXT

20 March 1996
By Parliamentary Staff, PA News
Health Secretary Stephen Dorrell, in the full text of his statement on BSE, told the Commons:
"I would like to make a statement about the latest advice which the Government has received from the Spongiform Encephalopathy Advisory Committee.

"The House will be aware that this committee, which is chaired by Professor John Pattison, was established in 1990 to bring together leading experts in neurology, epidemiology and microbiology to provide scientifically based advice on the implications for animal and human health of different forms of spongiform encephalopathy."

Mr Dorrell said: "The committee provides independent advice to Government. Its members are not Government scientists; they are leading practitioners in their field and the purpose of the committee is to provide advice not simply to Government, but to the whole community on the scientific questions which arise in its field.

"The Government has always made it clear that it is our policy to base our decisions on the scientific advice provided by the advisory committee. The committee has today agreed on new advice about the implications for animal and human health of the latest scientific evidence. Copies of the committee's advice, together with a statement from the Chief Medical Officer which is based on that advice, have been placed in the Vote Office.

"The committee has considered the work being done by the Government Surveillance Unit in Edinburgh which specialises in Creutzfeldt-Jakob Disease. This work, which relates to the 10 cases of CJD which have been identified in people aged under 42, has led the committee to conclude that the unit has identified a previously unrecognised and consistent disease pattern.

"A review of patients' medical histories, genetic analysis and consideration of other possible causes have failed to explain these cases adequately. There remains no scientific proof that BSE can be transmitted to man by beef, but the committee have concluded that the most likely explanation at present is that these cases are linked to exposure to BSE before the introduction of the specified bovine offal ban in 1989.

"Against the background of this new finding the committee has today agreed on the series of recommendations which the Government is making public this afternoon."

Mr Dorrell said: "The committee's recommendations fall into two parts.

"Firstly, they recommend a series of measures to further reduce the risk to human and animal health associated with BSE. Agriculture Minister Douglas Hogg will be making a statement about those measures which fall within his department's responsibilities immediately after questions on this statement have been concluded.

"In addition the committee recommended that there should be urgent consideration of what further research is needed in this area and that the Health and Safety Executive and the Advisory Committee on Dangerous Pathogens should urgently review their advice. The Government intends to accept all the recommendations of the Advisory Committee in full; they will be put into effect as soon as possible.

"The second group of recommendations from the committee offers advice about food safety on the assumption that the further measures recommended by the committee are implemented. On that basis the committee has concluded that the risk from eating beef is now likely to be extremely small and there is no need for it to revise its advice on the safety of milk.

"The Chief Medical Officer will be writing today to all doctors to ensure that the latest scientific evidence is drawn to their attention. In the statement by the Chief Medical Officer which we have placed in the Vote Office, Sir Kenneth Calman poses to himself the question whether he will continue to eat beef. I quote his answer: 'I will do so as part of a varied and balanced diet. The new measures and effective enforcement of existing measures will continue to ensure that the likely risk of developing CJD is extremely small.'

"A particular question has arisen about the possibility that children are more at risk of contracting CJD. There is at present no evidence for age sensitivity and the scientific evidence for the risks of developing CJD in those eating meat in childhood has not changed as a result of these new findings.

"However, parents will be concerned about implications for their children and I have asked the Advisory Committee to provide specific advice on this issue following its next meeting.

"Any further measures that the committee recommend will be given the most urgent consideration. As the Government has repeatedly made clear, new scientific evidence will be communicated to the public as soon as it becomes available."

Agriculture Minister Douglas Hogg, in the second BSE statement, told the Commons:

"I would like to make a statement about BSE.

"In view of the statement which Mr Dorrell has just made, the House will wish to know the action I propose to take to ensure the risk to the public is minimised.

"The additional recommendations just made by the Spongiform Encephalopathy Advisory Committee that most immediately affect agriculture departments are that carcasses from cattle aged over 30 months must be deboned in specially licensed plants supervised by the Meat Hygiene Service and the trimmings kept out of any food chain; and that the use of mammalian meat and bonemeal in feed for all farm animals be banned.

"The committee go on to state that if these and their other recommendations are carried out the risk from eating beef is now likely to be extremely small.

"The Government has accepted these recommendations and I will put them into effect as soon as possible. Any further measures that SEAC may recommend will be given the most urgent consideration.

"Also, and with immediate effect, I have instructed that existing controls in slaughterhouses and other meat plants and in feed mills should be even more vigorously enforced.

"I do not believe that this information should damage consumer confidence and thus the beef market. But I should say that support mechanisms exist in the Common Agricultural Policy and the Government will monitor the situation closely. I will naturally report developments to the House.

"I recognise that there will be public concern, but the Government's Chief Medical Officer advises us that there is no scientific evidence that BSE can be transmitted to man by beef. Indeed he has stated that he will continue to eat beef as part of a varied and balanced diet as indeed shall I. In view of what I have announced, we believe that British beef can be eaten with confidence."

2 A Diagnostic for Risk Communication Failures

Various prescriptions for communicating risks to the public:
- All we have to do is get the numbers right.
- All we have to do is tell them the numbers.
- All we have to do is explain what we mean by the numbers.
- All we have to do is show them that they've accepted similar risks in the past.
- All we have to do is to show them that it's a good deal for them.
- All we have to do is treat them nice.
- All we have to do is make them partners.
- All of the above.

Baruch Fischoff

Problems in communicating about risks originate primarily in the marked differences that exist between the two languages used to describe our experience with risks: the scientific and statistical language of experts on the one hand and the intuitively grounded language of the public on the other, as shown in figure 2.1. This contrast can easily be misunderstood: "expert assessment" simply means that some group or individual has brought specialized knowledge to bear on a risk issue, usually by referring to published scientific literature and by using technical terminology (toxicology, epidemiology, statistics and probability, and so on). In this sense people associated with all major groups – governments, academics, environmentalists, citizens, industry – use expert assessment and its technical languages. "Public assessment," on the other hand, simply means that people are referring to risk issues in ordinary language and in the context of their own everyday experiences, without necessarily being aware of the results of specialized knowledge.

In what follows we use "expert" and "public" as shorthand expressions for these two ways of talking about risks. This is most certainly not a case of being either right or wrong all of the time – a case where experts are always right and the public wrong, or vice versa. Rather, the contrast is a matter of which standpoint anyone decides to take in commenting on a risk issue.

However, people who have chosen one of these standpoints often express great frustrations with those on the other side. We can see some of the sources of those frustrations if we think of the many

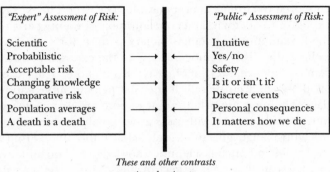

Figure 2.1
Some characteristics of the two languages of risk communication

controversies over risks associated with industrial chemicals. Experts expect the public to recognize, for example, that chemicals have quite different properties depending on their specific molecular structures; that the hazards associated with those properties vary widely even in "families" of closely related compounds such as dioxins; that our exposures to various compounds also vary greatly; that in all cases "the dose makes the poison"; that there can be great variation in the responses of different species, as well as different members of the same species to the same doses of compounds; that the harm which can be done is often distributed with apparent randomness in a population, so that we cannot tell which exposed individuals will be most affected; and so on.

On the other hand, members of the public expect experts to understand that it is harm to particular individuals that concerns them above all; that some ways of falling ill and dying are more feared than others; that, in view of the massive scientific databases on the familiar chemicals, there should be more certainty in expert judgments, as opposed to the familiar refrain, "more research is needed"; that lifestyle choices (with their attendant risks) voluntarily made are legitimate and may not be questioned, whereas risks involuntarily imposed on individuals are suspect; that the distributions of risks and benefits often do not appear to be equitable; that experts appear to be condescending and arrogant in their relations with non-experts; that experts employed by governments and industry obviously cannot be trusted to be forthright about risks; and so on.

Many of these contrasts are rooted in the difference between the experts' quantitative language and the qualitative terminology ordinarily employed by citizens in everyday life. The expert might say: "A lifetime exposure to aflatoxin at a concentration of twenty parts per billion in food, assuming an average dietary pattern for Canadians, yields an estimated excess carcinogenic risk to the exposed population (95 per cent confidence level) of one case in a million." The citizen might say: "Will my children be safe if they eat peanut butter sandwiches every day?" The most important point is: both are legitimate expressions of our attempts to deal with risks as we go about our daily business.

Neither language can entirely replace the other. From the citizen's standpoint, advancing scientific knowledge and quantitative risk assessments mean that every aspect of life soon can be described in these terms – but one will still not know for sure what to do, given the residual uncertainties. Consider the well-informed citizen who seeks to follow the ever-developing risk assessment of alcohol consumption. Alcohol is a carcinogen and has many other adverse effects at certain dose levels. On the other hand, a moderate daily intake of alcohol, perhaps varying with the type of alcoholic beverage, may offer a measure of protection against certain types of health risks (in particular, red wine in moderation may offer some protection against both heart risk and cancer). And yet, just how solid is the current scientific consensus on the relative risk numbers for alcohol consumption? And where exactly is the balance point in consumption between benefit and risk? Now consider that a modern citizen's dietary intake may involve thousands of identifiable chemicals and that dietary risk is one of hundreds of risk factors in everyday life. It is no wonder that we all seek and employ short cuts ("a couple of glasses of wine a day with meals is probably okay").

An expert in quantitative risk assessment might be preoccupied with other types of questions. How can regulators decide whether to allow industries to emit certain substances, for example, unless we have well-crafted quantitative risk assessments? How else could we decide whether or not to worry about the relatively small amounts of dioxins that some industries generate? Especially since – at the levels we are all ordinarily exposed to (the so-called "background exposure level") – no specific cases of current human illnesses or fatalities are attributable to dioxins, based on what is known to date from massive investments in scientific research programs. On the other hand, all around us, every day, many citizens are lighting up cigarettes and driving recklessly in their cars, and for those activities we have pretty good numbers: annually about forty thousand tobacco-related fatalities and four thousand auto accident fatalities in Canada, as well as serious illnesses and other impacts almost too extensive to measure. So: what risks are worth worrying about, and what risks should be put out of mind?

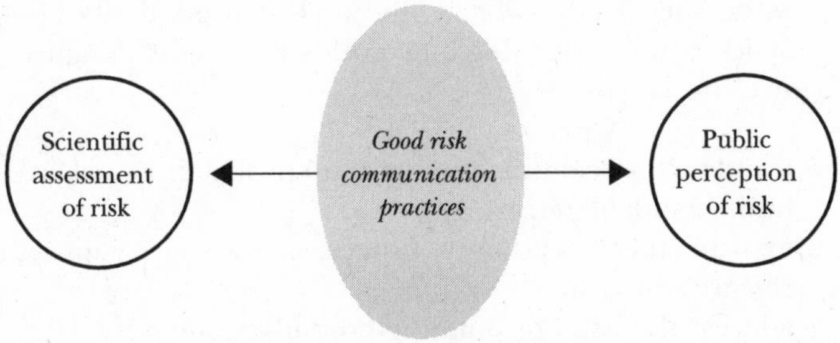

Figure 2.2
Function of good risk communication practice

The very examples used in the preceding paragraph will make some observers angry, because they appear to violate the boundary – sacred to some – between voluntary and involuntary risk. So be it: that is part of the inherently controversial nature of risk subjects in general, and risk communication in particular. The main point is that these two ways of analysing and speaking about the experience of risks, and the state of tension between them, will continue to exist. On the one hand, the expert assessment of risk is essential to the making of informed, reasoned choices in everyday life: to ignore the results of scientific risk assessments (ever-changing as they are) is merely to substitute a subconscious process for a conscious one. At the same time, citizens in a democratic society cannot allow experts to dictate lessons in risk management to them; on the contrary, their informed consent must form the basis of the collective allocation of resources for risk control and risk reduction. In general, therefore, society must manage the tension between these two profoundly different ways of representing risk, rather than try to eliminate the difference itself.

THE TASKS OF GOOD RISK COMMUNICATION PRACTICE

Good risk communication practice exists in the zone that separates the languages of expert risk assessment and public risk perception (fig. 2.2). According to the argument made above, both languages are necessary, because the daily business about managing risks – both the personal business of individuals and the social allocation of risk reduction resources – cannot be conducted in either one alone. But at the same time, the strong differences between the two languages constitute barriers to dialogue and cooperative understanding. Good risk communication practice seeks to break down those barriers and facilitate the productive exchanges between the two spheres.

More specifically, what is the work that good risk communication practice seeks to do? Reading from left to right in figure 2.2, it seeks (for example) to:

1 translate the scientific findings and probabilistic risk assessment into understandable terms;
2 explain the uncertainty ranges, knowledge gaps, and ongoing research programs;
3 address the issue of building credibility and trust.

And, reading from right to left, it seeks (for example) to:

1 understand the public's "framing" of the risk issue, especially its qualitative dimensions;
2 acknowledge the specific questions that arise in this domain (which may be, and often are, quite different from those posed by experts);
3 analyse the conditions needed for allowing the public to acquire needed information, skills, and participatory opportunities.

For governments and businesses, competence in good risk communication practice might be tested by examining the extent to which the organization has succeeded in earning the public's trust for its statements about the risks for which it is responsible, by learning to communicate effectively about the scientific basis of those risks, by being able to understand easily the public's framing of risk issues, and by being completely transparent and at ease in communicating with the public about risks.

At the level of social discourse the gradual spread of good risk communication practices might be expected over time to do the following: (a) nurture a facility for interpreting risk numbers, including the meaning of risk estimates and the uncertainties associated with them; (b) help people to put the whole assortment of risks affecting them into a broad framework (relative risk, comparative risk); (c) build institutional structures for arriving at a consensus on risk management options, and for allocating risk reduction resources effectively.

THE RISK INFORMATION VACUUM

We have located the work of risk communication in the gap that separates the unfolding scientific description of risks and the public understanding of those same risks. Further, we have suggested that the competing "expert" and "public" understandings of the same risks are equally legitimate and necessary. Indeed, it is inevitable that these

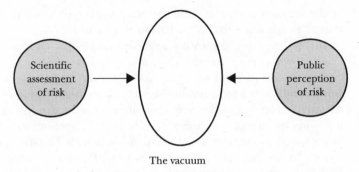

The vacuum

Figure 2.3
Risk information vacuum

competing perspectives should arise in a technologically advanced society, given the complexities inherent in our risk-taking behaviour.

We postulate that this gap will exist in most cases of publicly debated risks. In many cases the gap cannot be closed appreciably because the scientific and public apprehensions of a risk are framed by fundamentally different assumptions or values. But in all risk situations where some *public policy* response is called for – to ban a substance, to control emissions, to warn consumers about product hazards – what occurs in that gap can have huge consequences for institutions and the public alike. One of the most serious manifestations of these "gap dynamics" is the emergence of a risk information vacuum (fig. 2.3). The risk information vacuum arises where, over a long period of time, those who are conducting the evolving scientific research and assessments for high-profile risks make no special effort to communicate the results being obtained regularly and effectively to the public. Instead, partial scientific information dribbles out here and there and is interpreted in apparently conflicting ways, mixed with people's fears. In this connection the main theses of our book are, first, that failure to implement good risk communication practices gives rise to a risk information vacuum; and second, that this failing can have grave and expensive consequences for those who are regarded as being responsible for protecting the public's interests.

Society as well as nature abhors a vacuum, and so it is filled from other sources. For example, events reported in the media (some of them alarming) become the substantial basis of the public framing of these risks; or an interest group takes up the challenge and fills the vacuum with its own information and perspectives; or the intuitively based fears and concerns of individuals simply grow and spread until they become a substantial consensus in the arena of public opinion;

or the vacuum is filled by the soothing expressions beloved of politicians: "There is no risk of ... [fill in the blank]."

Among our case studies both dioxins and PCBs offer good illustrations of this phenomenon. The public had barely heard of dioxins before an EPA official in 1974 called them "by far the most toxic compound known to mankind." And, although an extensive scientific research effort got under way thereafter, no effective public communications occurred, and the risk information vacuum about dioxins was allowed to emerge to be filled subsequently by Greenpeace and others. In the case of PCBs a similar lack of effective communication of the scientific understanding created a vacuum that was subsequently filled by high-profile events such as the 1988 warehouse fire and community evacuation in St-Basile-le-Grand, Quebec.

In the case of "mad cow" disease, the legitimate public panic that began to spread in Britain in 1995 arose from an information vacuum created by the British Ministry of Agriculture Fisheries and Food: its stubborn refusal to give the public any inkling of the developing scientific suspicions about the transmissability of bovine spongiform encephalopathy (BSE) meant that the public was totally unprepared for the eventual revelation of the possibility, so long denied, that a dreaded human disease could be contracted by eating beef. The consequences for the European Union countries include a sharp decline in beef sales, a terrible risk control strategy in Great Britain (mass slaughter and incineration of cattle), and billions of dollars in compensation, price support payments, and the cost of the mass slaughter program – some of which might have been unnecessary, arguably, had the government been completely candid in its public statements about the evolving scientific research results on BSE.

In the case of silicone breast implants, the manufacturers failed to disclose in a timely fashion all the information in their possession relevant to the risks associated with the implants and failed to encourage a full and frank discussion of those risks among consumers and medical professionals. In this information vacuum grew fears of serious and dreaded types of immune-system diseases, which became key factors in successful personal-injury lawsuits – although later epidemiological research showed those fears to be almost certainly groundless. The final chapter in this episode has not yet been written but billions of dollars in compensation claims are "on the table," and whatever the ultimate outcome, the results will have been extremely damaging to the firms involved as well as to many women.

Our case studies include one in which this syndrome is still developing, namely, environmental risks associated with the agricultural applications of genetically engineered crops. These risks – for example,

the risk that the novel genetic material will "outcross" into the culti-
vated plant's wild relatives (known as "gene flow" or "gene escape" in
the scientific literature) – can cause legitimate concern, in large part
due to the unfamiliarity of this new technology. But neither the agricultural biotechnology industry in Canada nor the main regulatory
agency (Agriculture Canada) wants to talk about any of this with the
public. The operative philosophy appears to be "let sleeping dogs lie."
A vacuum is developing which almost certainly will be filled in the
future by worrisome events, possibly causing significant damage to the
industry.

Does any of this matter very much? We think that it does, and that
(as our case studies will reveal) there are substantial monetary and
other costs attributable to risk communication failures. Many of these
damages stem from what happens when a risk information vacuum is
allowed to develop – namely, a process of "amplification" whereby the
risk issues are "put into play" and develop in ways that might otherwise
never have happened.[1] This process of risk amplification is shown in
every one of the case studies to follow, and it is, we believe, one of the
most important inherent features of risk communication failures.

WHAT IS RISK COMMUNICATION?

Risk communication is the process of exchanges about how best to
assess and manage risks among academics, regulatory practitioners,
interest groups, and the general public. Risk is the probability of harm
in any given situation, and this probability is determined by two
factors: (a) the nature of a hazard and (b) the extent of anyone's
exposure to that hazard. For each person the risk of being injured or
killed in a traffic accident, for example, is first a function of the various
hazards inherent in using powered vehicles – mechanical failure,
driver's level of skill and care, actions of other drivers, state of mind,
road conditions, and so forth. The other factor is exposure, that is,
the amount of time any person spends on the road in the midst of
the above-mentioned hazards. The product of the two factors (hazards
and exposures) adds up to the overall risk.[2]

The sharp disagreements that can occur are sometimes based on
disagreements over principles or approaches, sometimes on differences in the information base available to various parties, and sometimes on a failure to consider carefully each other's position.
"Exchanges" can mean anything from a presentation of relatively
straightforward information to arguments over contested data and
interpretations, to sincere or disingenuous concern, to what is in the
eyes of some just plain misinformation (inadvertently misleading data)

or disinformation (deliberately misleading data). But systematically neglecting a responsibility to initiate conversations about risk – in other words, allowing a risk information vacuum to develop – may well be the most serious failing of all in the domain of risk communication practices.

In such situations the risk communication process itself often becomes an explicit focus of controversy. Charges of media bias or sensationalism, of distorted or selective use of information by advocates, of hidden agendas or irrational standpoints, and of the inability or unwillingness of regulatory agencies to communicate vital information in a language the public can understand, are common. Such charges are traded frequently at public hearings, judicial proceedings, and conferences, expressing the general and pervasive sense of mistrust felt by many participants toward others. Of course there are also genuine differences of principle, outlook, and values among the citizenry; disagreements will persist even with the most complete and dispassionate knowledge of others' views.

The phrase "risk communication" itself is not very old. It appears to have been coined in 1984[3] and arose out of a growing interest in risk perception, which draws on psychological research to help explain why various individuals and groups hold such sharply different views about risks. In particular, understanding the disparities between risks as assessed by "experts" on the one hand and as understood by non-expert members of the general public on the other has been a major preoccupation. Whereas risk perception studies have been concerned with explaining those disparities, risk communication has from the beginning had a practical intent: given that these disparities exist, are deeply entrenched in human awareness, and form the basis of strongly held attitudes and behaviour, how can we improve the quality of the dialogue about risk across the gap that separates experts from the general public? Second, how can we apply this improved dialogue about risk to achieving a higher degree of social consensus on the inherently controversial aspects of managing environmental and health risks?

In seeking to answer these questions, risk communication researchers married their knowledge about risk assessment and management issues with the approaches used in the field of modern communications theory and practice. Statements about risk by various parties are treated as "messages" intended to persuade others to believe or do something. Like all such messages circulating among persons, their effectiveness as acts of *persuasive communication* can be evaluated according to well-established criteria such as whether they gain attention, are understood, are believed, are acted on. This paradigm of communications research has developed since 1945 and has an enormous published literature to support it.[4] Risk communication research drew upon this resource and adapted its findings to the particular concerns of the risk studies area.

THREE PHASES

Three phases in the evolution of risk communication have emerged over the past fifteen years, with each of the later stages responding to and building upon the earlier ones, and with each contributing something of lasting value. Phase one (about 1975–1984) stressed the quantitative expressions of risk estimates and argued that priorities for regulatory actions and public concerns should be established on the basis of comparative risk estimates.[5] Phase two (about 1985–1994) stressed the characteristics of successful communications: source credibility, message clarity, effective use of channels, and, above all, a focus on the needs and perceived reality of the audiences.[6] Phase three (beginning around 1995) has emphasized the development of a long-term organizational commitment and competence in practising good risk communication.

Phase One (1975–84)

The enduring strength of what was accomplished in this phase is captured in the following statement: in order to function sensibly in a world of expanding opportunity, we must have the capacity to assess and manage risks at an exacting level of detail. The scientific approach to risk management offers an imperfect but indispensable tool for doing so. Through judicious risk-taking behaviour, individuals and society derive enormous benefits. For example, industrial chemicals are the basis of most consumer goods today, but these same chemicals are also dangerous; it is a matter of the dose. Prescription drugs are the best example: in the correct doses the benefits are substantial, and the side-effect risks, while always present, are minimized.

Some serious weaknesses emerged in this phase, the worst of which could be labelled the "arrogance of technical expertise." Faced with public scepticism about risk-based decision-making in areas such as the safety of nuclear power generating stations, and opposition to the results, many experts responded with open contempt towards the public and its perception of risk.[7] For such experts, "perceived risk" is often correlated with "false" understanding and is contrasted with "real risk," which is allegedly an "objective" ("true") account of reality. Fortunately one now encounters this invidious distinction less and less, since there is a greater appreciation of the errors in judgment that experts too are prone to making.[8] Partly as a result of the arrogance of expertise, there exists a profound public distrust of experts and the institutions they represent, which weakens the force of sensible contributions technical experts can make to the public discourse on risk-taking. Another weakness is that critical data gaps and ever-changing scientific research results are common in all significant risk management areas. The uncertainties introduced thereby produce legitimate concerns when "yes/no" decisions must be made.

The underlying message of permanent value in phase one is: for individuals as well as societies, managing opportunities and dangers on the basis of comparative risk information should be seen as an inescapable duty of intelligent life. However, this message could not be communicated effectively to a wide range of public audiences, partly because its authors were often so openly contemptuous of the fundamental beliefs about risk-taking held by the very audiences they were addressing.

Phase Two (1985–94)

The radical break which defines the transition from phase one to phase two was the realization that statements about risk situations ought to be regarded as acts of persuasive communication, that is, as messages intended to persuade a listener of the correctness of a point of view.[9] Guidance for this new approach was found in the history of twentieth-century marketing communications, which had demonstrated first in commercial advertising, then more broadly, the effectiveness of a strategy taking into account two key factors: (a) the characteristics of the audience itself, and (b) the intrinsic legitimacy of the audience's perception of the situation. The coinage of good communication is trust in the message source ("Will you believe me when I tell you something?"), and this is the underpinning for *credibility*, which is a perception of the intrinsic honesty of the message content itself as well as the entire institutional context within which the message is generated.

The great strength of this new approach was that the formulae of good communications practices adapted from modern marketing had been tested and refined over a long period and, for some purposes, were known to be highly successful. But there proved to be severe difficulties in adapting this marketing communications paradigm to risk issues. Slovic and MacGregor have diagnosed the main problem well:[10] "Although attention to communication can prevent blunders that exacerbate conflict, there is little evidence that risk communication has made any significant contribution to reducing the gap between technical risk assessments and public perceptions or to facilitating decisions about major sources of risk conflict (i.e. nuclear waste). The limited effectiveness of risk communication efforts can be attributed to the lack of trust."

The paradigm of persuasion in the marketing communications approach had identified a broad range of techniques for enhancing trust and credibility for messages. However, the early studies on propaganda recognized that too strong a focus on persuasive techniques alone (especially those that seek to manipulate audiences' emotions) was potentially dangerous, for it could result in the message's rational content being subverted by those excessively clever techniques. So in the more prosaic world of risk issues, emotive techniques of effective persuasive communications (such as techniques for convincing an audience that one is a credible spokesperson on risk issues) could take precedence over the informational content of the risk message itself.[11]

The underlying message of permanent value in phase two may be stated as follows: there is an obligation on the part of major institutional actors in society to communicate effectively about risks, not by simply touting the superiority of their own technical risk assessments but through making an honest effort to understand the bases of public risk perceptions and experimenting with ways to construct a reasoned dialogue around different stakeholder assessments of risk situations.[12] The residual weakness here is that trust in the communicator is often far too low for these experiments to succeed.

Phase Three (Current)

Phase three begins with the recognition that lack of trust is pervasive in risk issues; and because of this, risk communication practice must move away from a focus on purely instrumental techniques of persuasive communication. Phase three is characterized by an emphasis on social context, that is, on the social interrelations among the players in the game of risk management.[13] It is based on the presumption that, despite the controversial nature of many risk management issues, there are forces at work also that favour consensus-building, meaningful stakeholder interaction, and acceptance of reasonable government regulatory frameworks. When those forces are relatively weak, the field of risk management is exposed to wide-open confrontation among stakeholder interests.

Phase two remained incomplete because the key ingredient of successful persuasive communications (trust) cannot be manufactured by the use of techniques alone, no matter how artful the practitioners. A

EXPERTISE	Not viable in risk communication without trust
TRUST	Not viable without credible evidence of changes in long-term organizational commitment
ORGANIZATIONAL COMMITMENT	Requires credible criteria for "best practices"

Figure 2.4
Three phases of risk communication

working hypothesis is that trust in institutional risk actors (governments and industry) can accumulate, slowly, through the commitments by those institutions – as demonstrated by deeds, not words – to carry out responsible risk communication, and furthermore to do so consistently, as a matter of daily practice over the long term, not just in response to crisis events. The underlying message of permanent value in phase three may thus be stated: A demonstrated commitment to good risk communication practices by major organizational actors can put pressure on all players in risk management to act responsibly.

The evolution of risk communication practice to date through these three phases is summarized in figure 2.4.

METHOD FOR THE STUDY OF RISK COMMUNICATION FAILURES

Briefly described, the method for the case studies in this book is as follows. The material chosen for analysis is the record of a long-running controversy over health or environmental risks associated with substances such as dioxins. We track the scientific understanding and description of the risks associated with these chemical compounds, as documented in published and unpublished reports by industry sources, governments, and independent researchers. A special attempt is made to follow in detail the chronology of emerging scientific research on a new hazard, such as "mad cow" disease, and to track the reactions to this new knowledge at particular times by various constituencies (politicians, general public, environmentalists, industry, and so forth), in an effort to understand how and why a risk controversy grows.

In summary, the first step undertaken in the case studies may be characterized by the attempt to answer the following question: "What did the experts know, and when did they know it?" The next step traces the evolution of public understanding and controversy with an analogous question: "What did members of the public know, and when did

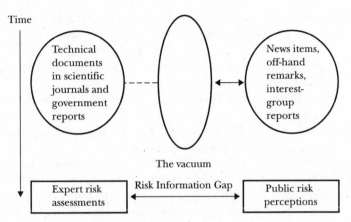

Figure 2.5
A method for the study of risk communication failures

they know it?" Here we are interested in how the public perception of risk and benefit was formed; what awareness there was of the evolving state of scientific understanding of the relevant issues; and precisely how a particular environmental or health hazard became controversial. The sources for this are newspaper and other media accounts, records of public hearings, the activities of public-interest groups, and so forth. In most of the following case studies we track meticulously the media coverage of developing risk controversies, taking this reportage as both a source of clues to the public understanding of risks as well as a primary filter through which the public learns about the scientific description of those risks.[14] Above all else, the exact chronology of events becomes very important in order to "match" the parallel tracks of the two dimensions (expert risk and perceived risk) to see when each is or is not influenced by the other, and why.

Finally we examine closely all of the main points of divergence between expert and perceived risk and look especially for the risk-communication exchanges, if any, that occurred at those points. We ask, for example: What effort, if any, did risk managers make to explain clearly to the public the risk and benefit assessments they had conducted? What effort, if any, did risk managers make to understand thoroughly the nature of public concerns? We also ask: What events fueled public concern? What was the nature of media reporting of relevant events? The following overriding question is posed: As the public awareness of the issue was developing, did any agency seek to take responsibility for the issue and to address the risk information gap? If so, what happened? Figure 2.5 shows all of the above components.[15]

In this model the possibilities for closing the risk information gap depend upon such factors as:

1 whether the type of risks involved have special characteristics of dread and unfamiliarity;
2 whether the public comes to believe that it has been misled by experts;
3 whether extensive media coverage of sensational events, attributable to a particular risk situation, occurs;
4 how scientific research findings are interpreted by various parties;
5 whether key stakeholders choose certain issues for special attention;
6 whether a competent agency assumes responsibility for implementing good risk communication practice at any time in the sequence of events.

TOWARDS GOOD RISK COMMUNICATION PRACTICE

Our primary purpose in documenting risk communication failures in our case studies is not to lay blame but rather to learn from the mistakes that have been made so far. Mistakes are inevitable, and seeking to learn from them is just about the only way of figuring out how to do things more wisely. In the first chapter and those that follow, we present seven extensive case studies in various dimensions of health and environmental risks. The concluding chapter synthesizes the conclusions from the case studies into a set of lessons that can lead the way towards better risk communication practices.

3 Dioxins, or Chemical Stigmata

WITH STEVE E. HRUDEY

[Dioxin is] by far the most toxic compound known to mankind.
Dianne Courtney, EPA official, 1974

Dioxins are the deadliest chemicals known to guinea pigs.
Clyde Hertzman, professor of Epidemiology, University of British Columbia

We've always believed dioxin is a killer.
Sheila Copps, minister of the Environment, 1994

We have targeted the mega-uglies [*les produits les plus menaçants*] – this
includes dioxin and PCBs – for virtual elimination.
Sergio Marchi, minister of the Environment, 1996[1]

PROLOGUE: MADAME MINISTER, WHERE ARE THE BODIES?

Our society's experience with understanding and managing risks associated with dioxins, in the period beginning with the early 1970s,
could teach us a great deal about how to handle risk issues in general.
But to date it has not done so. Consider the fate of the first epigraph,
from a statement by a U.S. regulatory scientist; her description of
dioxin as "by far the most toxic compound known to mankind"
inspired a kind of journalistic mantra in later news stories about events
associated with dioxins.[2] There are actually many different meanings
that could be implied by this phrase. Here are just three of them:

1 Dioxin poses a greater threat to human health than any other
substance that humans encounter.
2 Dioxin is the most toxic substance ever administered to laboratory
animals in scientific tests.
3 Dioxin is the most toxic substance that modern industry has ever
created.

Minister Copps chose the first meaning and carried it a few steps
further. For if dioxin represents the most serious known threat to
human health, it would be only reasonable to presume that there are
all kinds of dead bodies in our environment whose fate was attributable

to dioxin exposure. Of course this might conceivably be so, but, despite the implications of the minister's dramatic rhetoric, we cannot pinpoint any such cases, and we have other reasons to think that it would not make much sense to go looking for them. The second meaning is closer to the literal truth, although the animal test results show a great variation among species in reactions to dioxin and laboratory animal tests have confirmed several natural toxins (e.g., botulin) to be more acutely lethal. And since the implications of these lab study results for human health are not clear, at least not at first glance, it is also not clear whether citizens should worry about them or not.

The third possible meaning introduces further complications. Dioxins indeed are produced by various industries, but this is unintentional, because these substances have no useful properties. Happily, many industries are now fully committed to lowering steadily the emissions of dioxins from their facilities. There are also other sources for the creation of dioxins, such as combustion, and some of those processes occur naturally. Because there are many sources of dioxin compounds, we cannot eliminate our exposure to dioxins, at least not very easily. But is this something that citizens should worry about?

The statement by Minister Marchi on 10 December 1996 certainly would lead us to believe that citizens should still be worrying about dioxins. One cannot be entirely sure what the neologism "mega-ugly" means, but the phrase's connotations are perfectly clear, and they are decidedly negative. (The French version renders it as "the most menacing or threatening substances," which is no more comforting.) It certainly seems to suggest that citizens should be worrying about dioxins right now. But should they? Before deciding, it might be helpful for them to hear the tale of dioxins as a risk issue, starting with the evolving scientific understanding and then looking for clues to the public understanding of this issue. Among other things, they would discover the existence of a risk information vacuum, originating as in our other cases in a systematic failure of effective risk communication.

As we shall see, because the risk information vacuum for dioxins was allowed to develop and then be filled by the perspectives of a single interested party (Greenpeace), whose views went virtually unchallenged in the public domain itself (insofar as effective communication is concerned), dioxin was "put into play" as a risk issue. The quoted phrase comes from the financial sector and refers to the situation in which a corporation's publicly traded stock is made the subject of competing bids in order to secure control of the company. The analogy here is control over the positioning of a risk issue in the public's mind within a hierarchy of priorities, or "agenda setting." The desired outcome is to evoke a demand in the name of the public to "do something" about the issue, in such a way that politicians and their civil servants will find it impossible to ignore, or at least will find that lack of resistance to this demand is the easiest course of action.[3]

Having been put into play, dioxin became a stigmatized substance.[4] The social process of "stigmatizing" something is much like stereotyping, scapegoating, and witch-hunting. All amount to creating short cuts to resolve situations in which high degrees of fear and uncertainty exist among the population – and where some individuals or groups have been singled out by others and become victims in this process, paying the price for those sham resolutions. The short cuts appear to be good solutions for the general apprehensions in part because no more plausible answers for the fears have been forthcoming. The stigma that dioxins have borne is simply the sign for the sum total of all the potentially hazardous and health-threatening effects attributable to the products of a fecund industrial chemistry. The phrase "by far the most toxic compound known to mankind" was transmuted into many others, notably "the deadliest poison ever made by man," "more poisonous than cyanide or strychnine," "so deadly that 1/200 of a drop will kill a human" – phrases that conjure up images from detective fiction of a substance deliberately made to cause harm in minuscule doses being administered to innocent victims by cunning criminals.

This overly dramatic phraseology is part of the stigmatizing process in that it has the effect (intended or not) of creating a short cut for human understanding: we have at least a vague idea of what strychnine is and what it does to people, and now we know that dioxin is "like" strychnine. But the short cut is in fact most detrimental to our appreciation of what dioxins are, how and why they are generated in the first place and then end up in our environment, what effects they may have on different species, and what it is prudent to do about all this. Such an appreciation in the public mind can arise – in view of the enormous complexity in the scientific research on dioxins – only if a reasonable effort is made to convey that complexity from scientists to the public in understandable terms. On the whole this has not happened, not for the entire period of more than twenty years in which dioxin has been a risk issue in North America. *It is still not happening now,* despite the fact that controversy over dioxin risk was re-ignited six years ago, when "hormone mimicking" was first reported in the press.[5]

The process of stigmatizing something like a chemical takes root and flourishes in the vacuum created by the absence of other information that is sufficiently clear and compelling to make a difference in the public mind. In the sections that follow we will show how this happened.

1 RISK ASSESSMENT OF DIOXINS

We had a serious situation in our operating plants because of contamination of 2,4,5-trichlorophenol with impurities, the most active of which is 2,3,7,8-tetrachlorodibenzodioxin. The material is exceptionally toxic; it has a tremendous potential for producing chloracne and systemic injury. One of the things we want to avoid is the occurrence of any acne in consumers. I am particularly concerned here with consumers who are using the material on a daily, repeated basis such as custom operators may use it. If this should occur, the whole 2,4,5-T industry will be hard hit, and I would expect restrictive legislation, either barring the material or putting very rigid controls upon it. This is the main reason why we are so concerned that we clean up our own house from within, rather that having someone from without do it for us ... I trust you will be very judicious in your use of this information. It could be quite embarrassing if it were misinterpreted or misused.

> Dr Verald K. Rowe, director of toxicology for Dow Chemical Co. (u.s.),
> internal company memo addressed to Ross Mulholland,
> a product manager at Dow Chemical Canada, 24 June 1965

There is abundant evidence that 2,3,7,8-TCDD occurring as an impurity in 2,4,5-T is highly toxic.

> Dow Chemical Co., letter to Melvin R. Laird,
> u.s. secretary of Defense, 1970

Dr Johnson said that "since 1950 we have been keenly aware" that highly toxic compounds are formed from 2,4,5-trichlorophenol at high temperatures, and in 1965 [1957: WL] the chief offender was identified as 2,3,7,8-tetrachlorodibenzo-*p*-dioxin ... This [latter] material and its congeners are likely to attract a good deal of attention in the months ahead.

> Article in the scientific journal *Nature* (April 1970),
> citing Dr Julius E. Johnson, director of research, Dow Chemical

Yet there is no need to quibble: TCDD is unquestionably a chemical of supreme toxicity to experimental animals. Moreover, severe chronic effects from low dosages have also been demonstrated in experimental animals. Therefore the concern about its effects on human health and the environment is understandable ... Two years ago a conference on dioxin at Michigan State concluded that the TCDD case is relatively less important than a number of other issues and that the nation's limited scientific resources should be devoted to the issues posing a greater threat. On the basis of the evidence turned up so far, the conclusion is still valid.

> Fred H. Tschirley, *Scientific American* (February 1986)[6]

General Characterization of Dioxins

Dioxin has become the popular name variously for a specific and very toxic organic compound, 2,3,7,8 tetrachlorodibenzo-*p*-dioxin (2,3,7,8-TCDD) or for any of the family of seventy-five chlorinated dioxin compounds, which consist in the basic dibenzo-*p*-dioxin structure with varying degrees and location of the chlorine atom in the molecule. More recently, terminology has been expanded to dioxin-like compounds, which are those that behave similarly to dioxin in their ability to interact with a specific enzyme receptor in various living systems. The group of dioxin-like compounds includes some specific poly-chlorinated biphenyls (PCBs), the polychlorinated dibenzo-*p*-furans, chlorinated naphthalenes, diphenyl ethers, and other aromatic compounds.

These compounds are members of a larger group of chlorinated organic compounds that are relatively persistent in the environment and in organisms. In the environment, it is their resistance to micro-biological decomposition and their stability through abiotic degradation processes which causes them to persist. In organisms, their resistance to metabolism and their tendency to concentrate in fatty tissues impede excretion. These properties combine to make the compounds bioaccumulate in organisms and biomagnify through food chains. Because of these capabilities, very low level emissions of these compounds to the environment can build up through food chains and pose a potential health risk to organisms at the higher levels in the chain.

Dioxin differs from other notorious substances such as DDT and PCBs in that it has never been commercially produced. Rather, it is an unwanted contaminant, first recognized in the manufacture of trichlorophenol, primarily produced as a feedstock for the production of 2,4,5-trichlorophenoxyacetic acid (2,4,5-T). Dioxin was further distinguished from other industrial chemicals and environmental contaminants by the extremely low levels at which it could cause toxic effects (more than a thousand-fold lower than other toxic industrial chemicals and known environmental contaminants). The experience with human exposures to dioxin in the past fifty years has occurred in two major phases. The first phase (about 1950–80) involved accidental releases of sufficient quantities to cause characteristic skin reactions and other effects in humans or dramatic mortality among other animals. These incidents are summarized in tables 3.1 and 3.2.

The second phase, over the past twenty years, has been characterized by the detection of dioxin at substantially lower levels in a variety of emission sources and environmental media, largely because of the dramatic improvements in analytical detection limits for dioxin (over a one-million-fold increase in sensitivity), allowing the measurement of dioxin where it would have previously been non-detectable. This second phase has been accompanied by parallel advances in sensitive biological test procedures that demonstrate biological responses at the lower, ultratrace levels; but the toxicological significance of these sensitive biological measures remains uncertain.[7] Likewise, this second phase of discovering the pervasive presence of dioxin and dioxin-like compounds has not been accompanied by the direct human toxicological responses so apparent in the first phase of gross exposure.

Human Exposures, Phase One – Major Industrial Incidents

A series of industrial accidents in the chemical industry was responsible for the recognition that dioxins are capable of producing chloracne. A form of persistent and potentially disfiguring acne, chloracne was first recognized as an occupational disease in the German chemical industry in 1895; however, it was not until 1957 that dioxin was isolated as the cause by Dr Karl Schulz, a dermatologist at the University of Hamburg, consulting for the Boehringer Chemical Company, a manufacturer of trichlorophenol. He first demonstrated by testing on a rabbit's ear that dioxin was an impurity in trichlorophenol which caused the skin condition.[8] Several industrial accidents causing chloracne in humans and involving the manufacture of trichlorophenol or 2,4,5-T are now recognized as major dioxin exposure incidents. They are shown in table 3.1.

Human Exposures, Phase One – Major Incidents Involving a Broad Cross-Section of a Population

In addition to these industrial manufacturing accidental exposures, there have been several other major documented human exposures to dioxins. These non-manufacturing incidents are summarized in table 3.2.

In 1968 an epidemic of skin disease in Fukuoka, Japan, was ultimately traced to contamination of rice oil (Yusho) with PCBs used as a heating medium in the rice oil processing plant. The heating process was believed to have produced substantial quantities of polychlorinated dibenzofurans (PCDFs) from the parent PCBs, and some of these have toxicity approaching that of the most toxic dioxins. The incident caused widespread chloracne in most victims. Swollen eyes, eye discharges, and nail pigmentation were also common, while a substantial

Table 3.1
Documented Dioxin Exposure Incidents from the Manufacture of Trichlorophenol or 2,4,5-T[9]

Dates	Location	Description
1949	Nitro, W. Virginia, USA	Monsanto trichlorophenol plant 122 cases of chloracne
1953	Ludwigshafen, W. Germany	BASF trichlorophenol plant 55 cases of chloracne
1956	Grenoble, France	Rhone-Poulenc trichlorophenol plant 17 cases of chloracne
1963	Amsterdam, Netherlands	NV Philips 2,4,5-T plant 44 cases of chloracne
1964	Midland, Michigan, USA	Dow Chemical trichlorophenol plant 49 cases of chloracne
1965–69	Prague, Czechoslovakia	Spolana trichlorophenol unit in 2,4,5-T plant 78 cases of chloracne
1966	Grenoble, France	Rhone-Poulenc trichlorophenol plant 21 cases of chloracne
1968	Derbyshire, U.K.	Coalite trichlorophenol plant 79 cases of chloracne
1976	Seveso, Italy	ICMESA trichlorophenol plant release caused exposure of public; 134 confirmed cases of chloracne; more than 500 residents treated for presumed symptoms; an estimated 37,000 residents exposed

minority of victims suffered a variety of neurological symptoms. Over the two- to four-month period of exposure, Yusho victims were estimated to have been exposed to dioxin equivalents at ten thousand to 100,000 times the background population exposure. Tragically, this scenario was replicated eleven years later in Taiwan, with the so-called Yu-cheng poisoning of 1979. In this case two thousand people consumed rice oil contaminated with PCBs and PCDFs at levels about 10 per cent of those that had occurred in the Japanese Yusho incident. Similar symptoms and outcomes were observed in this later accident.[11]

Perhaps the most morally repugnant page in the dioxin story is that associated with the use of Agent Orange in Vietnam and Southeast Asia. This herbicide was formulated as a fifty/fifty mixture of 2,4,5-T and 2,4-D (2,4-dichlorophenoxyacetic acid); the former was manufactured from the 2,4,5-trichlorophenol in a manner that could yield significant contamination with 2,3,7,8-TCDD. Military use of Agent Orange began in 1962 and peaked between 1965 and 1969. Thereafter usage was scaled back and ultimately stopped in 1970 because of growing protests about engaging in chemical warfare and ecological damage arising from indiscriminant herbicide spraying. It is estimated

Table 3.2
Major Dioxin Exposures from Other Sources[10]

Dates	Location	Description (additional references)
1962–70	Southeast Asia	U.S. military use of Agent Orange, a herbicide mixture containing dioxin-contaminated 2,4,5-T; widespread civilian and military exposure
1968	Western Japan	Rice oil contaminated with PCBs containing polychlorinated dibenzofurans ingested leading to over 1800 individuals being classified as patients; called the "Yusho" or oil disease and caused a range of symptoms including chloracne (Masuda 1994)
1971	Times Beach, Missouri, USA	Waste oil hauler applied dioxin-contaminated organic sludges (still bottoms) from a hexachlorophene manufacturer as waste oil for dust control in an arena on a horse breeding farm, causing 48 deaths of 85 exposed horses along with deaths of hundreds of birds and several cats, dogs and rodents (Carter et al. 1974)
1979	Central Taiwan	Rice oil contaminated with PCBs containing polychlorinated dibenzofurans ingested leading to illness of over 2,000 individuals; called "Yu-Cheng" or oil disease and caused a range of symptoms including chloracne (Hsu et al. 1994)
1979	Love Canal, New York, USA	Declaration of emergency by President Carter because of hazardous waste exposures including dioxins in wastes buried in Hooker Chemical hazardous waste site and evacuation of residences
1981	Binghampton, New York, USA	Transformers containing PCBs burn in an office building and expose firefighters to dioxins and furans; building was abandoned and subjected to massive cleanup
1988	St-Basile-le-Grand, Quebec, Canada	PCB storage depot catches fire, causing evacuation of residents over concerns of dioxin and furan exposures, but no characteristic disease symptoms arose in the public (see further Chapter 8)

that a total of 11.5 million gallons of Agent Orange was sprayed over the territory of Vietnam.[12]

Vietnam veterans returned home to a growing controversy surrounding 2,4,5-T, in part because of concerns over dioxin contamination. These concerns resulted in a suspension of those 2,4,5-T uses leading to greatest human exposures in 1970 by the U.S. Department of Agriculture, and the beginning of a long campaign by the newly founded U.S. Environmental Protection Agency (EPA) – to which responsibility for pesticides had been transferred – to restrict and ultimately ban uses of 2,4,5-T on food crops.[13] Given the unprecedented proportion of disabled veterans produced by the Vietnam war and the poor reception and assimilation offered to returning soldiers from this unpopular war, growing speculation that Agent Orange exposure may have harmed those exposed led to a strong reaction by potentially affected veterans. This culminated in a massive toxic tort case involving fifteen thousand named individuals, a network of fifteen hundred law firms for the plaintiffs, defence preparation costs of $100 million, and an original settlement of $180 million in May 1984, the largest in u.s. history to that time.[14] In this case, however, evidence of substantial dioxin exposure among most claimants was not nearly as clear as had been the case for the earlier industrial accidents.

Just as the 2,4,5-T and Agent Orange issues were gathering strength, a salvage oil company sprayed a horse riding arena in eastern Missouri in May 1971. Within days, hundreds of birds normally resident in the rafters were found dead in the arena, followed by rodents and several cats and dogs. Of the eighty-five horses exercised in the arena, sixty-two became ill and forty-eight died. Soil was removed from the arena in October 1971 and again in April 1972, but horses continued to die until January 1974. Two other horse arenas and one farm were oil-sprayed by the same company, leading to several more horse deaths, as well as the death of seventy chickens at the farm. Three children and one adult were exposed, and all developed skin conditions consistent with chloracne.[15]

These incidents led to an investigation by the u.s. Centers for Disease Control (cdc) which was not completed until 1974. A determination finally was made that soil in the first horse arena had been contaminated by over thirty parts per million of the most toxic dioxin. These levels exceeded the levels of dioxin typically found in contaminated 2,4,5-T, and the source was ultimately traced to the distillation bottom sludges from a hexachlorophene manufacturer. The manufacturer had contracted with a waste disposal firm to dispose of 68,000 litres of the sludge estimated to contain more than twenty kilograms of dioxin in total. The firm in turn sold these organic sludges to the oil salvage company that disposed of them all over Missouri. The cdc finding ultimately led to a buyout in February 1983 by the federal and state governments of the entire community of Times Beach, where the waste oil hauler had sprayed twenty-three miles of roadways with dioxin-contaminated oils. The buyout of an entire town for almost $37 million attracted enormous national attention and made dioxin a household word in the United States.[16]

In the midst of the emerging decade-long dioxin disaster in Missouri, an explosion on 10 July 1976 at the icmesa trichlorophenol plant in Seveso, Italy, released a cloud of emissions containing an estimated one kilogram of dioxin, affecting a densely populated area of approximately eighteen hundred hectares. Small mammals, birds, and vegetation began dying within days, and signs of chloracne began to appear in exposed humans; eventually 733 people from the most exposed zone were evacuated from an area of 110 acres.[17] By the end of August over two thousand rabbits and twelve hundred small farm-yard animals had died, but no deaths were observed among any livestock (cattle, horses, pigs, sheep and goats).

The houses in the most heavily contaminated area were eventually purchased by the plant owner and destroyed.[18] Overall, 183 cases of chloracne were reported, with 85 per cent of these observed in chil-dren – 20 per cent of children from the most exposed zone contracted chloracne. Fortunately, only fifteen cases were classified as severe, and within five years the chloracne had virtually disappeared, except for scarring in the severe cases. Overall, these dioxin accidents showed a pattern of causing chloracne among substantial numbers of people following long-term or high-dose exposure, sometimes long after an encounter with the material, reflecting the persistence of the dioxin in the environment. It also caused obvious mortality among other exposed species.

An Overview of Dioxin Risk Assessment and the Animal Effects Studies

This is of course a detailed and highly technical matter, and we shall attempt only a sketch of the subject here. However, it is a key ingre-dient in our story for a number of reasons. First, as we shall see in part 2, beginning with the very first articles, the animal study results were often referred to in newspaper coverage of dioxins. This is interesting in itself, but what is more important is that the references to animal study results often were conflated with all kinds of specula-tion about presumed human health effects, so much so that sometimes it takes a keen eye to keep the two themes apart. It may be safely presumed that such a conflation had an impact on public understand-ing of dioxin risk. Thus although the animal study results are certainly important in and of themselves, they are also relevant to the analysis of the risk communication dynamics which is our particular focus.

The second reason for a brief review here is that the animal studies are the basis for the risk assessment exercise and, ultimately, for the calculation of what in Canadian regulatory practice is called the "allow-able daily intake" (ADI) of dioxins for humans. Our daily intake of dioxins is inadvertent, just as the creation and release of dioxins from industrial processes is. Most of it comes to us through the food we eat (along with a much smaller amount in the air we breathe), because dioxins circulating in the environment are deposited steadily on soil and plants, and the residues of these depositions remain on plant foods or are ingested in the meat from animals who have eaten plant materials. The ADI in Canada for some time now has been 10pg/kg-bw day (TCDD), that is, ten picograms (a picogram is one-trillionth of a gram) per kilogram of body weight per day. Health Canada has determined that, so long as that figure is not exceeded, our health should not be significantly affected by the dioxins we have taken in.

The allowable daily intake calculations have been a part of the dioxin risk controversy because the U.S. EPA's number (0.006pg/kg-bw day) is *1,700 times lower* than the number used by Health Canada and some European Union countries. Since the basis for this enormous difference has never been explained clearly and in understandable terms to the public, the regulatory process has sacrificed a part of its credibility in the risk management of dioxins.[19] The EPA apparently recognized the difficulty it had created with its 1985 dioxin assessment, which established its remarkably low number by assuming that dioxin was a carcinogen with no threshold and that a tolerable risk was a one in a million lifetime risk of cancer. Consequently, in 1987, noting the approaches used by other countries, EPA proposed to raise its number by taking a mid-point between its established value and those of the other countries. In so doing the EPA refused to accept the validity of the assumptions underlying the values used by other countries. As a result, it was criticized by almost everyone and its proposal was rejected even by its own Science Advisory Board. The EPA's attempt at regulatory sleight of hand exposed the huge amount of discretion typically involved in environmental risk assessment.

The relatively low U.S. number has not stopped others from saying that it should be lower still, perhaps zero, if in fact there is no (or zero) threshold for the harm that dioxins may do to us. This is the third reason why the risk assessment has opened an area of contention: taken in its literal meaning, the idea of "no threshold" is that a single molecule may be sufficient to set off a cascade of biological events culminating in an adverse health effect, whether it be cancer or something else, such as harm to an individual's immune, endocrine, or reproductive systems. Considering that there are about two billion molecules of TCDD in one picogram, the implications of a zero threshold position for those charged with the protection of public health and safety is ambiguous, to say the least.

All of this began in the late 1960s with the first laboratory studies (or at least the first ones leading to publications in peer-reviewed scientific journals) using different animal species and looking for various types of harmful effects.[20] Acute effects from relatively high doses of TCDD include weight loss, atrophy of the thymus gland, liver damage, and immune system suppression. Chronic or long-term effects include reproductive toxicity and teratogenicity, and in rats, for example, these effects occur at what can only be described as astonishingly low doses. The effects are also wide ranging; indeed, there is no organ that is not affected in some way when all of these experiments are considered. Scientist Stephen Safe once summarized it thus: "With laboratory animals, it seemed as if dioxin caused just about any effect you can think of. You name it, it did it, and at extraordinarily low doses. But one of the mysteries has been that unlike most toxic chemicals, it didn't cause all of the effects on all species, or even on all strains."[21]

But it was the cancer effects and acute lethality in animals which received the most attention. The first was summarized recently as follows: "2,3,7,8-TCDD is a potent animal carcinogen and has tested positive in 19 different studies in four different species."[22] It remains the most potent carcinogen ever tested in an animal bioassay. Because dioxin is not genotoxic, it has been generally regarded as a cancer promoter rather than a cancer initiator; however, there is continuing scientific debate about this point, and the difference has no significance so far as public perception of risk is concerned. Acute lethality studies use what is known as the "LD_{50}," the dose at which 50 per cent of the test animal population dies. The guinea pig results – LD_{50} at 0.6pg/kg-bw – were shocking to scientists, but the later results across a spectrum of species were noteworthy: acute lethality varies five thousand-fold from guinea pigs to hamsters. The general finding, however, is very straightforward: dioxin is acutely lethal at extremely low doses in a wide range of animal species. Moreover, most chemicals do not display the same range of toxicity values that TCDD does, and this in itself was surprising when the TCDD results were first recorded.

Thus the notorious phrase "by far the most toxic compound known to mankind" was a reference to the animal study results. This was not noted when that phrase was reported in the popular media. Considering that we are dealing with material that is "exquisitely lethal," as an article in *Science* once put it, the fact that naturally occurring botulin toxin is even more potent (LD_{50} of .01pg/kg) may be regarded as hair-splitting.[23]

There is much scientific contention about whether *any* of these kinds of effects may occur in humans exposed to comparable doses, that is, comparable to the average animal result for acute lethality (excluding the extremes of guinea pig and hamster), cancer, reproductive toxicity (effect on sperm production), or any other. Because of the many industrial accidents and ongoing occupational exposures, as well as one notorious series of experiments with prison "volunteers," there is substantial human experience with dioxin exposures vastly greater than any arising from current environmental exposures. The experiments on prisoners, for example, involved extremely high levels of controlled and intentional exposure (up to 7,500 micrograms – which is 7,500,000,000 pg).[24]

Epidemiological studies for workers exposed to high levels of dioxin and including those where serum levels of dioxin were measured in sub-groups have suggested that dioxin may cause a measurable increase in cancer risk.[25] However, even these highly exposed workers failed to demonstrate the remarkable cancer potency found in laboratory animals which determined the EPA risk assessment number (0.006 pg/kg-bw day). The follow-up results from Seveso are even more puzzling.[26] Excess cancer rates were not apparent among the most highly exposed or those who suffered chloracne (widely regarded as a reliable indicator that substantial dioxin exposure has occurred), but these observations were attributed to the small number of individuals (about seven hundred) resident in the most highly exposed zone. Yet, estimates of the dioxin doses received by children who developed chloracne at Seveso were over 3,000,000 pg/kg, a level 500 million times higher than the EPA safe level (300,000 higher than the Canadian safe level) and even three to five times higher than the level found to kill the average guinea pig.[27] This is puzzling because we know that individuals exposed to massive doses of radiation will either die quickly from acute damage or will be substantially more likely to contract cancer if they survive the acute effects. The analogy with radiation underlies the logic for low-dose, no-threshold cancer risk assessment, yet any analogy of dioxin with radiation clearly fails at the documented high level exposures to dioxin.

The Seveso studies did provide some evidence of increased cancer risk in the moderately exposed zone, with a larger number of individuals (about 4,800) resident, which contrasts with the absence of excess cancer risk in the highly exposed zone. Although these results can be subject to conflicting interpretations because of inevitable limitations in the epidemiologic method, they clearly fail to justify the remarkable cancer potency predicted by the EPA from the rodent experiments.

The current emphasis on what are called "receptor-mediated responses" in dioxin studies has turned debate entirely away from directly observed effects towards theoretical models of low-dose mechanisms. This refers to a sequence of events first observed in 1976, whereby the dioxin molecule, having entered a cell, binds to an intracellular protein receptor (the "Ah" or aromatic hydrocarbon receptor), a process which can be represented by the analogy of a key fitting perfectly into a lock. The result of their union is called a TCDD-receptor complex, and this complex in turn can bind to the cell's DNA at specific sites ("dioxin recognition sites"), causing the DNA to "bend." This bending, in turn, makes that part of the DNA sequence more accessible to other proteins; other effects follow. The most important part of this finding was that *all* currently known toxic effects of TCDD are a function of this single process. No less important for the controversy over "endocrine disruptors" now building was the conclusion that TCDD "may be analogous to a hormone."[28]

Some scientists have argued that the new Ah receptor-mediated approach confirms the existence of a threshold for dioxin as a carcinogen (i.e., an exposure level below which there is no risk of cancer causation). This is because dioxin is known *not* to act by causing DNA mutations which can be subsequently amplified when the mutated cells replicate to produce a clone of tissue which can ultimately become a tumour. Others have argued for the absence of a threshold because of experiments showing no threshold for a particular biological effect (that is, TCDD binding to the Ah receptor and then the binding of the Ah receptor complex to DNA). But a "biological effect" does not *necessarily* mean a "toxic effect" and certainly does not have to be a cancerous effect. This point has been conceded by the authors of a 1993 paper that has been widely cited by others who claim there is no threshold for dioxin toxicity: "It is important to note that changes in these proteins simply indicates that a receptor-dependent response has occurred; the relationship of these changes to toxic response such as cancer is unclear."[29] One explanation for this is that, since there are about ten thousand such receptors in the cell, a large number may have to be bound with dioxin before a biological response is triggered. In any case, this is a typical point on which it would be understandable for the non-expert citizen to become confused, a confusion that could only be dispelled by effective and credible risk communication, which is of course noteworthy by its absence.

Low-dose effects through receptor-mediated responses are now the key feature of dioxin risk assessment, a development that was powerfully reinforced by the EPA's elaborate reassessment which appeared in 1993 and 1994.[30] The rubric under which the huge 1994 studies were issued – "review draft (do not cite or quote)" – is amusing since, as anyone might have guessed, these quickly became some of the most frequently cited documents in the history of modern risk assessment. The 1993 study of risks to wildlife contained information that "TCDD residues in fish appear to have decreased over the past decade," but this piece of good news was swamped by the apparent implications of the human health assessment, namely, that background human exposures were at or near the levels at which serious adverse effects are documented in the animal studies (using standard extrapolation methods from animals to humans).[31] The new emphasis on immune, reproductive, and endocrine system effects, and the extremely low doses at which such effects are hypothesized to occur, meant that the dioxin risk controversy would begin all over again.

We shall return to these themes in section 2 in discussing Greenpeace's publications on dioxin. What will become evident is that three special features of dioxin's scientific history predisposed the issue of dioxin risk to special controversy:

- In the first phase of discovery, there was evident surprise among scientists and regulators at the acute lethality and carcinogenicity of dioxin in animal tests and at the range of its effects in organisms.
- In the second phase, the observations about the "hormonelike" activity of dioxin within cells, in the process of receptor-mediated responses, flowed easily into the wider concerns about endocrine disruptors beginning about 1995.
- A special feature of the second phase is the integration of concerns about human health effects on the one hand, and impacts on wildlife species on the other, which among other things creates a situation where some wildlife can be seen as "sentinel species" for impacts, especially reproductive failure, that may also show up later in humans.

All of these features are premised on complex scientific results that, on the surface level of apprehension, are of a kind that unsurprisingly and easily can raise "alarm bells" among the citizenry. To moderate that sense of alarm – say, by emphasizing the reductions in environmental burdens of dioxins over the preceding two decades – would have required a determined effort in effective and credible risk communication. No such effort was made.

2 WHAT DID THE PUBLIC HEAR ABOUT DIOXINS?

[Dioxin is] so deadly 1/200 of a drop will kill a human.
    Expression frequently found in articles in the *Globe and Mail*, 1980–82

It's a nasty material to have around.
    J. R. Hickman, Health Canada, 1982, as reported in the *Globe and Mail*

This most toxic of man-made chemicals was used in the Vietnam War in a defoliant called Agent Orange.

> Article in the *Globe and Mail*, October 1987, dealing with
> trace amounts of dioxin found in consumer paper products
> made from chlorine-bleached pulp[32]

Newspaper Coverage

In view of the extent of the subsequent controversy over dioxin risk, which continues to this very day, it is terribly ironic that in the first article ever published in the *New York Times* (16 September 1972) in which the word "dioxin" was prominently mentioned, it was a North Vietnamese medical scientist who referred to it.[33] The irony is that for much of the next decade the extensive use of herbicides by the United States as a form of chemical warfare in Vietnam was the main context for dioxin references. The Agent Orange context overshadowed everything else, including the two other most notorious events of this period, the evacuation and demolition of the town of Times Beach, Missouri, and the chemical factory explosion in Seveso. This context, in which the dioxin story itself was identified with chemical warfare and an unpopular war, and which slowly metamorphosed into bitter controversy and class-action lawsuits against chemical manufacturers by Vietnam veterans, framed the dioxin issue from the outset in exceptionally contentious terms.

Added to this association with chemical warfare and alleged injustices to war veterans was the fact that dioxin was a contaminant of a very widely used pesticide, the herbicide 2,4,5-trichlorophenoxyacetic acid (2,4,5-T). Pesticides have always been the most controversial class of chemicals, because of course they are deliberately designed to poison things and, beginning in the 1950s, new generations of pesticides based on chlorinated compounds were dispersed in the environment in enormous quantities. The first monument of modern environmentalist literature, Rachel Carson's *Silent Spring*, published in 1962, fingered DDT and other pesticides as the main culprits in causing adverse impacts on species that were not intended to be harmed. When the definitive public label was hung on dioxins – "by far the most toxic compound known to mankind" – by an EPA scientist testifying before a committee of the U.S. Congress in August 1974, the context was a failed attempt by EPA to ban 2,4,5-T on the grounds that its use as an agricultural herbicide on food crops was leading to dioxin contamination of foods consumed by people.[34]

Two weeks later, the story of Times Beach hit the newspapers: "Dioxin, the deadly chemical contained in a herbicide once used to defoliate forests in South Vietnam, has been identified as the agent that killed many horses and scores of other animals in Missouri. Two young girls, one 6 years old and the other 10, became ill because of exposure to the substance. The younger suffered such severe kidney damage that she was hospitalized for four weeks at St Louis Children's Hospital ... More than 50 horses, 70 chickens, several dogs, a dozen cats and hundreds of wild birds were killed."[35]

Now the ante had been raised significantly, with the death of both domestic and wild animals and serious injury to children added to the elements previously mentioned. Thus in a short period of two years dioxins had accumulated more intensely negative associations than many other chemical substances do over the course of a century.[36]

The initial *New York Times* story about Times Beach offered the first mention in the press of the acute lethality of dioxins to guinea pigs (0.6pg/kg-bw) – or, as it was expressed more clearly two years later in the context of Seveso: "A dose of less than a billionth of a gram is fatal to guinea pigs." But the very first story at all, the report from Vietnam in September 1972, had initiated the blending of references between animal study results and fears of human health effects from exposure to dioxins, as well as the parallel conflation of items associated with 2,4,5-T on the one hand and with dioxins on the other. Thus that first story referred to animal experiments as showing effects ranging from "liver injury, to chromosomal changes, to embryonic tumors called teratoma, and to cancer," and immediately moved on to allegations of unusual numbers of cases of primary hepatoma, or liver cancer, in human patients. The first story on Times Beach (August 1974) dealt with human injury in Missouri, suspicions of birth defects among the Vietnamese, and the animal study results (birth defects, acute lethality). The first story on the Seveso explosion also mentioned human illnesses, animal deaths, birth defects in Vietnam, and the guinea pig acute lethality number. This theme continued in *New York Times* coverage throughout the decade; the June 1980 article of the important National Cancer Institute dioxin studies (animal cancer bioassays) discussed the lab animal findings in connection with Vietnamese birth defects as well as alleged cases of "cancer, loss of sex drive, personality changes and inexplicable weaknesses of the limbs" among American Vietnam war vets.[37]

Although there are not a lot of press stories about dioxin in this period, by 1976 the phrases "one of the most toxic chemicals known" and "one of the deadliest chemicals known" were firmly entrenched in journalistic usage. What was missing, however, was a way of making these expressions more meaningful to the ordinary understanding of citizens; this lack was repaired by the common device of analogy or comparison. The first had been supplied early on, by the Harvard University biologist Matthew Meselson, who had gone to Vietnam in 1973 to test for dioxin residues in fish. Meselson remarked then that dioxin was "a nasty poison that is 100 times more toxic than the deadliest nerve gas."[38] The graphic notion of dioxin as a "poison" resurfaced five years later and stuck fast, again prompted by specific events, in this case the discovery of large quantities of buried toxic waste in Love Canal and Hyde Park in northern New York State. Referring to the trichlorophenols in the waste, a long article in the *Times* published in late 1978 noted, "One of the byproducts is dioxin, a poison as virulent as botulism or shellfish toxin. A millionth of a gram is said to be potent enough to kill a rabbit, and 3 ounces, minced small enough into New York City's water supply, could wipe out the city. Experts calculate that the 200 tons of chlorophenol in the Love Canal may contain about 130 pounds of dioxin."[39]

In addition, both of the initial context-setting themes returned again and again: the Agent Orange story kept resurfacing as Vietnam veterans pressed for recognition and compensation for what they believed to be their herbicide-caused health problems, and the EPA kept trying to restrict more and more the uses of 2,4,5-T for herbicide applications. In a lengthy 1979 *Times* article on allegations of serious adverse health effects attributed to both the wartime and domestic agricultural uses of phenoxy herbicides, Matthew Meselson was quoted again: Dioxin is "the most powerful small molecule known and it is now beginning to appear that it is the most powerful carcinogen known. Nobody argues about the toxicity of this poison."[40] Over the next three years the following characterizations appear in articles in the *Times*: "a poison 100,000 times more deadly than cyanide," "dioxin, a highly poisonous chemical," the "virulent poison and carcinogen dioxin," and the "deadly poison dioxin."[41]

The powerful and emotive "poison" characterization was picked up by the environmental reporters for Canada's *Globe and Mail* in late 1980, in the first story ever published on dioxin in this newspaper, and was recycled faithfully over the next two years. In addition to finding the rubric "the deadliest man-made chemical" in that first article, readers were told that dioxin is "so deadly 1/200 of a drop will kill a human." The reference to possible or probable human deaths was always latent in the poison analogy, but the expression "1/200 of a drop" made it much more vivid. The reporters (Jock Ferguson and Michael Keating) were very fond of it, and it is found in every one of the five articles that they wrote for the *Globe* between 29 November and 10 December 1980 and in a number of their other pieces published in the first half of 1981. By the time an editorial on dioxin, entitled "Slack Rules for a Poison," appeared in August 1981, it is clear that the phrase had attained the status of conventional wisdom: "Lest we forget, about 1/200 of a drop will kill a human being."[42]

The poison analogy predominated. Dioxin is "the most poisonous substance made by man" or "the deadliest poison ever made by man. It is more toxic than cyanide or strychnine." Another article expanded the analogy in an informative way – TCDD is "far more toxic than curare, strychnine or cyanide though less toxic than botulism, tetanus or diphtheria" – although one cannot know whether readers derived any reassurance from dioxin's relative placement on this list of horrors.[43] Coverage of dioxins in the *Globe and Mail* faded thereafter, but it would be hard to imagine that this barrage of consistent and dramatic terminology, dominating a dozen articles over a period of about eighteen months (representing the initial spate of coverage in this newspaper), would not have made some lasting impression on the Canadian public. With the exception of a single article in 1984, again dealing with the U.S. veterans' lawsuit about exposure to Agent Orange, dioxins stories then disappear from the *Globe and Mail* for fully five years. The issue resurfaced in 1987 in an entirely new context: the generation of dioxins in the bleaching of pulp, dioxin releases to the environment in effluent from pulp and paper mills, and dioxin residues in consumer paper products (tissue and toilet paper, tampons, milk cartons, etc.) made from bleached pulp. And there was a new principal actor – Greenpeace – which would transform once again the basic rules of the game for dioxin risk issues.

For the past decade Greenpeace and other environmentalist organizations that have followed its lead have been in firm control of the public agenda on dioxin risk. Current indications are that the endocrine disruptors context will, if anything, strengthen their hold on the issue agenda. And in this entire period there are no exposure episodes, involving either industrial workers or the public, that are comparable in any way with those summarized in tables 3.1 and 3.2. Indeed, it would be fair to say that dioxin risk as a public issue has escalated in direct proportion to the falling level of both directly evident human effects from dioxin exposure and falling levels of total dioxins burden in the environment of industrialized nations. What can explain this paradox?

Greenpeace and Dioxin: From Pulp Mills to PVC

In 1986 the EPA and the American Paper Institute had agreed to collaborate on what was called the "Five Mills study," sampling for dioxin releases at five pulp mills in different parts of the country.

Neither the collaboration itself nor the nature of the shared responsibilities had been publicly announced when it was implemented. In
September 1987 Greenpeace released some preliminary findings from
the study that had been leaked to the organization from sources inside
the industry. At the same time Greenpeace took effluent samples
(unauthorized, of course) from a British Columbia pulp mill and sent
them to a private laboratory for analysis. The samples had been taken
by the two Greenpeace members who had scaled Macmillan Bloedel's
Harmac facility in Nanaimo on 21 September, unfurling a banner
reading "Dioxin Kills." Greenpeace warned the public not to eat
seafood caught in the vicinity of the mill. The Canadian federal
government responded – predictably – by announcing that a study
would be conducted and that sampling results in hand did not exceed
permitted levels. Greenpeace's rejoinder came a few months later with
its release of a leaked government document suggesting that dioxin
contamination of seafood taken in the vicinity of another B.C. mill
exceeded permitted levels. In 1988 the federal government closed the
shellfish grounds around B.C. coastal pulp mills and issued a health
warning about dioxin contamination. In the United States Greenpeace
engaged the EPA in high-profile legal and public-relations battles over
the Five Mills study and EPA's regulatory stance.

Greenpeace complemented its direct action and media activities with
the preparation and wide circulation of a two-hundred-page document,
*No Margin of Safety: A Preliminary Report on Dioxin Pollution and the Need
for Emergency Action in the Pulp and Paper Industry.* This is Greenpeace's
initial documentary foray into the dioxins issue, and it was followed by
many others in the decade to come. The product of authors who have
both legal and scientific qualifications, it is extensively footnoted and
reproduces in full the leaked government documents with which this
episode in dioxin controversy began. *No Margin of Safety* opens with a
series of chapters providing background for the pulp-and-paper issue:
a highly technical section on dioxin chemistry and the results of
experimental studies on animals; the long story of regulatory struggles,
including fights between government and industry as well as internal
bureaucratic moves; and some of the legal battles over 2,4,5-T. The
document then turns to the issue at hand, with long accounts of the
run-up to the "secret" Five Mills study and associated industry-
government negotiations related to potential regulation. It provides a
basic account of the technology of kraft pulp mills and paper bleaching
and concludes with a chapter on alternatives to bleaching and an
argument for the elimination of dioxins in pulp mill effluent.

No Margin of Safety and Greenpeace's later publications and activity
on dioxins made it by far the leading environmentalist player on
this issue. It first broadened its focus to take in the entire chlorine

industry, arguing for a complete phase-out of chlorine chemistry, and in recent years has narrowed it again, zeroing in on PVC (polyvinyl chloride) and the connection between PVC and dioxins. For the entirety of the preceding decade Greenpeace's voice was rarely absent from any notable news dealing with dioxin, whether generated in North America, Western Europe, or elsewhere.[44] During this time the chemical industry's own communications effort on dioxin appears to have been largely a scramble to respond to each new Greenpeace foray, while governments, for the most part, have retreated either behind the wall of bureaucratic silence or to the comforting sanctum of scientific research. But, ironically, the latest scientific analysis, and especially EPA's 1994 dioxin re-assessment, served only to reinvigorate the dioxins issue by folding it into what will be undoubtedly the hottest risk issue of the coming decade – endocrine disruptors.

In fact, the rest of the story shows clearly the full consequences of the risk information vacuum for dioxin, which we maintain is what allowed Greenpeace to keep the dioxin issue in play after 1985. Greenpeace has used dioxin as the linking theme in a series of high-profile campaigns beginning in 1987 and continuing to the present day. Starting with pulp-mill effluent, Greenpeace has taken the dioxin issue into chlorine chemistry generally, then to incineration, then to PVC (polyvinyl chloride, which is now the largest single segment of the industrial chlorine market), and finally to hormone disruptors.

Greenpeace's activities are an effective amalgam of "actions" (sometimes complex and meticulously planned, such as the 1995 occupation in the North Sea of a Shell oil-drilling platform slated for marine disposal), staged events and press briefings, participation at international scientific and policy-oriented meetings, collaborative research, publication, and dissemination of print materials. The fact that these activities take place on a world stage, combining contributions from chapters based in North America, Western Europe, and elsewhere, gives added scope to their impacts. Major interventions have taken place on issues in climate change, fossil fuels, ozone, toxic substances, pulp and paper, plastics, chlorine, waste management, nuclear power and radioactive materials, marine ecology, forests, and biotechnology. Here we shall use the publications record as a surrogate for this activity as a whole, a large percentage of which consists in a risk communication exercise directed at a broad spectrum of the public. Following are selections from a list of dioxin-related publications appearing in the period between 1987 and the present:

- *No Margin of Safety*, 1987, approximately 200pp.
- *Hazardous Waste Incineration*, 1993, 20pp.
- *PVC – Dioxin Factories*, 1993, 19pp.

- *Achieving Zero Dioxin*, 1994, 57pp.
- *Dioxin and the Failure of Canadian Public Health Policy* and *Dioxin and Human Health: A Public Health Assessment of Dioxin Exposure in Canada*, both 1994, 6pp., 13pp.
- *Dow Brand Dioxin*, 1995, 41pp.
- *Polyvinyl Chloride (PVC) Plastic: Primary Contributor to the Global Dioxin Crisis* and *PVC: Poison via Chlorine*, 1995, 22pp., 2pp.
- *Body of Evidence: The Effects of Chlorine on Human Health*, 1995, 21pp.
- *Taking Back Our Stolen Future: Hormone Disruption and PVC Plastic*, 1996, 38pp.

All the publications after *No Margin of Safety* are shorter and thus less intimidating to a reader. (Also in recent years Greenpeace has adopted the practice of summarizing its longer analyses in one-page or two-page documents.) *Body of Evidence* is a colour-printed, beautifully illustrated pamphlet, based on a longer document prepared by Greenpeace U.K., covering a wide range of human health and ecosystem issues, including endocrine disruptors.

As the titles indicate, all of the individual major themes are connected with the others, and dioxin serves as the primary connective tissue. The case for such connections is made in a series of publications (most of them listed above) that take up the following set of relationships, for example: (1) pulp and paper – chlorine, (2) pulp and paper – dioxin, (3) dioxin – chlorine, (4) chlorine – incinceration, (5) dioxin – incineration, (6) PVC – incineration, (7) PVC – dioxin, (8) PVC – chlorine, (9) chlorine – hormone disruptors, (10) PVC – hormone disruptors. The arguments and selection of evidence to support them in many of the individual publications overlap with the linked themes followed up in others, so that each separate set of arguments appears to reinforce the others, building overall momentum towards support of the action recommendations for "dioxin elimination," "chlorine phase-out," and "PVC phase-out." The concept of complete phase-outs is based on the contention that there are alternative products and practices which are affordable and acceptable to consumers and which pose less risk to human health and the environment.

The longer documents pay homage to a scientific discourse, in that they are framed in terms of evidence gleaned from scientific studies; many are elaborately footnoted and referenced. Unquestionably these are biased accounts, using selective quotation and reference to achieve a rhetorical effect. But there are better and worse examples of such bias, and Greenpeace's are almost always in the former category, largely because the construction of arguments around the selected evidence is generally sophisticated and the issue coverage is comprehensive.

Achieving Zero Dioxin, for example, is composed of five short chapters: an overview of the history of dioxin risk assessment, three chapters on formation and sources of dioxin in the environment (primary and secondary sources), and a concluding chapter of recommendations for "a national strategy for dioxin elimination." The tone is relentlessly scientific, but in addition a considerable effort has gone into the presentation of the science in well-organized, clear, and readable form. All of this leads smoothly up to the sharply focused conclusions, which are in a form likely to be remembered.

One of the positive features of much of Greenpeace's literature is that, although there is a tough and uncompromising "action" line flowing from the prior effort in constructing supporting evidence, neither the representation of science itself, nor the recommended policy actions derived from the analysis, stray very far from what we might call the outer boundary of prevailing scientific consensus. On many specific points in these texts there could be found some "reputable" scientists who would agree, or at least concede the plausibility of the construction. This is also consistent with Greenpeace's strategy in at least some international meetings where actions on chemical pollutants are being debated, namely, to participate in less-than-perfect solutions that can win broad support, including support from the chemical industry.

This writing strategy is adhered to even when it requires the authors to draw modest rather than earthshaking conclusions in the scientific argument, conclusions that can appear curiously at odds with the dramatic style of the action recommendations. For example, *Achieving Zero Dioxin* uses the 1994 EPA reassessment in commenting on human cancer risk associated with the background exposures to dioxin, and then affirms EPA's conclusion as its own: "According to EPA's risk estimates, dioxin would cause from 350 to 3,500 cancers each year in the U.S. – up to 3 percent of all cancers."[45] Considering that this is a (theoretical) estimate arrived at through elaborate calculations, and that the larger number is the highest possible value that could be derived from the calculations – after making very pessimistic assumptions to maximize exposure estimates – the result is not all that impressive. This is especially so when we also know that nearly two-thirds of cancers are attributable to lifestyle factors (smoking, diet and exercise, alcohol, UV radiation, and a few other factors) that individuals could control if they were worried about cancer and wanted to do something about their chances.[46]

This commitment by Greenpeace in its publications to what could be called a partisan yet plausible construction of science, arrayed in support of dramatic and easy-to-grasp "solutions" and communicated with a remarkable facility (given the inherent complexity of the material), serves the organization well. It provides a rational underpinning for the more direct actions and staged events: the reasoned contents of these publications provide substantial credibility for what might otherwise appear as simple publicity-seeking. Greenpeace is nothing if not strategically astute in its public communications. Unfurling a huge banner that reads "Dioxin Kills" on the side of a pulp mill facility stretches the truth to the breaking-point – assuming that the members of the public who saw it had read its tacit reference to mean that humans were regularly dying of dioxin exposure! (Dioxin certainly kills animals of many species at very low doses in laboratory experiments, but it is unlikely that this is how the audience would have interpreted the message.) On the other hand, the carefully constructed account of dioxin risk in Greenpeace's series of publications pulls the organization back into the accepted circles of civil discourse, with the resultant publicity becoming an asset in recruiting and fund-raising.

We are aware of no other products in dioxin risk communication that even attempt to supply a comparable synthesis of scientific sophistication plus effective rhetorical construction. For ten years Greenpeace has been without peer in this domain, and its reward has been to exert a major continuing influence on our society's risk agenda. To some extent this has been too easy a victory, because the other actors who might have been expected to enter the lists in some fashion (governments and industry) have for the most part not even tried. They may reply that they cannot act as Greenpeace does, which is true enough but irrelevant. Of course they would have to find a mode of credible risk communication very different from Greenpeace's, which requires the devotion of time and resources – but then, their resources exceed Greenpeace's by a considerable margin. The main obstacle is that still, after so much buffeting in the ugly controversies over risks, with few exceptions neither governments nor industry senior managers charged with risk management are much inclined to assume responsibility for credible risk communication with the public.

3 WHY IS DIOXIN RISK CONTROVERSIAL?

Imagine that a scientifically literate visitor from outer space landed on earth and, for want of something better to do, engaged some humans in a conversation about dioxins. Detecting an element of anxiety in the conversation, the visitor asked her interlocutors if there were any points about dioxins on which everyone agreed. Yes, they said, and the following list was produced:

1 Dioxin is an extremely toxic substance on the basis of animal studies, showing a wide range of adverse effects at various doses.
2 Although human health effects are not as clear, all responsible agencies agree that exposures should be kept to very low levels.
3 Although no public scientific agency can identify specific adverse human effects from dioxins at current average levels of exposure, massive and expensive research programs are under way to try to ensure that nothing of relevance is being missed.
4 Anthropogenic contributions to dioxin releases are an important source of environmental dioxin levels, and unflagging attention is given to reducing such releases from major point sources.
5 Dioxin levels in the environment appear to have peaked and are slowly declining, but there is a strong desire to ensure that this trend continues.

The visitor, considering what she had heard and observing other aspects of human behaviour with respect to risk factors, began to annoy her hosts considerably by persisting in wondering why dioxin risk was regarded as something particularly noteworthy for earthlings. Judging discretion to be the better part of valour, she departed early for the return trip.

Since the rest of us are stuck here on planet earth for the time being, we must make the effort to explain the controversial nature of dioxin risk. There are at least two reasons for doing so. The more important is that the problem is still with us, since dioxins are implicated as endocrine disruptors, and the latter are definitely high on our risk issue agenda now and for the foreseeable future. The second is that we should try to learn from our previous failures, all the more so in this case because dioxin carries the mark of so many aspects of chemicals risk issues in general, and chemicals of one sort or another always seem to be prominent on that same agenda.

In the preceding section we identified this paradox: dioxin risk as a public issue has escalated in direct proportion to the falling level of both directly evident human effects from dioxin exposure and falling levels of total dioxins burden in the environment. Is there a good explanation for this paradox? We think that it may be found in the multi-dimensional character of dioxin risk perception, including certain unique aspects of the way in which the issue originated and developed. Although these unique aspects play a role in the place of dioxins on the risk issue agenda, other aspects are generic: in those other aspects dioxin became the chief bearer of the stigmata of industrial chemistry as such, eliciting in many persons a set of ambiguous reactions to the interplay and inseparability of risks and benefits and the dependence of our lifestyle on modern technologies. We may summarize the dimensions of the dioxins risk issue as follows:

- *Agent Orange:* Its attachment to this controversy, which among other things played out over an extended period of time (about 1965–85) because of the drawn-out legal battles, kept dioxins in the public eye.
- *Pesticides:* Its connection with endemic controversies over pesticide use generally, and a very contentious substance (2,4,5-T) in particular, had the effect in newspaper accounts of weaving together the reports of alleged adverse human health affects of 2,4,5-T with those of dioxins.
- *Dramatic Incidents:* This is the series of high-profile accidents or unexpected discoveries at Times Beach, Seveso, Love Canal, and Hyde Park.
- *Dramatic Language:* A unique stereotyping in language ("most toxic," etc.) did not discriminate between the intrinsic hazard of the most toxic dioxins and the relative human exposures to them.
- *The Risk Information Vacuum:* An enormous scientific research effort, yielding results (such as the variations in observed effects among species) the meaning of which are inherently difficult for non-specialists to comprehend, was not matched by any reasonable effort to communicate credibly, in a publicly understandable language, the ever-changing and sometimes inconsistent interpretations of that research.
- *A Dramatic Turn in the Science:* After twenty years of being framed primarily in terms of cancer risk (and where some later analysis had begun to lower estimated human cancer risk), the emphasis in public awareness shifted in 1990 to an entirely new dimension, first called "hormone mimicking," and to molecular-level biological events, which virtually started the dioxin risk controversy all over again.
- *A Capable New Actor:* Greenpeace's leap into dioxins issues in 1987 brought to the ongoing controversy an organization capable of reaching broad audiences and attracting media attention, with both high-profile "actions" and effective technical analysis in its publications.

In our view only the sum total of all these dimensions, and not any one or any subset of them, can explain the paradox represented by the persistence of our society's dioxin risk controversy.

Moreover, the specific temporal sequencing of these dimensions contributes in no small measure to the controversy's intractable nature. The initial framing of the issue in the context of chemical warfare, an unpopular war, and aggrieved war veterans cast it in exceptionally bitter terms which inevitably seeped into all subsequent aspects. Second, the extreme toxicity of 2,3,7,8-TCDD in animal tests was itself newsworthy, but in the coverage of the series of dramatic incidents in the 1970s the newspaper accounts often conflated the discussions of experimental animal effects with both actual and alleged human health effects, blurring the otherwise important distinctions between the two types of findings. The animal results had shown some remarkable effects at comparatively low doses, but by the mid- to late 1980s the relevance of those effects for human impacts was widely questioned by many scientists. It was at that point that the new turn in the science, focusing on more subtle molecular-level events in the receptors within cells, became publicly known. In these and other respects, therefore, not only the multiple dimensions themselves but also the sequence of particular events within them had a part to play in the outcome.

Brief mention will be made here, to be elaborated further in the afterword to this chapter, about the nature of the risk information vacuum for dioxins. So far as governments are concerned, they appear to believe that, in cases (like dioxins) where they throw huge amounts of resources at scientific research and risk assessment programs, the *meaning* of the results from these efforts will somehow be diffused serendipitously throughout the public mind. In Canada, so far as one can tell, those in government who are in charge of environmental and health protection programs simply do not believe that constructing an effective risk communication dialogue with the public is a part of their responsibilities. It may be only a slight exaggeration to consider the one-liner on dioxin attributed to Roy Hickman in a 1982 newspaper article – "It's a nasty material to have around" – as the only statement on dioxin ever issued by Health Canada to the Canadian public in clearly understandable language throughout the entire history of the risk controversy over dioxins.

In 1988 Health Canada released a four-page information bulletin on dioxins (updated with only minor wording changes in 1990). So far as we know, this is the only document intended for a broad public distribution, ever issued by Health Canada on the subject. We examine this document in the afterword. Also in the late 1980s the Canadian Council of Resource and Environment Ministers issued a ten-page pamphlet summarizing the scientific database on dioxins and furans, including sources and exposures and listing some government policies for the same.[47] While this document is better than nothing at all, it is extremely tentative in its conclusions and has the usual emphasis of government publications on the need for more research. It even complains about how expensive a proposition it is to test for dioxins!

For further information the reader is referred to a list of technical scientific publications issued by various Canadian government agencies since 1981.[48]

In the United States the EPA devotes so much energy to battling with both industry and environmentalists over regulatory agendas, both in and out of courts, that there does not seem to be much left over for public communication. Given the evident complexity and changing character of the scientific research program results for dioxins and the corresponding lack of appropriate public communication, just how an informed understanding of the risk assessment and management issues is supposed to take root and influence attitudes among the citizenry is one of the great mysteries of our time.[49]

Industry's share in creating and maintaining the risk information vacuum for dioxins is different in nature but no less weighty. Here again the issue framing was critical, because the decade of high-profile legal battles with Vietnam vets over Agent Orange set the tone for much of the subsequent period. This meant that industry would not say publicly what was said privately and that the public messages would be largely ones of denial and stonewalling. Moreover, it was an era when industries relied heavily on public-relations firms for "issue management" and the crafting of elaborate strategies for dealing with the public, politicians, and the press. In retrospect, had industry taken but a small fraction of the monies it paid out to PR firms over the years and spent it on finding a way to create a credible risk communication dialogue with the public, the dioxin issue might not be today as intractable as it still is.

The afterword to this chapter looks a bit more closely at the actions and inactions that created the risk information vacuum for dioxins. And we should recall here the reasoning advanced in our introductory section to this chapter about the importance of the information vacuum in this case. We contend that it was this vacuum that in the period after 1985 allowed Greenpeace to put dioxin risk into play as a significant element in society's overall risk agenda and indeed pretty much allowed Greenpeace to control the agenda-setting for dioxin risk from then to the present.

Michael Gough's comprehensive account of the controversy over Agent Orange and dioxin, published in 1986, closed with the following sentences: "After a decade and a half of studies and debates, harm from environmental exposure to dioxin has been assessed as nondetectable. Although concern about risk remains, exposures have been reduced, so that the level of risk has decreased. The consensus among most scientists [is] that harm has been limited to highly exposed

industrial populations and that none has been shown from environmental exposures ... We are putting the dioxin problem behind us."
He had reckoned without Greenpeace.

4 TRAPPED IN THE RISK INFORMATION VACUUM

On 25 March 1996 in Toronto a combined public sitting of the City Services Committee and the Toronto Board of Health heard an extraordinary eleven-hour debate starting at 7 P.M. and lasting through the night. The meeting was held to consider a motion from the Board of Health to institute a phase-out of purchases by the city of PVC-based products (most of which is sewer pipe), on the grounds that PVC materials posed unacceptable health risks, including dioxin risk. It is unlikely that there had been any comparable meeting on any subject associated with concerns over public health risk in the city's entire history.[50]

Greenpeace's global campaign against PVC had won over some of the city councillors on the Board of Health. The campaign is summed up in the following sentences from one of its publications: "Extremely toxic byproducts, including but not limited to dioxin, are generated throughout the PVC life cycle. PVC, more than any other product, is the source of persistent, toxic poisons that are now present in the air, water, soil, food, and tissues of living beings around the globe." Greenpeace also sought to strengthen its case in this regard by preparing detailed and highly technical analyses of available alternative products for all uses, including health care uses, where PVC currently has significant markets.[51] To counter both the proposed action and the reasoning against PVC, interested parties in the industrial sector mobilized deputations and submissions from vinyl industry and chemical industry association officials based in Canada, the United States, and Europe; technical consultants in toxicology, epidemiology, and incineration technologies; and representatives of the Ontario and American Water Works associations.[52] The City Services Committee voted unanimously against the motion, but the Board of Health voted narrowly in favour. When the joint recommendations came before Toronto City Council on 1 April the motion to limit the use of vinyl pipe was defeated eleven against and six in favour.

At least some participants must have felt that they were attending a play staged in the theatre of the absurd – in the sense that such an extensive sitting on *this* issue in *this* jurisdiction at *this* point in time is odd, to say the least. Certainly we do not take the position that the issues about PVC (and more generally about chlorine chemistry and dioxin) raised by Greenpeace and its supporters are trivial or unworthy of discussion: quite the contrary. But we do wonder about how those who organized that official City of Toronto session on PVC risk could have placed this issue so high in their priority list of risk issues affecting city inhabitants. We think that they could not have spent very much, if any, time and energy on thinking about ranking risk priorities at all. Because if they had, almost certainly they could have found some other issue – say, accidents and deaths related to the use of bicycles on city streets – where, based on a fair reading of the risk numbers, the application of their intelligence and concern might lead to practical risk reduction measures and health benefits.

Such a ranking exercise was not on the table, for dioxin is in play as a risk issue in a way in which most other such issues are not. Although Greenpeace lost the vote, it achieved a significant victory in having this session held at all. There will be other opportunities. So its importance lies not in the outcome of the vote but rather in another domain entirely: namely, as an illustration of how a risk information vacuum permits the leap from single-party diagnosis (PVC is the source of serious human health problems) to a definitive solution (eliminate PVC products) without transiting an intermediate step: a reasoned debate among citizens well informed about the competing scientific and policy analyses of a very complex risk management issue.

The poison analogy illustrated earlier provides the most dramatic instance of the unfortunate consequences stemming from an inadequate public dialogue on dioxin risk and – insofar as these are the stigmata of risks associated with industrial chemicals generally – on environmental and health risk issues more broadly considered. The notion that dioxin may be described appropriately as a "virulent poison" so deadly that "1/200 of a drop will kill a human" is odd for a number of reasons, perhaps most so because "technical" dioxin – that is, TCDD isolated as a pure chemical – has never existed in any form resembling a "droplet" or indeed in any pure form at all outside of controlled laboratory settings. In this respect it differs from the more familiar poisonous substances related to it by analogy, namely, cyanide or strychnine or curare, all of which have been actually employed as such for nefarious purposes. In other words, this is the wrong category or "mental slot" entirely, and putting it in that category, although it attests to a vivid imagination on the part of those who did so, inhibits others from understanding what type of material it is and how one is likely to encounter it in the environment.

Other aspects of the risk communication failure in the case of dioxins are more prosaic but no less influential. We may appreciate them best by asking: What major themes should have been communicated effectively and credibly to the public by industry and government researchers and officials in order to forestall the emergence of a risk information vacuum for dioxins? Here are some of them, none of which in fact was communicated clearly and unequivocally:

- Clear and candid statements over the years, first from the chemical industry, and later from other industry sectors as well (including pulp and paper, metal smelting, iron and steel, and plastics) – to the effect that they were and are very concerned about the production of dioxins in their facilities, due to the "supreme toxicity" of these substances and the evidence that they can cause serious adverse human health effects at higher doses.
- Similarly clear and candid statements over the years from these same industries that controlling dioxin emissions from their facilities is a high priority for them, and that they are working hard at reducing those emissions to the lowest feasible levels.[53]
- A clear statement from regulators as to why different regulatory agencies, all of which have highly competent scientists on their staffs, could come up with such widely disparate numbers for tolerable intakes of these substances.
- A similarly clear explanation from regulators about the nature and possible consequences of the cellular-level biological effects (called "hormone mimicking"), both for humans and other species, resulting from exposure to very low doses of dioxins and similar substances.
- A good news statement from governments, to the effect that the attention paid to dioxins over the last twenty years has paid off in sharp reductions in industrial emissions and in cases of extreme human exposure, as well as in generally falling environmental burdens, and that, if we just keep going down this fairly straightforward path, dioxin exposures probably will not represent a major risk factor in the lives of our citizens.[54]

These are all, we believe, (roughly) true statements. Our citizens have not heard them, on the whole, certainly not with a clarity sufficient to command their attention, whether or not their content may be found here and there in occasional government press releases or in the carefully worded productions of the public relations firms labouring on behalf of industry associations.

We close with a curiosity. The fact that this issue remains in play after so long is, we have tried to show, the outcome of both a specific chronology of events and the persistence of a substantial information vacuum. This means, among other things, that the issue is driven by a number of accidental features, including the skilled interventions by Greenpeace. But another one of those accidental features is that, even as environmental dioxin levels have been dropping, our analytical capability for measuring these levels has been increasing in sensitivity by leaps and bounds. To some extent, therefore, so long as it remains in play the dioxin issue will be carried along simply by our ability to measure dioxin at progressively lower levels in the environment, regardless of whether or not toxic effects are found at those levels.

All of which makes the most recent Canadian federal government actions pointless and indeed self-defeating. As noted at the outset, the minister of the Environment, upon tabling the new Canadian Environmental Protection Act in the House of Commons in December 1996, labelled dioxin and PCBs "mega-uglies" and said that they and similar substances were destined for "virtual elimination" through resolute action by his government. The labelling was bad enough, but what is worse, the draft legislation actually defines virtual elimination in terms of no detectable level.[55] Since it is certain that dioxins *will* be found in the environment at progressively lower levels, what the minister and his officials have done is to guarantee that the dioxin risk issue will remain in play in Canada for many years to come.

AFTERWORD:
GOVERNMENT AND INDUSTRY
(MIS)COMMUNICATION ON DIOXIN

The Canadian Federal Government

From those responsible for health and environmental risk assessment in the Canadian government, citizens have heard very little about dioxins, except for episodic announcements such as the closing and reopening of shellfish grounds around pulp mills on the coast of British Columbia, or actions taken to reduce dioxin contaminants in bleached paper products below currently detectable levels. The great international scientific effort to which Canada has contributed, and the risk assessments that form the basis of regulatory positions, are contained in a series of highly technical documents issued since 1981.[56]

As mentioned earlier, in this entire period only a single short document on dioxins intended for broad public distribution was produced (in November 1988) by Health Canada. It makes the following points; we have added questions about the wording of various passages within parentheses:[57]

- "Dioxins and furans can significantly damage the health of laboratory animals. The impact of these substances on humans is less certain. Dioxins and furans are therefore the subject of considerable controversy, both in the public realm and within the scientific community." (What is the nature of the controversy?)
- "This compound [2,3,7,8-TCDD] has been referred to as the most toxic chemical known to man – a statement that is unsubstantiated by scientific evidence." (Is this and the statement above – "can significantly damage the health of laboratory animals" – a fair representation of the remarkable acute lethality and carcinogenicity impacts of TCDD in laboratory studies?)
- "Because dioxins and furans are products of incomplete combustion, they are found in very minute levels throughout the environment." (What about trichlorophenol production?)
- "All Canadians (and people living in industrialized nations around the world) are constantly being exposed" to them, primarily through foods. (How do they get into foods?)
- "No long term effects have been found in fish, wildlife or domestic animals exposed to levels of dioxins and furans typically found in the environment. The remarkable loss of reproductive capacity in fish-eating birds in the Great Lakes area in the 1970s may have been associated with dioxins and furans." (This is at best confusing, at worst apparently inconsistent.)
- "No conclusive link has been established between human exposure to dioxins and furans and effects such as cancer, coronary disease or abnormal reproduction." (What does the qualifier "conclusive" indicate?)
- "Establishing levels of exposure to dioxins and furans which might be considered acceptable for the general population is however a topic of controversy. Most countries ... have derived tolerable exposure guidelines similar to Canada's." (The guidelines number is not mentioned.)
- "However, using different approaches for assessing the risk to human health of exposure to 2,3,7,8-TCDD, some agencies in the United States have arrived at widely contrasting conclusions, the extreme being one agency which accepted a risk 2,000 times greater than another. These agencies are reviewing their risk assessments in light of other, international standards." (Is this supposed to be clever? Is EPA not recognized by name by Health Canada? Whose approach is wiser, and why?)
- "The Government of Canada recognizes that these compounds are undesirable environmental contaminants and that, where possible, their unintentional production should be limited." (There are two

qualifiers in a single sentence – "where possible"; "limited" [rather than "stopped"].)

Greenpeace would not have needed to be concerned by the competition for public attention from this source.

Since 1992 the whole issue of endocrine (hormone) disruptors, including the implication of dioxin and "dioxinlike" compounds in this issue, has taken hold ever more widely in the public imagination. But there is no document or activity from the Canadian federal government in this entire period in which a serious attempt has been made to explain to a broad spectrum of citizens, in a comprehensible language, the great and changing complexities in dioxin science and risk assessment which have evolved from the early 1970s to the present. But if these agencies do not even attempt this task, who is supposed to do it?

In fact, Greenpeace is the only organization in Canada which has a publicly accessible document available that provides a critical overview of the human health effects issues. *Dioxin and Human Health: A Public Health Assessment of Dioxin Exposure in Canada* is written on Greenpeace's behalf by Tom Webster, who holds an appointment at the Boston University School of Public Health. Like the related publications, this one is replete with scientific citations and has the tone throughout of a careful, reasoned analysis. Of course it criticizes Health Canada for what is regarded as its too-lax guideline for dioxin intake and suggests a more stringent one. But this perspective is less important, in our view, than the simple fact that the document stands alone as a publicly accessible risk communication exercise about Canada's public policy on dioxin.

The Chemical Industry

The chemical industry has been in a much more difficult position, because it has so little perceived public credibility when it speaks about risks on matters in which it has an economic interest. And yet it has not helped its own cause in at least some of its public communications. To illustrate this point we shall refer to one document, released in late 1994 by the u.s. Chlorine Chemistry Council (ccc), a group formed under the auspices of the Chemical Manufacturers Association, entitled *20 Questions and Answers about Dioxin* (abbreviated *Q&A* below). There are many reasons why this cannot be considered to be an effective risk communication document in the context of the long history of dioxin controversy. Here are just a few of them:

1 *Lack of straight talking:* Statements that TCDD is "exceptionally toxic" or "highly toxic," cited above among the earlier epigraphs in the first section of this chapter, were made by officials at Dow Chemical Co. in internal memos and in a private communication to the U.S. secretary of Defense in 1970. So far as we know, to this day there is no comparable public statement from the chemical industry, and there is certainly nothing as clear and straightforward in the *Q&A*. Why not?

2 *Sources of dioxin in the environment.* A press release dated 12 September 1994 from the office of the CCC's managing director, designed to accompany the *Q&A*, states that "we do not believe that our industry is a major dioxins source." This is a most unfortunate assertion, for numerous reasons:

First, because it is by no means certain that it is true.[58] A major 1994 scientific review article concluded: "Numerous studies have thus correlated the environmental loading of PCDD/Fs with chloro-aromatic production this century, indications that global PCDD/F contamination is primarily a contemporary development associated with anthropogenic activities."[59] It is even quite possible that the chlorine industry itself is no longer the primary industrial originator of dioxins at the present time. On the other hand, given their long persistence in the environment, much of the anthropogenic environmental dioxin burden undoubtedly produced by this industry in the past is still with us.

Second, because it is irrelevant even if it is true. This is because, even if the chlorine industry contribution were relatively small, in comparison with both other industries and with the "natural" background, *any* incremental addition could still be important. (The current global climate change debate is going on in these terms right now.)

Third, the general trajectory of environmental dioxin levels – showing a gradual increase beginning in the 1920s and a very sharp rise through the 1960s and '70s, then peaking and starting to fall in the 1980s – correlates well with the rapid increase in industrial organochlorine production earlier in this century and then with the impact of control programs designed to restrict industrial releases of dioxins. This is *prima facie* evidence that the industrial contribution is significant.

Fourth, the reference in the *Q&A* to the finding of some of the less toxic dioxin forms (octachlorodibenzodioxin) in ancient human tissue is subject to different interpretations[60] and is also irrelevant so far as the issue of the sources of the most toxic dioxins is concerned. The *Q&A* does not mention that octachlorodibenzo-dioxin is three orders of magnitude (one thousand times) less toxic than TCDD.[61]

3 *Trivializing health effects.* The *Q&A* identifies chloracne as "a skin disorder so named because it mimics adolescent acne." Although one would not learn this from the *Q&A*, chloracne is a contraction for "chlorine acne," and its naming has nothing to do with adolescent acne. And as one medical text puts it: "Chloracne ... is far more disfiguring than adolescent acne."[62] The ill-advised "mimicking" statement in the *Q&A* makes one think of television commercials pitching remedies to teenagers desperate for social approval. While the mildest forms of industrial chloracne may resemble common acne, the more serious forms are disfiguring ailments that may persist for long periods of time. Other debilitating effects also accompany the relatively high exposures that give rise to chloracne.

In these and other respects there is a fundamental lack of candour in the industry communications directed at the public: after perusing them one wonders why anyone would think that dioxin risk is controversial. They have the tone of someone suggesting that we all "put the issue behind us" and move on, or hoping simply that, finally, the issue will just go away. That is unlikely to happen.

4 Hamburger Hell: Better Risk Communication for Better Health

WITH LINDA HARRIS

> Eating is one of the great sensual pleasures of life, the place where mystical at-oneness with the world meets, demystifies and celebrates biological necessity ... Eating is more than bodily nourishment, and a meal is more than food ... Eating is an essential ingredient in our understanding of ourselves, a literal coming to our senses. For this reason, eating is intimately bound up with our sense of being, individually and culturally. Not only eating: the food poisonings we suffer are direct reflections not only of hygiene and agricultural practices, but, at a very deep level, of who we are and who we are not. You can tell who a person is by what she chooses to make her sick.   David Waltner-Toews[1]

On 11 January 1993 two-year-old Michael Nole ate a cheeseburger as part of a "$2.69 Kid's Meal" at the Jack-in-the-Box restaurant on South 56th Street in Tacoma, Washington. The next night Michael was admitted to Children's Hospital and Medical Centre in Seattle, and ten days later he died of kidney and heart failure.[2] Two more children in the Pacific Northwest, as well as another child in California, subsequently died after being exposed to someone who ate at a Jack-in-the-Box restaurant. When it was all over, there were over 700 confirmed and probable cases in this outbreak of food-borne illness connected with Jack-in-the-Box restaurants. Of these, 125 people had to be admitted to hospital and at least twenty-nine suffered kidney failure, twenty-one of whom were required to undergo kidney dialysis. Dean Forbes, a spokesman for Children's Hospital in Seattle, summarized public sentiment in the wake of this food poisoning outbreak: "This has been a nightmare for the parents," he said. "To think that something as benign as hamburger could kill a kid is just startling to most people."[3]

To the food microbiologist hamburgers are anything but benign. In fact they can be teeming with microorganisms that, under certain conditions, can lead to significant health problems, or at least to a session of penance on the porcelain goddess of food-borne illness.

The hamburgers eaten by Michael Nole and thousands of other patrons of the Jack-in-the-Box fast food chain in the western United States in early 1993 were found to contain *Escherichia coli* O157:H7, a variant of normal human gut bacteria found in undercooked beef, municipal water, raw milk, and even apple cider.[4] First identified as a cause of human disease in 1982, the Jack-in-the-Box incident, as it has come to be known, is to date the largest and most serious outbreak of *E. coli* O157:H7 infection in North America, and it has sparked a surge in the public awareness of bacterial risks in food and has catalysed political reform of the entire meat inspection system in the United States.[5]

But even with this dramatic increase in public awareness (see figure 4.1), outbreaks continue to occur in North America and abroad. During the summer of 1996 over 9,500 Japanese, largely schoolchildren, were stricken with *E. coli* O157:H7; twelve died. How the bacterium was distributed so widely has still not been determined, although school lunches are suspected. In November 1996 in Scotland over four hundred people fell ill, twenty of whom – mostly pensioners who had attended a church supper – died. That same month, sixty-five people in four u.s. states and British Columbia fell ill after drinking juice manufactured by Odwalla Inc. of Half Moon Bay, California. The product was found to contain *E. coli* O157:H7. One of those victims, a sixteen-month-old girl, died in Denver. The juice contained unpasteurized cider, which became contaminated, possibly through cattle or deer feces on fallen apples, which were insufficiently cleaned.

This chapter tells the story of *E. coli* O157:H7 in order to demonstrate how scientific information can fill the risk information vacuum and lead to suitable risk management changes by responsible institutions. It will also demonstrate the magnitude of such a challenge, as well as the need to couple risk assessment, management, and communication activities tightly in an overall risk analysis framework – and the almost inevitable failures entailed by such challenges.

THE RISK EMERGES

In 1977 researchers at Health Canada laboratories in Ottawa first identified a subset of the *E. coli* family that produces a toxin – called verotoxin – which can lead to diarrhoea and serious illness in humans.[6] In 1982 a particularly virulent strain of these verotoxigenic *E. coli* or VTEC, called *E. coli* O157:H7, was found to be responsible for outbreaks of human illness in Oregon and Michigan after customers at McDonald's outlets ate contaminated hamburgers. There have since been dozens of documented outbreaks involving *E. coli* O157:H7 – and several involving other members of the VTEC family – in North America.[7]

At the heart of *E. coli* O157:H7 outbreaks is a simple question that is almost impossible to answer: Has the food supply become more hazardous in recent years? Dozens of dangerous microorganisms are now part of the North American lexicon – salmonella, shigella, campylobacter, vibrio, cryptosporidium, and listeria. The discourse about these pathogens is no longer confined to scientific circles but can be heard in a wide variety of public forums from television sitcoms to presidential speeches. This is almost entirely due to the notoriety of the Jack-in-the-Box outbreak.

Health Canada estimates 2.2 million cases of food-borne illness (largely microbial in origin) each year in Canada, resulting in a social cost – including medical treatment, productivity loss, pain and suffering of affected individuals, and lost sales – of $1.3 billion annually.[8] The most widely quoted figures in the United States peg the incidence of food-borne illness at 6.5 to 33 million cases each year, accounting for an estimated five hundred to nine thousand deaths.[9] Precise figures are difficult to come by because most cases of food poisoning exhibit mild, flu-like symptoms which are not reported or are not confirmed with laboratory testing. For each case of confirmed food poisoning, there may be anywhere from thirty to 350 undiagnosed cases.[10] The social cost of food-borne illness in the United States has been estimated at anywhere from $4.8 billion[11] to $8.4 billion[12] to $23 billion,[13] including the costs of medical treatment, productivity loss, pain and suffering of affected individuals, industry losses, and losses within the public health sector.[14]

While millions of cases of food poisoning are suspected annually in North America, there are still relatively few deaths, as a general rule, which is one reason why cases of *E. coli* O157:H7 infection are particularly worrisome. In 1991 a U.S. Food and Drug Administration (FDA) official stated that *E. coli* O157:H7 may become recognized in the 1990s as the cause of the greatest incidence of severe food-related illness of the known food-borne pathogens.[15] It was a prophetic statement, but one that was barely heeded. Scientists are only now beginning to understand how *E. coli* O157:H7 gets into the food supply and why certain people are affected by the toxin which the bacterium produces in the human body. The U.S. Centers for Disease Control and Prevention (CDC) estimates that each year in the United States, *E. coli* O157:H7 kills 250 to five hundred people and sickens another twenty thousand. In Canada the incidence of VTEC-related illness peaked in 1989 with 2,432 cases; in 1995 the total was 1,643.

Upon human ingestion, the bacterium can attach to the surface of the intestines but does not invade the cells; rather, it forms colonies and excretes a toxin which is absorbed through the intestinal wall. The toxin, first identified in 1983 by Herme Lior of Health Canada's Laboratory Centre for Disease Control, accumulates in kidney cells, and this can result in a spectrum of diseases. The most serious is a severe illness known as hemolytic uremic syndrome (HUS), the leading cause of acute kidney failure in children. Two to ten days after eating food contaminated with VTEC, people may experience severe stomach cramps, vomiting, and mild fever. Most will recover, but some will develop a watery or bloody diarrhoea; several studies have shown that *E. coli* O157:H7 is a major cause of bloody diarrhoea.[16] About 10 per cent of those with hamburger disease, especially children, the elderly, or people who have a suppressed immune system, will develop HUS. Fifteen per cent of those children will need permanent dialysis or a kidney transplant. What is worse, HUS is often misdiagnosed, and surgeons will sometimes unnecessarily operate and remove sections of the bowel.[17]

Dr Mohamed Karmali, microbiologist-in-chief at Toronto's Hospital for Sick Children and a professor of microbiology at the University of Toronto, who first established the link between HUS and VTEC in 1983, says there are currently about 150 new cases of HUS each year in Canadian children under five years of age. In Canada, HUS admissions peak during summer months. Health officials think that this is due to two factors (although they have good research data for only the first of these): first, to the summertime ritual of barbecuing hamburgers, which are sometimes undercooked, leaving any VTEC present available to infect the unsuspecting diner (hence the term, hamburger disease); and second, to an increased shedding of VTEC by animal carriers during the summer months. Researchers at the University of Alberta have conducted several clinical trials of a drug they have developed which can mop up and neutralize *E. coli* O157:H7 toxins in the intestines. However, Dr Karmali stresses the need for preventative measures.[18]

Ruminants such as cattle, sheep, and deer have been identified as a reservoir of *E. coli* O157:H7. In cattle the bacterium is most often found in intestines and on the surface of hides. One Canadian abattoir survey found that over 10 per cent of cattle carry *E. coli* O157:H7, where it is apparently part of the normal bacterial population. Current thinking is that ground beef is contaminated during slaughterhouse processing. Because the actual number of organisms required to cause disease is quite low, because VTEC appears in meat in a random or sporadic fashion, because VTEC can survive refrigeration and freezer storage, and because the bacterium is difficult to detect rapidly, large batches of hamburger potentially can be contaminated with *E. coli* O157:H7.

In the Jack-in-the-Box outbreak the contaminated burgers were traced back to a processing plant in California where an afternoon lot of approximately 500,000 hamburger patties was found to be contaminated. Separate surveys in Canada and the United States have found that about 2 per cent of raw hamburger sold in supermarkets carries *E. coli* O157:H7. Two per cent may not sound like a lot, but considering that the United States produces 33 million beef carcasses annually, yielding 23 billion pounds of beef and 6.9 billion pounds of ground beef, 2 per cent distributed around North America becomes quite a large amount.[19] The American Meat Institute (AMI) has estimated the incidence of *E. coli* O157:H7 on beef carcasses at 0.2 per cent and in raw ground beef at 0.1 per cent. In the United States the value of annual sales at wholesale of ground beef was pegged at $9 billion in 1994, with an average annual per person consumption of thirty pounds of ground beef. Canada and the United States remain nations of meat-eaters.

WHO SAID WHAT WHEN?

Governments, scientists, and professional health associations are faced with a dilemma: At what point does sufficient evidence exist to justify changes in policy or the issuance of public warnings about the potential dangers of a hazard? As mentioned earlier, VTEC was first identified in 1977; *E. coli* O157:H7 was first identified as a cause of human disease in 1982, after forty-seven people in White City, Oregon, and Traverse City, Michigan, developed severe stomach disorders after eating hamburgers at McDonald's outlets.[20] Reporting on *E. coli* O157:H7 in the *New York Times* began on 8 October 1982 with prompt coverage of this first known outbreak.[21] Researchers at CDC said that the bacterium associated with the outbreaks was normally killed by cooking. The next day federal epidemiologists characterized the disease as an intestinal ailment that had not proven fatal and was not a major public health hazard;[22] yet within a month, by 5 November, another twenty-nine cases were reported.

In 1983 CDC issued a report on the Oregon and Michigan outbreaks and by 1984 the first report on the behaviour of the organism and possible control measures appeared.[23,24] At that time a minimum internal cooking temperature of 140°F (60°C) for hamburgers was recommended by the U.S. Food and Drug Administration (FDA) and applied to restaurants and other food service establishments – but as a recommendation only. Although not specifically stated in the paper, calculated lethality based strictly on this internal cooking temperature suggested that even reaching an internal temperature of 60°C might not have destroyed all *E. coli* O157:H7 possibly present.

A search of the InfoGlobe database revealed the first mention of *E. coli* O157:H7 in a *Globe and Mail* story on 4 October 1983, describing three stricken children who ate burgers at fast-food outlets in Calgary.[25] However, there is probably an even earlier case in Canada, a 1980 outbreak linked to unpasteurized apple cider in southwestern Ontario, which sent twenty-three children to hospital suffering from HUS. In retrospect this incident was probably caused by VTEC, but because *E. coli* O157:H7 was not linked to human disease until 1982, investigators at the time were concentrating on chemical, viral, or known bacterial causes.

The term "hamburger disease" was first used in the *Globe and Mail* on 2 August 1991 to describe a large outbreak of VTEC in the Northwest Territories resulting in 521 cases, twenty-three of which resulted in HUS; two persons died. In reporting the 1983 Calgary outbreak, the city health department noted that while the O157:H7 serotype was relatively new, the bacterium "appears (to) be transferred from person to person." This was an astute observation, because even ten years later health inspectors were reported to be surprised to find that during the Jack-in-the-Box outbreak, *E. coli* O157:H7 could be spread from person to person. In response, the Calgary health department ordered inspections to check grill temperatures at fast-food outlets and to collect samples for laboratory testing.

Throughout the 1980s, reports on the epidemiology, physiology, pathogenicity, and control of this relatively unusual and newly recognized pathogen began to appear in the scientific literature. The scientific accounts of *E. coli* O157:H7 identified in the three scientific article databases increased slowly from 1982 to 1992. Several review articles had been written by the late 1980s, and two international conferences that focused solely on these organisms had been held by that time. However, information about *E. coli* O157:H7 was not widely disseminated beyond scientific circles; there was little information in either food trade publications or those aimed at physicians.[26]

It was a full decade after its discovery before *E. coli* O157:H7 achieved the status of being reviewed in a non-specialty journal, all previous reviews having been published in epidemiology, microbiology, and infectious disease journals.[27] No articles specifically related to *E. coli* O157:H7 were found in the specialized trade publication *Dairy, Food and Environmental Sanitation* prior to 1993 (although several review articles about pathogens in food mentioned the organism).

One article, for example, stated that *E. coli* O157:H7 was an emerging pathogen in the food supply which could be controlled by adequate cooking. Another noted that little was known about the source and prevalence of *E. coli* O157:H7, but that control could be achieved by adequate cooking and prevention of cross-contamination.[28] Similarly, in the more widely read journal *Food Technology*, no article specifically related to *E. coli* O157:H7 was published prior to 1993, although a 1986 article by Kvenberg and Archer described *E. coli* O157:H7 as an example of a newly discovered pathogen associated with beef, and an article by Genigeorgis mentions outbreaks involving *E. coli* O157:H7 and points to under-cooking as a contributing factor.[29]

Searches of two journals that may be more widely read by quality control or production people in the meat industry, *Food Processing* and *Meat Technology*, revealed no articles specifically focused on *E. coli* O157:H7 from 1990 to 1993. However, specific food-borne bacterial pathogens such as *Listeria monocytogenes* were mentioned in more than one article, indicating that these journals were not devoid of information on the microbiologial safety of foods.

Although the trade journal *Beef* was not systematically searched, an article was found in 1989 dealing with changes in cooking temperatures implemented by the U.S. Department of Agriculture (USDA) after an 1988 outbreak in schoolchildren involving pre-cooked hamburger patties prepared in a USDA-inspected plant. That 1988 outbreak led to a quickly formulated policy change announced on 27 December 1988, requiring an increase in cooking temperature from 140°F to 160°F (60°C to 71.1°C), which prompted complaints that the high temperature would result in a dry, unpalatable hamburger. After considering further comments from the industry, as well as research results (eventually published in 1991),[30] these policy changes were modified on 5 June 1990 to allow somewhat lower temperatures and to provide more cooking options.

Consumer information available from U.S. government agencies, especially USDA, indicated as early as 1989 that consumers should fully cook hamburger (employing the slogan "Why Experts Say Cook It"). A similar warning was included in consumer information from Health Canada beginning in 1991. A 1990 USDA booklet entitled *Preventing Foodborne Illness* recommended the thorough cooking of hamburger meat. Also about that time USDA began to expand the Hazard Analysis Critical Control Points (HACCP) model – a systematic way to identify those points in a food processing system where risks are present, and to determine how to best manage those risks. The model goes beyond the confines of processing facilities and restaurants to include the farm at one end and household consumption at the other. The notion of a "farm-to-fork" or "gate-to-plate," comprehensive food safety system began to be advocated. The USDA Hotline with a consistent message for thorough cooking of hamburger meat was also available to consumers.

While discussion of *E. coli* O157:H7 had remained confined to select scientific circles throughout the 1980s, both the *New York Times* and the *Globe and Mail* had continued to report outbreaks and suggest possible remedies. On 17 July 1985, the *New York Times* reported the results of a U.S. National Research Council committee which called for modernization of federal meat and poultry inspection to improve detection of microbial and chemical contaminants.[31] The story noted that the report endorsed the creation of an identification system to track livestock back to their original farm and feedlot, where much of the exposure to infectious organisms and chemicals occurred. These issues were revisited once the Jack-in-the-Box episode thrust meat inspection back onto the public agenda in the United States.

In 1985 nineteen out of fifty-five affected people at a London, Ontario, nursing home died after eating sandwiches apparently infected with VTEC.[32] In its subsequent coverage the *Globe and Mail* noted that "in 1982, researchers found that the microorganism could also cause disease in humans" and that "its occurrence is frequently linked in the medical literature to consumption of hamburgers." An inquest into the outbreak yielded numerous stories about the "obscure but deadly bacterium, *E. coli* O157." On 12 October 1985, in response to the ongoing inquest, the Ontario government announced a training program for food handlers in health-care institutions, "stressing cleaning and sanitizing procedures and hygienic practices in food preparation."[33] The province also required nursing homes to develop "a comprehensive contingency plan for controlling outbreaks of infectious diseases." The remainder of coverage in the *Globe and Mail* (figure 4.1) reported sporadic outbreaks.

In 1986 and 1988 the *New York Times* carried general stories warning about possible risks from food-borne illness, especially during summer cook-outs.[34] In 1989, after two months in which dozens of stories appeared about the risks from daminozide (Alar) and from Chilean grapes contaminated with pesticides, a story appeared quoting food experts who insisted that microbes, rather than chemical pesticides and food additives, posed the biggest food safety threat.[35] These same scientific experts said there had been a marked increase in microbial contamination and, at the same time, constantly diminishing contamination by pesticides in the food supply. Fear of chemicals, they said, had obscured low and decreasing risks associated with both natural and man-made pesticides. On 18 September 1990 the *New York Times*

number of stories

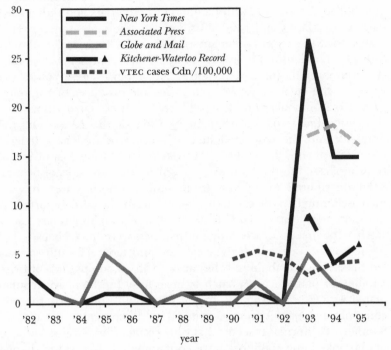

Figure 4.1
Specified media coverage of *E. coli* O157:H7, 1982 to 1995, and incidence of
verotoxigenic *E. coli* in Canada per 100,000 population, 1990–1995 (Health Canada)

covered the release of a National Academy of Sciences report that
urged USDA to go further than it had proposed to do in reforming its
beef-inspection system, primarily to protect consumers from the growing incidence of food-borne disease.[36] Again, these warnings, while
they may have been acted upon internally at USDA, were under-
reported in the public domain until the Jack-in-the-Box episode. It
appears that, all too often, fundamental change is carried out only
after a catastrophe has occurred.

THE JACK-IN-THE-BOX OUTBREAK

On 13 January 1993 a physician in Washington State reported a cluster
of children with hemolytic uremic syndrome and an increase in emergency room visits for bloody diarrhoea in people of all ages.[37] Laboratory tests on the stools of infected patients revealed the presence of *E.
coli* O157:H7. Most infected people had eaten hamburgers from local

outlets of Jack-in-the-Box, a nationwide fast-food chain. Epidemiologists linked the illnesses with hamburger patties labelled with a use-by date of 19 March 1993 and distributed to the restaurants by Foodmaker Inc., the parent company of Jack-in-the-Box. (Jack-in-the-Box, with 1,170 outlets in the western United States, represented two-thirds of Foodmaker's 1992 revenue of $1.29 billion.) These patties were traced to the meat-packer Vons Inc., the sole producer of hamburger patties for Foodmaker, and to a production date of 19 November 1992. CDC informed USDA on 18 January 1993 of the *E. coli* O157:H7 outbreak and the suspected link to meat produced at a federally inspected plant.[38] *E. coli* O157:H7 was isolated from lots of ground beef implicated in the outbreak. Meat from the same lots of beef had been distributed to at least three other western states in which increased numbers of cases of bloody diarrhoea were reported. An interstate recall was initiated by Jack-in-the-Box on 18 January 1993.[39]

After the first reports of food-borne illness were traced back to Jack-in-the-Box, subsequent analysis by state and federal health scientists led the restaurant chain to voluntarily recall 28,000 pounds of frozen hamburger patties from a batch of meat found to be heavily contaminated with *E. coli* O157:H7. In the meantime, some forty thousand contaminated patties were consumed in Washington, Nevada, and Southern California. It seems that only certain hamburgers had been undercooked and therefore were contaminated, due to variations in cooking procedures. Although the FDA had set a national minimum internal cooking temperature for ground beef of 140°F, Washington State had raised its standard to 155°F in mid-1992, after earlier outbreaks of *E. coli* O157:H7. The change was made by Washington State in response to the 1991 USDA proposal discussed above, although it allowed the requirement to be waived if a customer specifically requested an under-cooked hamburger. (McDonald's, the world's largest fast-food restaurant, has long cooked its burgers to 157°F and adopted a unique cooking method following outbreaks of *E. coli* O157:H7 traced to burgers served at McDonald's). Robert Nugent, president of Jack-in-the-Box, said company outlets cooked its meat below the 155°F Washington State standard because it was not aware that a change in the regulations had been made – an astonishing statement from a company doing close to a $1 billion in annual sales.

It took the company one week to publicly admit its responsibility, from the initial establishment of a link between food-borne illness and Jack-in-the-Box's hamburgers. Nugent initially blamed regulators and suppliers; however, once responsibility was admitted, the company responded by destroying twenty thousand pounds of frozen patties, changing meat suppliers, installing a toll-free number to field calls, and telling employees to increase the cooking temperature. An offer to cover victims' hospital costs came two weeks after the news of the first poisoning. Subsequently, government investigators discovered that not only had the 155°F standard been ignored but that in some cases, hamburger patties had been undercooked in some outlets to internal temperatures as low as 135°F.[40]

As shown in figure 4.1, the Jack-in-the-Box outbreak led to a large increase in national reporting on *E. coli* O157:H7. The story was first carried in the *New York Times* on 23 January 1993 after the first child died, and in the *Globe and Mail* on 29 January 1993, using an *Associated Press* (*AP*) wire story after a second child had died.[41] However, almost immediately thereafter, the way the story was told changed between Canada and the United States. The *New York Times* and *AP* published a series of articles critical of the entire meat inspection system; no such criticism appeared in the *Globe and Mail* or *Kitchener-Waterloo Record*. Instead, the Canadian stories often focused on a drug developed at the University of Alberta which could apparently "mop up" the toxins secreted by *E. coli* O157:H7.[42] This is a classic case of "Canadianizing" a story originating in the United States.

Because of the severity of the Jack-in-the-Box incident, the congressional hearings that ensued, and continual media investigations, the FDA finally issued its notice on the national recommended cooking temperature of 155°F which had been first proposed two years earlier. On 20 January 1993, two days after CDC informed USDA of the outbreak, newly appointed Secretary of Agriculture Mike Espy announced immediate plans to implement organic acid sprays to kill bacteria on meat, coupled with increased inspection.[43] "If any child dies as a result of something we have done or haven't done, it's just not good enough," said Espy. "As a parent and a consumer, I can well understand the fears and anguish this has caused." These initial actions were followed in mid-March with announcements that the entire meat-inspection system in the United States would be overhauled. "We can't inspect meat in 1993 the same way we inspected it in 1933," Espy said. "We have to change to a system not based on sight and touch but one based on microbiology."[44] Highlights of the proposals included the temporary stationing of scientists and some federal inspectors on farms and feedlots to collect data and determine whether modern mass-production techniques were tainting the meat supply; new research to develop quicker diagnostics; more careful processing of meat; and mandatory safety labels to inform restaurant employees and home cooks how to handle meat safely. These changes "would affect every level of the $80 billion U.S. beef, pork and poultry production system, from the farm to the kitchen." On 2 April 1993 the *New York*

Times ran an editorial hailing Espy's willingness to confront the problem as "a refreshing break from Agriculture's traditional laxity in consumer protection." Espy's plan was praised as the most ambitious updating of the nation's meat inspection system since its establishment eighty-seven years earlier.[45]

Media interest stimulated by the Jack-in-the-Box episode continued to reverberate. An outbreak of hamburger disease that struck dozens of people and was traced to two Sizzler restaurants in Grants Pass and North Bend, Oregon, was widely reported.[46] The source of the infections was determined to be salad dressing and sauces containing mayonnaise contaminated by bad meat. More importantly, a number of articles specific to *E. coli* O157 began to appear in food trade journals.

THE EFFECT OF JACK-IN-THE-BOX

From April 1993 to December 1996, interest in the Jack-in-the-Box outbreak continued, but reports of previous food-borne illnesses involving *E. coli* O157:H7 were also recollected. Any such illness became news material, accounting for part of the continued coverage. The story went on developing differently between the United States and Canada. Outbreaks relating to unpasteurized milk, fresh (unpreserved) apple cider, other fast-food restaurants, and salami were reported by the American media. Several television documentaries were broadcast on news-magazine shows such as ABC's *20/20* and *Turning Point*, CBS's *48 Hours*, and NBC's *Dateline*.[47] Researchers and physicians began to call for improved national surveillance and screening of stool samples for *E. coli* O157:H7.[48]

Criticism of the U.S. meat system continued in the wake of the Jack-in-the-Box episode and, after efforts to implement safe-handling labels on uncooked meat and poultry products in the fall of 1993 failed, USDA was presented as a typical bureaucracy unable to bring about change, even if young children died.[49] (Safe-handling labels eventually were adopted.) Articles produced on the first anniversary of the Jack-in-the-Box outbreak were largely critical of the lack of reform in meat inspection. Favourable opinions of USDA in the press had been transformed into traditional cynicism because actions failed to match words; change in risk management procedures – in this case meat inspection – had not been implemented. For example, *Reuters* reported on 11 January 1994 that consumer groups and food activists said "little has been done by the U.S. Agriculture Department to ensure that last January's deadly outbreak of food poisoning in Washington State never happens again." Robert Greene of the *Associated Press* said that in January 1993 "the government's system of protecting consumers from unsafe meat and poultry collapsed. After a year of promises, public hearings and news conferences, the Agriculture Department can offer consumers no assurances that raw meat and poultry is any freer of *E. coli* or other foodborne pathogens. And there's no guarantee that labels warning shoppers to store, handle and cook raw meat properly will appear soon."[50]

Typical also was a quote in the Robert Greene story from the mother of Michael Nole, Diana Nole of Tacoma, Washington: "There hasn't been anything done," she said. Greene noted that Nole was "expecting a second but only child next month. Her firstborn, Michael, died last Jan. 22 at age 2, 12 days after eating a tainted hamburger."

Other stories focused on what had been learned in the previous year and how little was still known about *E. coli* O157:H7.[51] Even among victims who had recovered, the extent of the bacterium's devastation continued to surprise medical scientists. "Studies in Utah show that 11 per cent of survivors have serious lingering problems, such as high blood pressure. And fully half show traces of mild abnormalities, such as subtle kidney injury." "Other kinds of food poisoning you can treat," said Dr Patricia Griffin, an assistant chief in the bacterial disease division at the u.s. Centers for Disease Control and Prevention. "With O157, you're in the hands of God."[52]

The Jack-in-the-Box story even garnered the attention of satirists. During the news portion of a 1994 broadcast of the television show *Saturday Night Live*, the anchor stated: "Dr Kervorkian helped with two more suicides this week. He went to the drive-through at the local Jack-in-the-Box."

The USDA continued to conduct and publicize basic research about the ecology of *E. coli* O157:H7. On 9 March 1994 *AP* reported that in a survey of seven thousand cattle from 1,811 dairy operations in twenty-eight states, *E. coli* O157:H7 was found in feces from 3.6 of every thousand sucklings (i.e., an incidence of less than four-tenths of 1 per cent). However, because this was the first time such a baseline study had been conducted, scientists were unsure whether this amount is relatively high or low.

In August 1994 u.s. Agriculture Secretary Mike Espy announced the development – after more than a year of work by USDA scientists – of a new, rapid test that could detect bacteria on meat and poultry.[53] "The test, an adaptation of bioluminescence technology, takes five minutes to get results as opposed to a forty-eight-hour test now used by some plants," stated the *Washington Post*. But there were limitations.

The test could not identify specific bacteria such as salmonella or *E. coli* O157:H7, or low levels of bacteria.

James Marsden, vice-president of science and technical affairs at the American Meat Institute, criticized the fact the test did not distinguish between types of bacteria or determine whether they are harmful: "It just verifies what you already know, that you have microbiological populations on raw carcasses." Consumer groups also doubted the test would improve the safety of the nation's meat supply. And Espy himself had to deny suggestions that the announcement was designed to assuage concern over his ethical conduct. Earlier that month Attorney General Janet Reno had asked "that an independent counsel investigate whether Espy accepted gifts from Tyson Foods Inc., the nation's largest poultry processor, in violation of the 1907 Meat Inspection Act."

Indeed, changing to an inspection system based on science rather than sight and smell, while providing a comfortable soundbite for media purposes, is an exceedingly difficult proposition. Industry rightly complained that end-product testing was contrary to basic HACCP principles, because the control points are supposed to occur earlier in the processing chain, and testing might give a false sense of security to consumers. But industry groups also failed to come up with a compelling alternative vision, one that could capture the public imagination, such as "changing to an inspection system based on science rather than on sight and smell." For even if the proposed end-product tests were appropriate, such quick and cost-effective tests for slaughterhouses simply are not available. Although large numbers of samples can be screened and all serotypes of VTEC and all toxin types of verotoxin can be detected using African green monkey cells, tissue culture presents serious limitations and results in a large number of false positives. New immuno-assay tests and the use of genetic probes coupled with polymerase chain reaction (PCR) technology are being developed to provide a more accurate and timely assay for VTEC, but such work remains largely confined to the laboratory at this time.[54]

The Jack-in-the-Box outbreak also increased calls for food irradiation as a solution to the *E. coli* O157:H7 problem. Health columnist Jane Brody wrote that food irradiation is simply misunderstood, just as milk pasteurization was at the turn of the century.[55]

In mid-August 1994 Michael R. Taylor was appointed chief of USDA's Food Safety and Inspection Service, and in late September USDA said it would now regard *E. coli* O157:H7 in raw ground beef as an "adulterant," a substance that should not be present in the product. "Adulterated" food products must be recalled, reprocessed (which might include cooking), or destroyed. By mid-October Taylor had announced plans to launch a nationwide sampling of ground beef to assess how much contamination existed from *E. coli* O157:H7.[56] The five thousand samples would be taken during the year from supermarkets and meat processing plants alike "to set an example and stimulate companies to put in preventive measures." Positive samples would prompt product recalls of the entire affected lot, effectively removing it from any possibility of sale. (The sampling revealed almost no instances of meat contaminated with *E. coli* O157:H7.)

In response, the American Meat Institute (AMI) filed a lawsuit to prevent the testing and issued a press release entitled "Fact Sheet: *E. Coli* O157:H7, Microbiological Testing and Ground Beef."[57] And while the AMI said it supported microbiological testing as part of a comprehensive safe food production program, it also said that it "questions the effectiveness of USDA's *E. coli* testing initiative." Instead, the AMI called for a comprehensive overhaul of the inspection system, including the development of a gate-to-plate HACCP system. "The fact is, you cannot test your way to a safer food supply," stated the AMI release. "That supply can only be built through safe food production processes at all stages of the food production chain … Reducing or eliminating pathogens, such as *E. coli* O157:H7, requires building preventive measures into food production from farm to table."

This angered consumer groups such as the Safe Food Coalition, which issued their own release.[58] According to coalition coordinator Carol Tucker Foreman, "Beef is heavily advertised as a staple of American family dining. But from the fast food restaurant to the kitchen table, beef products can bring disease and death to the family dinner. While the industry is happy to use the USDA inspection seal as part of its marketing strategy, the industry is now trying to kill effective inspection methods that would make that seal stand for safer beef products."

The brouhaha received coverage in the *New York Times* and the *Associated Press*.[59] The *New York Times* even weighed in with an editorial slamming the American Meat Institute and six other food-industry and supermarket groups for filing suit. The editorial concluded, "It is not consumers the lawsuit seeks to protect but the industry's right to sell tainted beef."[60]

In early December 1994 another outbreak, this time involving salami, received widespread publicity.[61] At least eighteen people were stricken in California and Washington. Dr David Swerdlow of the CDC said it was the first time *E. coli* O157:H7 had been found in a cured meat; the AMI immediately pledged to test whether *E. coli* O157:H7 could survive the process used to make dry sausages like salami, which involves only meat curing, not cooking. (The high acid levels were previously thought to kill bacteria like *E. coli* O157:H7.) On 15 January

1995, as part of a comprehensive proposal to revamp the U.S. inspection system, USDA said that salami and other fermented dry sausage products would be routinely tested for *E. coli* O157:H7.

The VTEC-in-salami story garnered attention again in March 1995 after the CDC issued its report on the outbreak.[62] The story surfaced again in the *New York Times* on 25 June 1995 when food writer Marian Burros revealed that a scientific paper published three years earlier had reported that *E. coli* O157:H7 could survive the processing of dry-fermented sausages.[63] She wondered why USDA had not notified processors of the potential risk. Michael Doyle, director of the Center for Food Safety and Quality Enhancement at the University of Georgia and one of the researchers on the project, said that the researchers had not been inclined to publicize the information at that time because there had been no reports of outbreaks caused by fermented sausages. "The epidemiology wasn't there and we didn't see any problem," said Doyle. "As a scientist, I think it's prudent and useful to share all this information generated in the lab, but what you find in the lab may not relate to reality or what is practical." Dr James Marsden, senior scientific advisor to the American Meat Institute, said: "You can't advise the public to cook these, because they come ready to eat. For years we've been accused of blaming the victim, but the victim has no role in this. The responsibility lies squarely with the industry."

As the second anniversary of the Jack-in-the-Box outbreak approached, the USDA issued a massive overhaul of meat inspection regulations, dubbed "mega-reg," including microbiological testing and the mandatory adoption of the HACCP system.[64] However, with the Republican party controlling Congress and the Senate, a moratorium on any new regulations was adopted and the future of mega-reg seemed in doubt through much of 1995. Newspaper columnists representing both the political right and left used mega-reg as, respectively, evidence of bureaucrats out of control or the callousness of the free market. Nationally syndicated cartoon strips such as "Doonesbury" (19 August 1995) satirized Republican attempts to implement cost-benefit analysis as part of regulatory proposals such as mega-reg:

"What's an American life worth? Meat industry?"
"Senator Dole, we put that figure at about $35."
"Really? We [tobacco industry] got it pegged at 12 cents."

In the midst of this debate the CDC released a report concluding that *E. coli* O157:H7 sickened as many as twenty thousand people annually in the United States, up to five hundred of whom, mostly children and the elderly, die.[65] The report said that as more laboratories test for the bacteria, they are discovering more and more isolated victims who are not part of an outbreak.

Meanwhile, the Republican-led battle against mega-reg assumed centre stage on the national agenda. In the first of three columns,[66] *New York Times* op-ed columnist Bob Herbert began with an exemplar, recounting the death of six-year-old Alex Donley, who ate a hamburger and died four days later. "He died horribly. 'Nearly all of the organs in Alex's body were destroyed,' said his mother, Nancy Donley. 'Portions of his brain were liquefied. That's how virulent a pathogen this is. My husband and I wanted to donate his organs, and have him live in another child, but we couldn't. We were able to donate his corneas. That's all.'" Herbert went on to say of the House Appropriations Committee vote to shelve the new mega-reg and order USDA to negotiate new rules with the meat industry, "that, of course, is like negotiating prison rules with convicts ... Two things will happen to anyone who takes a close look at the way meat is processed and inspected in this country: they will wonder how it is that even more people are not made sick by tainted meat, and they will get sick to their stomachs themselves." In a later column, Herbert painted a revolting picture of meat production in the United States:

The bacterium *Escherichia coli* O157:H7 is a nightmare embedded in millions of hamburger patties ... *E. coli* O157 micro-organisms are so virulent there can be no guarantee – short of burning a burger to a cinder – that cooking has warded off the danger ... This is a problem that the Federal Government can do something about. *E. coli* O157 is found in the intestines and fecal matter of cattle. Its journey to the dinner table begins with grotesquely sloppy practices in some of the nation's slaughterhouses and meat-packing plants. Before they are slaughtered the cattle are kept in small holding pens where they often stand in excrement and dirt up to their bellies. They are then moved – with large clumps of filth clinging to their hides – to the slaughter facility ... Then the animals are gutted, often by inexperienced, careless workers who allow the fecal matter to spill onto the meat. That is the most common point of contamination.

Meanwhile, another VTEC outbreak was documented in a CDC report, this time *Escherichia coli* O104:H21, which sickened eighteen people in Montana in 1994 who had drunk contaminated milk.[67]

Finally, President Bill Clinton "used the *E. coli* word," telling the story, during his regular Saturday radio broadcast, of Eric Mueller, a thirteen-year-old California youth who was "poisoned by an invisible bacteria, *E. coli*, that contaminated the hamburger" he had eaten a few days earlier. "How did this happen?" Clinton asked. "Because the federal government has been inspecting meat the same old way since the turn of the century."[68] Not unexpectedly, the president's political opponents described him as "employing rhetorical germ warfare" in this story. Senator William Roth dismissed Clinton's criticisms when he delivered the Republican response an hour later: "As a regular hamburger eater, I can tell you the opponents of this reform are full of baloney." Three days later, Agriculture Secretary Dan Glickman and Republican congressmen agreed on a compromise that would let new meat safety rules go ahead while addressing industry worries.[69]

Foodmaker Inc., the operator and franchiser of the Jack-in-the-Box chain, reported on 1 August 1995 its first profitable quarter since the January 1993 outbreak.[70] Several stories also noted that the company had settled about seventy lawsuits linked to the outbreak, including a $15.6 million settlement for twelve-year-old Brianne Kiner of Seattle after the bacterial infection left her with kidney, pancreatic, and intestinal damage. Media coverage also noted that Jack-in-the-Box had introduced a HACCP system that had become the model for the industry.[71]

In June 1996 the proposed USDA recommendation of a mandatory HACCP-based system was agreed to by the Republican Senate and Congress. On 6 July 1996 President Clinton announced that for the first time in ninety years of federal regulation every slaughter plant would have to test its raw products for bacterial contamination, while Agriculture Department inspectors would begin conducting regular tests for salmonella.[72] By January 1997 all meat-processing plants, regardless of size, were required to implement sanitation plans and begin testing for *E. coli* to monitor how well their HACCP systems were working. (Generic *E. coli* are indicators of fecal contamination, but their usefulness as an indicator of VTEC contamination is a matter of debate.) Ronnie Rudolph of Carlsbad, California, whose six-year-old daughter, Lauren, had died in the Jack-in-the-Box outbreak, was quoted as saying: "Until the end of my life I will not give up this fight because today is just the beginning of getting this right."[73] The *New York Times* again praised the move as a "historic transformation," citing the 1985 report by the U.S. National Academy of Sciences as evidence of the recognized need for change, and stated that the "public's demand for safer food in the wake of well-publicized food poisoning cases won out."[74]

Throughout this time discussion of food-borne illness had begun to infiltrate popular North American culture. Sensational papers and magazines routinely began to cover outbreaks and risks. Comic strips such as "Herman" and "Cathy" satirized the feeling that "everything will make you sick," and the television sitcom *Frasier* featured a discussion of risks from campylobacter and listeria growing in dirty kitchen dishrags. When reports of food-borne illness were combined with stories about the Ebola virus, flesh-eating disease, and antibiotic resistance, there was a huge increase in "killer-bug" stories. Manufacturers have kept pace. Dial soap is now advertised as "killing more bacteria" than competitors' brands. Clorox bleach is shown in television commercials as the only effective way to rid the kitchen countertop of salmonella. And anti-bacterial sponges are flogged as harbouring fewer bacteria than dirty dishrags.

Canadian coverage of *E. coli* O157:H7 in the *Kitchener-Waterloo Record* and the *Globe and Mail* was much more muted, limited largely to the occasional wire story highlighting an aspect of American coverage, although the *Kitchener-Waterloo Record* did carry several reports highlighting research into the causes of *E. coli* O157:H7 contamination and the risks faced by small children on dairy farms in Ontario.[75] Questions were also raised about the Canadian meat inspection system, but these were confined largely to agricultural trade magazines.

THE RISK CONTINUES

Upton Sinclair's *The Jungle*, his famous exposé of the horrific conditions in Chicago's meat-processing plants, was published in 1906, and within two years the U.S. Congress had enacted the Federal Meat Inspection Act as an amendment to a USDA appropriations bill. Ninety years later the same pattern was repeated. Hamburgers and apple pie are at the heart of American food traditions and mythology, and yet, within the past decade, the wholesomeness of both has been called into question through the controversies over hamburger disease and the use of Alar on apples.[76]

In general, the media coverage reviewed here highlighted the risks posed by *E. coli* O157:H7 and discussed how the deaths of many children and massive illness could have occurred. Scientific uncertainty, regardless of how minor an element it was in a story, was often a focal point of print media coverage. The reports were generally accurate and ultimately captured public outrage, helping to create the political pressure necessary to catalyse reforms to the meat inspection system (at least in the United States).

Consumer behaviour also appears to have been affected. The recent increase in perception of spoilage as the most dangerous food safety risk, with the caveats discussed above, offers a rough estimate of increased consumer perception following media coverage. Further evidence is shown in figure 4.1. As the number of media reports about *E. coli* O157:H7 increased in both the United States and Canada, the incidence of reported VTEC infections decreased per 100,000 people in Canada, even as surveillance efforts were increasing. The rise in media and scientific interest in *E. coli* O157:H7 since January 1993 has increased physician reporting of cases of bloody diarrhoea to public health officials. Such reporting helps identify clusters of cases.[77] In light of the Jack-in-the-Box outbreak, MacDonald and Osterholm made several recommendations to bolster detection of *E. coli* O157:H7 at the clinical level and to expand national surveillance of the bacterium.[78] They also recommended increased consumer education about the need to cook hamburger thoroughly and the risks associated with drinking raw milk: "This can be accomplished through media efforts by state and local health departments." Results presented here suggest this has already happened.

The Jack-in-the-Box outbreak had all the elements of a dramatic story which catapulted it to the top of the public agenda – at least in the United States. Children were involved; the risk was relatively unknown and unfamiliar; and a sense of outrage developed in response to the inadequacy of the government inspection system and the identifiable target in Foodmaker Inc.[79] The same sense of outrage at the inadequacy of antiquated meat inspection techniques in Canada did not occur, but it could do so at any time.

A more fundamental question arising out of this work is: When should officials "go public" with warnings? At what point does sufficient evidence exist to justify public warnings about the potential dangers of a specific pathogen in a specific food? The protection of public health and the right of citizens to information that can affect their health is often balanced against the economic and social effect of such warnings through decreased sales. In retrospect, with *E. coli* O157:H7, there was a lack of communication and flow of knowledge from the scientific realm to the trade journals where information could have had an impact on quality control procedures. And even with the dramatic increase of both media coverage and public awareness related to microbial food-borne risks, ignorance flourishes.

Sometime in late September 1996 sixteen-month-old Anna Gimmestad of Denver drank a glass of Smoothie juice manufactured by Odwalla Inc. After her parents noticed bloody diarrhoea, Anna was admitted to Children's Hospital on October 16. On 8 November 1996 she died after going into cardiac and respiratory arrest. Anna had severe kidney problems related to hemolytic uremic syndrome and her heart had stopped several times in previous days. The juice that Anna – and sixty-five others who got sick – drank was contaminated with *E. coli* O157:H7, linked to fresh, unpasteurized apple cider used as a base in the juices manufactured by Odwalla. Because they are unpasteurized,

Odwalla's drinks are shipped in cold storage and have only a two-week shelf life. Odwalla was founded sixteen years ago on the premise that fresh, natural fruit juices nourish the spirit. As well as the bank balance: in fiscal 1996 Odwalla's sales had jumped 65 per cent to u.s. $60 million. Company chairman Greg Steltenpohl has told reporters that the company did not routinely test for *E. coli* because it was advised by industry experts that the acid level in the apple juice was sufficient to kill the bug. Just who these so-called "industry experts" are remains a mystery. Odwalla insists they were the u.s. Food and Drug Administration. The FDA isn't sure who was warned and when.[80] Despite all of the academic research and media coverage concerning VTEC cited above (even all of the stories involving VTEC surviving in acidic environments), Odwalla professes ignorance.

In terms of crisis management – and outbreaks of food-borne illness are increasingly contributing to the case study literature on crisis management – Odwalla responded appropriately. Company officials reacted in a timely and compassionate fashion, initiating a complete recall and cooperating with authorities after a link was first made on October 30 between their juice and the illness. They issued timely and comprehensive press statements and even opened a website containing background information on both the company and *E. coli* O157:H7. Upon learning of Anna's death, Steltenpohl issued a statement which said: "On behalf of myself and the people at Odwalla, I want to say how deeply saddened and sorry we are to learn of the loss of this child. Our hearts go out to the family and our primary concern at this moment is to see that we are doing everything we can to help them."

But for Odwalla – or any food firm – to say in 1996 that it had no knowledge that *E. coli* O157 could survive in an acid environment is simply unacceptable. When one of us called this $60-million-a-year company with the great public relations to ask why they didn't know that *E. coli* O157 was a risk in cider, it took over a day before the call was returned.[81] That's a long time in crisis-management mode. More galling was the company spokeswoman's explanation that she had received the message but that her phone mysteriously couldn't call Canada that day: great public relations, lousy risk management. What the Odwalla outbreak – along with that of cyclospora in fresh fruit in the spring of 1996 and with dozens of others – demonstrates is that vigilance along the entire trail "from farm to fork" is an inescapable requirement in a global food system. Risk assessment, management, and communication must be interlinked to accommodate new scientific and public information. And that includes those who make and sell funky natural fruit juices.

More recent research has uncovered additional risk factors for VTEC infection. More than two hundred different VTEC serotypes – members of the same bacterial strain but with different proteins on their outer shell – have been isolated from humans, foods, and other sources. About 150 of these have been isolated from humans and over fifty have been shown to cause disease in humans. While *E. coli* O157:H7 is the most familiar strain, and the one now more routinely tested for in laboratories, about 20 per cent of VTEC illness in Canada is now believed to be caused by non-O157:H7 strains.[82] Yet rarely are non-O157 strains of the bacterium tested for, due to time and expense.

Person-to-person contact is increasingly recognized as a source of infection. Both a nurse and a police officer investigating the 1996 Scottish outbreak have come down with the illness. A study of Ontario dairy farm families found VTEC in 6.3 per cent of the individuals on 21 per cent of the farms tested. More importantly, 70 per cent of children under ten years of age were seropositive, indicating exposure to VTEC. A separate study of children from Toronto in the same age group found only 5 per cent carried VTEC antibodies.[83] The authors conclude that people living on dairy farms have much higher exposure to VTEC but that exposure may confer some immunity, much like vaccines. However, this also means that members of farm families – say, children going to an urban day-care centre – could be a source for VTEC infection of others.

Researchers are also trying to reduce the bacterial load on cattle entering slaughterhouses, as well as on the final meat products, attempting to determine through experiments what conditions reduce the numbers of VTEC bacteria in cattle before they are slaughtered. Changes in diet, feed withdrawal times, and transportation conditions are all being examined. Other research questions are being posed: For example, can techniques such as steam pasteurization or acid rinses used in the plant reduce the bacterial numbers in raw meat?

In light of this unfolding scientific story, the overriding question remains: What organizations or individuals will assume responsibility to enter into a public dialogue about such risks? In the United States a collection of interest groups, politicians, regulatory agencies, and consumers themselves have eagerly engaged in a public debate about VTEC risk. Once again, Canadian authorities are largely quiet.

5 Silicone Breasts:
The Implant Risk Controversy

CONRAD G. BRUNK, WITH
THE ASSISTANCE OF
WILLIAM LEISS

In May 1995 Dow Corning Corp. announced that it was seeking bankruptcy protection in response to rapidly escalating numbers of compensation claims for alleged harms suffered by women who had been surgically fitted with the silicone breast implants manufactured by the company. The company had been found liable for large awards by juries who were convinced by the testimony of women and their physicians that a whole range of health problems was caused by the implants manufactured by Dow Corning and several of its competitors.

One of the first of these lawsuits had been brought over ten years earlier in 1984 when a California jury awarded Maria Stern $1.7 million in damages for illnesses it was convinced had been caused by Dow Corning's implants. The court found Dow Corning guilty of fraud in its handling of information the company possessed concerning the risks to women from its implants.[1] The flood of litigation against Dow Corning did not really begin until 1991, however, when a San Francisco jury awarded Mariann Hopkins $7.3 million because of its findings that Dow Corning implants were defective and that the company was guilty of fraud.[2] After the *Hopkins* decision the u.s. Food and Drug Administration announced a moratorium on the sale of the implants, reinforcing an avalanche of court suits filed against Dow Corning. By the end of 1992 the number of pending suits had increased from 137 to 3,558. A year later the number had reached more than twelve thousand,[3] and by 1994, 19,092 cases had reportedly been filed against Dow Corning.

After many of these suits had been consolidated into a class-action proceeding, an Alabama judge approved a tentative u.s. $4.5 billion settlement between several implant manufacturers and women who filed injury claims with the court, the largest class-action settlement in history. Dow Corning, which manufactured nearly 30 per cent of the over two million breast implants placed in women's bodies, agreed to pay nearly half of this $4.5 billion.[4] The other half of the liability was shared among several other companies, Bristol-Meyers Squibb, 3-M Company, and Baxter International among them. But the Alabama settlement was not the end of Dow Corning's liabilities, since the court left the door open for claims from additional women to be brought against the company. More claims were forthcoming, including actions on behalf of an estimated fifty thousand Canadian women, most of whom had been excluded from the Alabama settlement.[5] At some point in the proceedings, plaintiffs included Dow Chemical in the legal action, alleging that this parent company of Dow Corning shared liability because it had carried out some of the early studies on the potential effects of silicone on the immune system.[6] By 1995 over 440,000 women had registered in the global settlement against all the implant manufacturers including Dow Corning.

The Risk Communication Angle

If a final class-action settlement confirms Dow Corning's bankruptcy declaration, this will mean the loss of their company by existing shareholders as a result of litigation over a product that represented only 1 per cent of the company's total sales. The tentative class-action settlement entailed unprecedented court awards for alleged damages for which there was, and remains, little reliable scientific evidence. Despite the scarcity of scientific evidence for many of the alleged risks, juries had been accepting the contention that silicone breast implants posed clearly unacceptable risks for a wide variety of autoimmune and connective tissue diseases, as well as other severe disabilities suffered by women. This public perception of the risk supported the willingness of numerous juries and judges to be persuaded that Dow Corning was guilty of "injuring" many women and consequently ought to be liable for high levels of punitive damages.

The Dow Corning case raises fundamental issues about the relationship between science and public regulatory policy, as well as between expert and lay perceptions of risk. Risk communication is, in part, the art of effective bridge-building across the often wide spaces that separate these domains. If this artistry is maladroit, there can be disastrous repercussions on various levels, economic, political, and personal. One of the features is timeliness, and the question is whether Dow Corning assessed the human health risks of silicone implants and effectively communicated the nature of these risks – and the uncertainties associated with them – in a timely fashion. The story of Dow Corning's handling of the risk issues associated with silicone breast implants illustrates how easily a company can become the victim of its own mismanagement of risk and risk information.

Some prominent members of the medical-scientific community hold that the implants pose little or no risk of the type of ailments ascribed to them by public opinion and the courts. We believe that Dow Corning's management of the risk issues is in large part responsible for this discrepancy. As later discussion shows, it was the public revelation of Dow Corning's apparent failure to conduct a fully sufficient risk assessment, and the damaging evidence within its own internal files suggesting suppression and misrepresentation of the risk information in its possession, that led to the erosion of public trust in the company.

Scientific Support for Dow Corning

Dow Corning has steadfastly maintained that its silicone implant products did not pose risks of the kind that led judges and juries to award large settlements to the alleged victims. Despite claims brought by plaintiffs in these court cases that the company suppressed or falsified in the regulatory process clear scientific evidence of various systemic health risks such as cancer, autoimmune disease, and connective tissue disease, Dow Corning argues that it did not have significant scientific evidence of any of these risks. Moreover, it maintains that it had conducted sufficient research to warrant the conclusion that its products were safe. As time goes by and additional studies of the systemic effects of silicone implants are reported, Dow Corning appears to be more and more vindicated in its claims that the risks of its product have been grossly overestimated and that the trial settlements were wrongly imposed upon the company.

The scientific attack against the courts, lawyers, and plaintiffs' groups has been led by the editor of the *New England Journal of Medicine* (*NEJM*), Dr Marcia Angell. Soon after the controversy broke in 1994, the *NEJM* published the first major epidemiological study of breast implant patients. This eight-year retrospective study of 749 women who had received breast implants at the Mayo Clinic found no significant differences in the incidence of connective-tissue and other diseases among these women than among a non-implant control group twice the size.[7] In an editorial accompanying the publication of the study, Angell wrote that the study showed the decision of the FDA to remove silicone implants from the market in 1992 to be "overly paternalistic and unnecessarily alarming." She also claimed that the FDA decision, which was based on the fact that the manufacturers "had not fulfilled their legal responsibility to collect data on the question" (not because implants were known to pose a risk), was construed by the public as an indictment of the implants. Frightening stories of autoimmune and connective-tissue diseases swept through the public and were, she said, "reified by repetition ... The accumulated weight of anecdotes was taken by judges and juries as tantamount to proof of causation."[8]

Angell pursued this argument in a 1996 book *Science on Trial*,[9] in which she reported additional studies strongly corroborating the Mayo Clinic findings.[10] Angell argues that this story shows that the standard of scientific proof in the litigation of tort claims should be changed. In her view only scientific evidence based on a "factual standard" (i.e., published in peer-reviewed scientific journals) should be admitted as "expert testimony." However, the U.S. Supreme Court earlier had considered and firmly rejected this demanding "factual standard" in a 1993 case, *Daubert v. Merrell Dow Pharmaceuticals Inc.*[11] Instead, the court in *Daubert* empowered judges to make their own determinations about the scientific credibility of expert witnesses. Angell argues that such a legal standard permits the courts to base decisions upon scientifically unreliable foundations, and this, in her opinion, was clearly what happened in the breast implant cases.

Although some of the media commentary initially reinforced the allegations against Dow Corning and contributed to the public perception of the extensive risks associated with breast implants, in the wake of the evidence from the scientific studies the media interpretation also shifted dramatically. Stories with titles such as "The Great American Breast Implant Hoax,"[12] "A Confederacy of Boobs,"[13] and "Lawyers from Hell,"[14] appeared in major American magazines. Newspapers carried headlines such as "Dow Corning and the Courts: A Case of Justice or Total Travesty?"[15] "Why, to Science, the Law's an Ass," and "Can Science Free Women and Dow Corning?"[16] On 17 August 1995, the ABC show *Nightline* expressed a *mea culpa* for all the media with the comment that "it seemed we had it all wrong."[17]

As a result of the growing consensus in the scientific and journalistic community, even the widespread view among business ethicists that Dow Corning acted unethically has undergone revision.[18] The company has undertaken a vigorous public relations campaign to restore its image, which appears to be meeting with a great deal of success. The many groups who represent the alleged victims of silicone breast implants, led by the lawyers who so successfully managed the lawsuits, have responded with complaints about the way the company is spending "their" money to restore its image after a bankruptcy declaration. They have claimed that Dow Corning has in fact used millions of dollars to "buy" the scientific studies that fail to find significant systemic health risks. The company has admitted to having funded several of these studies but points out that the funding of more research is precisely what its critics have demanded; it adds that the research was carried out at respected, independent scientific-research centres.

The lawyers' and victims' groups have also pointed out that even these most recent studies have failed to rule out the possibility of significant risk for the systemic complications they believe are caused by breast implants. For example, the Mayo Clinic study involved too small a sample to rule out as much as a three-fold increase in the risk. One of the recent major studies did find a slight increase in reports of connective tissue disease among women with breast implants.[19] The most recent scientific review of all the epidemiological studies found that, while none has indicated a greatly increased rate of well-defined connective tissue disease or breast cancer in women with silicone breast implants, none has ruled out a moderately increased risk for these diseases either. This meta-analysis concluded: "Information is insufficient to adequately advise women who currently have or are seeking to obtain breast implants about the overall risk of these devices."[20] Thus, the most salient aspect of the science for these non-scientific groups is not the fact that the risks appear low but that this assessment itself is fraught with significant uncertainty.

DOW CORNING'S ASSESSMENT AND MANAGEMENT OF THE RISKS

The Alleged Systemic Health Risks

Medical devices companies began producing silicone-filled breast implants in the early 1960s. The product was hailed as a major advance on the original method of direct silicone injection into the breast, since the silicone was contained in a protective pouch designed to isolate it from body tissue, dramatically decreasing the risk of adverse effects from silicone migration. The implants were introduced to the North American market years before the u.s. government enacted the Medical Devices Amendment to the Federal Food, Drug and Cosmetic Act in 1976, giving the FDA the authority to review and approve the safety and effectiveness data of new medical devices. Because silicone breast implants had been on the market for almost fifteen years by that time, they were "grandfathered." This meant that no safety and effectiveness data on the implants were necessary unless and until the FDA requested them.

Nevertheless, Dow Corning undertook to conduct and sponsor research on the potential health effects of both the silicone itself and the breast implants. Included among these were toxicological studies of the effects of silicone and implants on laboratory animals, including whether silicone was "biologically inert." Some of these studies suggested that the silicone might not be as biologically inert as first assumed and that implants could produce inflammation and other responses that are consistent with immune response. Others suggested that silicone could enter the immune system of rats and mice and that these animals could develop sarcomas in response to injected silicone.[21] After the 1984 *Stern* lawsuit, Dow Corning had informed surgeons to whom they sold the implants of "reports of suspected immunological responses." But the company also added the following evaluation: "A review of the published experimental findings and clinical experience shows that convincing evidence does not exist to support a causal relationship between exposure to silicone materials and … rheumatic and connective tissue disorders."[22]

Clearly, Dow Corning scientists were convinced there was little, if any, risk of systemic health effects from their product. Because in their view the evidence of risk was meagre and public acceptance of the product during the first twenty years was high, and because the FDA did not (until 1988) request any safety studies from the industry, Dow Corning did not conduct extensive risk research. Nor did the company voluntarily make available the study results it did have to either the final consumers of the product or to the FDA. The company considered the initial studies it had conducted or sponsored to have failed to establish any scientifically significant evidence of systemic health effects. Even though some toxicological studies were consistent with that possibility, the observed effects were attributed to other factors.

Thus the recognized uncertainties in the toxicological studies led to a decision to discount the potential risks rather than a decision to conduct further research. This decision was supported by existing, though minimal, epidemiological evidence, which gave no indication of systemic health risks associated with the silicone implant. Dow Corning faced a situation fairly typical for health risk assessments, where the toxicology indicates some risk (usually in animal studies) – in the sense of *potential* harm to humans – that is not confirmed by the available epidemiological evidence. Dow Corning also made the typical choice in these contexts: to prefer the indicators of low (or zero) risk to the other indicators of potentially significant risk. This

choice underlay the decision not to conduct further studies and probably also the choice to withhold certain evidence from the regulators,
the consumers, and the public.

However, the failure to conduct more adequate risk research, especially given the growing allegations of systemic problems, is now seen
even by some of the strongest defenders of breast implant safety as
one of Dow Corning's major failures. For example, even Marcia Angell
admits that although the company "was right about the lack of evidence that the implants were dangerous ... there was also little evidence that they were safe, because the manufacturers had not fulfilled
their responsibility to look for it."[23] This is a damning statement,
considering its source. The decision not to conduct further research
with silicone and implants became one of the major factors in per-
suading juries and the general public that Dow Corning had subjected
women implant recipients to unacceptable risk.

The Risks of "Local Complications"

While the risks of systemic health effects from implants such as cancer
or autoimmune and connective-tissue disease seemed to be remote
during this period, other kinds of more immediate risks to women
were becoming clear to the company. Dow Corning knew in the early
1970s that the silicone could "bleed" or leak out of the envelopes in
which it was enclosed. Although most leakage was thought to be
contained in the capsule of scar tissue the body naturally formed
around the foreign implant, there was evidence that it could migrate
to surrounding tissue and to other areas of the body via the lymphatic
system.[24] Most of the evidence of silicone bleed came not from the
recipient women (who had no means of detecting it) but from their
surgeons. The sales personnel who dealt directly with the plastic
surgeons received a barrage of complaints from those surgeons that
Dow Corning's implants felt "oily" when they were removed from their
packaging.

This problem intensified in 1975 when, in response to pressure
from other manufacturers whose product was considered to have a
more "natural" shape and feel, Dow Corning developed an implant
with a thinner envelope filled with silicone of thinner consistency,
rushing the implants to market before adequate studies of their reliability could be carried out. Surgeons complained that the new
implants were bleeding and even rupturing during implantation, and
whole shipments were returned to the company.[25] Dow Corning did
not remove the implants from the market, nor did it warn recipients
of the risk. It did issue to the surgeons who implanted them warnings

about certain risks. These included warnings about fibrous capsule formations and the possibility of implant rupture during implantation, as well as recommendations of certain implantation techniques to prevent such rupture.[26]

Evidence of additional health risks with the implants emerged. Not only did the implants tend to rupture and spill during implantation, they were doing so after implantation as well. The result was that the breast would lose its shape and the contents would escape into the surrounding tissue, which could and did produce high levels of trauma for the recipient, requiring surgical removal and sometimes re-implantation. The rate of rupture has been a matter of wide disagreement between the industry and its critics. For most of this period Dow Corning claimed it was in the vicinity of 1 to 2 per cent; early scientific estimates were over 5 per cent. Implant victims' groups have claimed it to be higher than 50 per cent and have predicted that when enough time passes it will likely prove to be 100 per cent.

In testimony before a congressional subcommittee in August 1995, FDA Commissioner Kessler stated: "Published studies to date suggest a rupture rate between 5 and 51 percent – an enormous range – and unfortunately, we do not know with any confidence where within that range the real rupture rate lies." He also cited two studies indicating that the risk of rupture increases as the implants age. A published 1996 study by the FDA also reports that the rupture rate is still unknown but clearly increases with age. The National Breast Implant Task Force claims that in a meeting in September 1995 FDA officials informed them that its MedWatch reporting system indicated a 50 per cent rupture rate. These high estimates appear to be based upon studies done among women who report complications with their implants, and they may not accurately reflect the rupture rate among all implanted women. One of the problems in determining the exact rate was due to the fact that if the surrounding scar tissue capsule did not break, most of the silicone would be retained, and the rupture would not be noticed or reported. One study of women with implants who had mammograms showed that 5 per cent had unnoticed ruptures.[27]

Recent scientific studies lend support to the higher figures in the ranges. One study of three hundred women treated for implant problems at the University of Alabama found that 214 (71.3 per cent) of them had disruption (actual rupture or severe silicone bleed or both) of one or both implants.[28] Despite evidence of significant rupture rates, Dow Corning nevertheless continued to advise women in its product promotional literature during the 1970s and '80s that they could expect the implants to last a "natural lifetime."[29]

Further, Dow Corning learned early on that a normal body reaction to the insertion of the implant, as with any foreign object, was the formation of a fibrous capsule (a kind of scar tissue) around it, called "capsular contracture." This produced a hardening of the breast which led to other complications, such as chronic soreness and reduced sensitivity of the nipples. The therapy of choice among surgeons for post-operative amelioration of this problem was "closed capsulotomy" procedure. This involved a forceful squeezing of the breast by hand in order to break up the scar tissue and soften the breast – until the capsule formed again, which it usually did. Often the procedure was only partially successful, leaving the breast malformed. But more importantly, the procedure regularly produced an even worse result – the rupture of the implant itself, spilling its silicone contents into the surrounding tissue. By 1980 the company included in the package a warning to surgeons about this risk.[30] However, no similar warning was given to the women who received the implants.

Between 1985 and 1995 the FDA received over 91,000 adverse reaction reports associated with silicone breast implants.[31] These reports included cases of leaking and rupturing as well as of the painful hardening, deformation, and desensitization of the breasts, which are now widely recognized and uncontested on all sides, including scientists and the industry. But they included as well claims of adverse effects still not proven to be linked to them. However, it was not the risks of these "local complications" but rather those of the systemic diseases of the immune system and connective tissue that courts used to justify the huge damages awarded to the plaintiffs who sued Dow Corning.

DOW CORNING'S RISK COMMUNICATION

Dow Corning argues that the storm of criticism the company received for not informing patients or the public about the known complications of breast implants is without merit. It has steadfastly maintained that it honestly and forthrightly communicated to the appropriate stakeholders the risks of its implants as it became aware of them. The appropriate stakeholders, according to Dow Corning managers, were primarily the surgeons who were the direct customers of the company's product, and not the women who were the recipients of the implants and the bearers of the risks. The company argued that, like most medical device manufacturers, it relied on patient information being conveyed through physicians, and "physicians strongly maintained that direct communication by the company to patients was

inappropriate and potentially interfered with the doctor/patient relationship."[32] Further, as the company's health-care business manager
put it to a reporter who questioned the company's view of disclosure,
"We don't know who the patients are."[33]

If patients agreed to be fitted with silicone breast implants without
being fully informed of the known complications, it was the fault of
the physicians who recommended the devices and who profited from
the implantation. After all, it is the physicians who know each individual patient, and whose role it is to discuss benefits and risks of alternative therapeutic and cosmetic interventions. If Dow Corning
informed these physicians of the risks as they became known, had it
not fully discharged its responsibilities to its stakeholders?

In summary, Dow Corning argues that it managed the health risks
of its silicone implant products in a scientifically and ethically responsible way. It conducted preliminary studies of the potential systemic
health effects (cancer, autoimmune, and connective-tissue diseases),
which provided an adequate assurance that there were no significant
risks for these effects, and this assessment has been corroborated by
subsequent risk research. With respect to the "local complications"
risks, the company argues that, as it became increasingly aware of
these, it communicated them through the most appropriate channels,
namely, the surgeons who implanted the products in their patients,
knowing their individual health histories and the medical indications
for the implants. If the company "failed" to communicate the systemic
risks, it is because there were no significant risks to communicate. The
other known risks of local complications it did not conceal or misrep-
resent. If these risks were unacceptably imposed upon naive patients,
it was not a risk communication failure of Dow Corning's but of the
health professionals whose responsibility it was to communicate the
risks.

The Damning Internal Dow Corning Memos

Most of the awards of the courts following the 1991 *Hopkins* case were
not for the acknowledged local complications of silicone breast
implants – deformations of the breasts, development of painful capsular contractures, silicone bleeding, and implant ruptures. Instead,
most of the women received awards for a wide variety of ill-defined
systemic diseases which the scientific studies have failed to connect
with their implants. What led the judges and juries to find in favour
of these plaintiffs was not primarily the scientific evidence, which was
limited to the claims of a few scientists and the hypotheses of the
physicians (usually not the plastic surgeons) who testified on behalf

of their sick patients. Rather, it was the allegations the lawyers made that Dow Corning had irresponsibly withheld from the public and the government regulatory agencies the information it possessed about the known risks of silicone implants.

The allegations having the greatest impact upon judges and juries very likely were those stemming from internal memos discovered by Maria Stern's attorneys in the first big settlement against the company in 1984. These were discovered by Dan Bolton, a young law clerk (later the attorney in the *Hopkins* case), while digging around in boxes at Dow Corning's Michigan headquarters. These memos have become the focus of the storm of criticism directed at Dow Corning and are the basis for the allegations that the company suppressed, misrepresented, and even falsified scientific data on the risks of silicone implants.

There is some justification for company officials' claims that the memos were seriously blown out of proportion and that they do not support the serious allegations of misrepresentation and fraud claimed by their opponents in the courtrooms. Yet there is also no doubt that they call into question the company's claims that it acted responsibly in the assessment and communication of silicone implant risks. The internal documents gave the impression of a disregard for health risks, or at least appeared to put company interests ahead of genuine concern for its customers.

Among the documents Bolton discovered were memos from physicians to the company complaining about defective and ruptured implants, and detailing the effects of leaked silicone on the bodies of the women. Some claimed there was evidence that the silicone was not biologically inert and was causing severe foreign body reactions in some individuals. Letters from surgeons complained about the poor quality of the implants. In response to the complaint that the implants felt "oily" with silicone when they were removed from their packages, salesmen were urged by their managers to wash and dry the samples in washroom sinks immediately before using them in sales demonstrations, and to change the demonstration samples often, so that the silicone would not be evident.[34]

In one memo that received much attention from plaintiffs' attorneys, a salesman who had heard many of the complaints wrote to his Dow Corning boss: "To put a questionable lot of mammaries on the market is inexcusable. I don't know who is responsible for this decision but it has to rank right up there with the Pinto gas tank."[35] Another memo strongly suggested that a Dow Corning marketing executive made deliberately misleading assurances to complainants that the company was undertaking studies of the silicone migration and the contracture problems, in response to complaints about the product. He wrote: "I assured them, with crossed fingers, that Dow Corning too had an active 'contracture/gel migration' study underway. This apparently satisfied them for the moment, but one of these days they will be asking us for the results of our studies ... In my opinion, the black clouds are ominous and should be given more attention."[36] The warnings for the most part went unheeded by company management. Rather than undertake a serious research project on the risks of the product, the company chose to take the route of maintaining a strong public relations and marketing approach to the problem, based on assurances to the public there were no problems the company was not solving.

Most damning of the internal Dow Corning documents revealed at the *Stern* trial, however, was a report on a study co-authored by Silas Braley, the chemist who was in many ways the father of the silicone implant at Dow Corning. The study, which had been published in a medical journal in 1973,[37] involved four dogs with small implants observed over two years. The study largely reported the results at the end of the six-month mark (even though it was published after the end of the two-year period), finding only minor inflammation in some of the dogs. The internal report which had been kept within the company, however, revealed that at the end of the two-year period one of the dogs had died, and the other three had varying degrees of severe chronic inflammation. Two dogs suffered thyroiditis – evidence of autoimmune response – and spots on the spleen.[38]

During the *Stern* trial an expert witness named Marc Lappe, called by the plaintiff to comment on the study, pointed out the discrepancies between the published study and the internal reports. Dow Corning lawyers tried unsuccessfully to have Lappe's testimony excluded. The judge then asked to see the documents both Lappe and the Dow Corning lawyers brought into court, and noticed that the identifying numbers on the dogs had been altered on the documents Dow Corning had given the attorneys. It looked suspiciously as if the company had altered the data to make it more difficult to get at the full two-year results of the study.[39]

The revelation of these internal documents, especially the allegedly misreported dog study, was the key reason why the *Stern* jury found Dow Corning guilty of fraud and awarded Maria Stern $1.7 million. Subsequent developments in the case led to the continued suppression of this information. Dow Corning appealed the jury's decision, and during the appeal reached a settlement with Maria Stern for an undisclosed amount of money and an agreement that all the internal Dow Corning documents disclosed at the trial would remain confidential. This secrecy agreement won by the company may have been one of the most important contributions to its later troubles with the courts, for it made much more plausible the later charges that the company had withheld important risk information from the FDA as well as from its consumers and the public.

DOW CORNING AND THE FDA

Two years before the 1984 *Stern* decision the U.S. Food and Drug Administration had proposed to place silicone breast implants into a Class III medical devices category, which would require manufacturers to prove their safety in order to keep them on the market. It was not until 1988, however, that the FDA finally carried out the reclassification and asked the manufacturers to submit Pre-Market Approval (PMA) applications, which require the submission of scientific data showing their devices to be safe and efficacious. The PMAs were due by July 1991 and in that month Dow Corning submitted 329 studies. By September the FDA had responded to the manufacturer that the studies were inadequate to show that silicone implants were safe (or harmful), and therefore requested more data.

In the previous December the breast implant controversy had exploded into a full-scale public issue when CBS Television broadcast the program *Face to Face with Connie Chung*. For the first time on national television a medical specialist associated with the trial proceedings claimed that leaked silicone from breast implants "gets right into the heart of the immune system" and could be the cause of autoimmune-system diseases like lupus. This program produced an avalanche of public allegations about problems with the implants from women and their doctors. The following June, *Business Week* published an article entitled "Breast Implants: What Did the Industry Know, and When?"[40] The article charged that for at least a decade Dow Corning had been aware of animal studies linking implants to cancer and other illnesses, and accused top FDA officials of ignoring for more than ten years what their own scientists were telling them about concerns with breast implants.

In December 1991 the *Hopkins* court awarded Mariann Hopkins $7.3 million against Dow Corning. FDA head David Kessler was under intense pressure to do something in response to public concern. In the month following the *Hopkins* decision, Kessler received the information he needed to act. Hopkins's lawyer had won the case with the help of the internal memos and studies from the *Stern* lawsuit, in addition to new studies he subsequently obtained from Dow Corning. By January copies of these still-confidential documents turned up at Kessler's home in a package placed on his doorstep.

Kessler was apparently shocked by the contents. The package contained the older memos and studies suggesting risks which company personnel wanted to suppress and which, of course, had not been submitted with Dow Corning's PMAs. The newer documents were also disturbing, for among them were reports of internal Dow Corning studies suggesting that silicone was not inert and could affect immune systems. The package included dog studies which showed that dogs injected with silicone developed inflammation of the thyroid. Other studies in Kessler's package suggested that silicone could move into the immune systems of laboratory rats and mice. Included also were the letters written by doctors complaining about the reactions they were seeing to the implants.[41]

Three days after receiving the documents Kessler asked the manufacturers to place a voluntary moratorium on the sale of the silicone implants pending further study of their safety, and he recalled the FDA advisory panel to consider the new evidence. The advisory panel concluded that this evidence did not show that silicone implants were unsafe, and recommended that the moratorium be lifted to allow breast implants to be used for reconstructive surgery only, and then only under scientifically controlled conditions, so that their effects could be carefully studied. Kessler agreed, and in April 1992 he lifted the complete moratorium, allowing the sale of implants only under these conditions. The Health Protection Branch (HPB) of Health Canada followed the FDA action with a similar moratorium on sales in Canada.

HOW SHOULD IMPLANT RISK BE EVALUATED?

Certainly the FDA/HPB moratoriums contributed significantly to the perception that the implants were unsafe. The barrage of court settlements which followed appeared to confirm that Dow Corning had suppressed, and even falsified, clear scientific evidence that its product put its customers at risk of systemic diseases as well as known localized complications. In addition to marketing a product widely thought to be the cause of a host of diseases suffered by thousands of women, Dow Corning now was considered to have engaged in a conspiracy to conceal all this from the public and its regulatory agencies.

Dow Corning maintains that it has been the victim of a malicious smear campaign by greedy and unscrupulous lawyers who are making millions from court settlements. Even the revelation of the "damning internal memos" does not establish, Dow Corning claims, either that the company knew its implants were risky or that it unethically suppressed or falsified the scientific information it had. The so-called scientific studies reported in these documents were too incomplete and uncertain to establish any clear risk of systemic disease, so there was nothing scientifically reliable to report, either to the regulators or to the public. Even the decision to withhold the additional information in the infamous dog study, so influential in the *Stern* and *Hopkins* cases, had been distorted, according to Dow Corning. The company defends its decision on the grounds that its scientists had good reasons for believing that the death of the one dog, as well as the other observed but unreported effects, was unrelated to the silicone implants. But it admits that the original published versions of the paper "failed to include sufficient information on interim study results" and that "this was inappropriate."[42]

The more recent scientific studies cited earlier have largely supported Dow Corning's claim that there was little scientific reason, even in its own early studies, to suspect that silicone implants could cause systemic diseases. They argue that if there was little substantive data to report, it is also unfair to charge the company with suppression or falsification of relevant data. At worst the "damning internal memos" show that there may have been a few people in the company who *thought* there was a problem and who thus may also have *thought* there was a cover-up.

This is a very difficult case to evaluate, in part because the legal setting polarizes evidence as favouring one side versus another and all the nuances are ruled out. Moreover, now that the case is being fought out by Dow Corning and its adversaries in the court of public opinion as well as before the bar, every key piece of documentary material, in a record that goes back about thirty years, has been the subject of hotly contested interpretations. Nevertheless, we shall try to identify an evaluative position, unattached to the judgments of guilt or innocence made in the courts, that respects the nuances in the evidence we have looked at here.

In our review we have tried to be scrupulously fair, because all of the contending parties feel aggrieved and because the stakes in the ultimate outcome (still uncertain at the time of writing) are so high. So we will start with this statement that from the standpoint of our interest in good risk communication practice, the silicone breast implant episode appears to be a story about two major failings by a company. First was the failure to disclose to its customers *everything* of material relevance that it knew about the risks associated with its product, even though this did not violate any established code of practice at that time – it was not then the practice of manufacturers of drugs or devices to supply information to the patient or ultimate user. Second was the failure to pursue thoroughly the full range of scientific studies that would have shed more light on those risks. In our opinion these failures turned out to be crucial. They allowed others to draw certain conclusions about the more serious types of health risks on the basis of what had become known about Dow Corning's handling of information about the less serious types.

As we see it, this is the critical point in understanding the formation of opinion about the perceived safety of silicone breast implants in relation to Dow Corning's management and communication of the risks associated with those devices. Partly at issue here are two competing approaches to the question of silicone breast implant safety. Using one approach, three apparently reasonable conclusions could be reached:

1 There is a significantly high risk of localized complications from silicone breast implants (such as silicone bleed and migration, rupture, capsular contraction, desensitization). As more research is done, the estimates of these risks have increased.
2 These risks may be regarded as acceptable if they are clearly outweighed by the benefits women receive from the implants or if those women have given their informed consent to the risks. Perhaps Dow Corning should have supplied consumers with information about these risks directly rather than relying on the surgeons to provide it. But this is a question of the acceptability of the "local complications" health risks, and has no relevance to the quite different issue of the magnitude and acceptability of other alleged systemic risks.
3 There is a very low risk of systemic disease (autoimmune and connective tissue disease), although the remaining uncertainties in the studies are consistent with the possibility of some small increase in these risks associated with silicone breast implants.

Using a second approach, one that may be more appropriate for the actual bearers of the risks, essentially the same information leads to a quite different end-point:

1 There is a significantly high risk of localized complications from implants. The increasing evidence about these risk factors only serves to underline the importance of the early indications Dow Corning had about them.
2 These risks could be regarded as acceptable only if there had been full, informed consent on the part of the risk bearers. There was no such consent because the company did not perform the studies needed to confirm the indications it had of these problems and did not inform consumers of the risk information it had. Further, it

appears that the company had deliberately misled both the public and government regulators about these risks. There is even evidence that the company tried to withhold risk information (e.g., the "oily implants" memo) from surgeons. Furthermore, whether or not the company adequately informed surgeons about the risks, that it did not also communicate risks to patients themselves is problematic. Taken together, all these factors could lead to the conclusion that Dow Corning's handling of directly relevant information in its possession was unethical and injurious to the risk bearers.

3 Evidence revealed at trial and in the "Kessler package" created a *prima facie* case that Dow Corning had ignored and suppressed the known risks of local complications from breast implants. This raises a reasonable suspicion that it may also have ignored or suppressed information about systemic risks. The FDA's 1991 decision that Dow Corning's studies on implant safety were inadequate could be seen as reinforcing the suspicion, already formed, that Dow Corning had not carried out reliable studies showing the absence of significant risks of systemic disease. This creates the appearance of a company that does not have sufficient regard for protecting the health of its customers. Therefore, because these risks are being managed by an untrustworthy agent, they are unacceptable, even if they are now thought to be very low.

In contrast to the first approach, the second sees conclusion 3 as directly dependent upon (indeed, following from) conclusions 1 and 2. The risk of systemic diseases posed by silicone implants is unacceptable, not because its magnitude is above a certain threshold but because the producer of the risk is perceived to be untrustworthy. The producer of the risk is perceived as untrustworthy in this case in large measure because it failed to communicate openly and forthrightly to the public the known risks of local complications in the silicone implants. This failure to communicate the known risks induced, quite understandably, a perception that the company was not assessing, managing, or communicating responsibly all of the risks associated with its product, including the risks of systemic disease.

IS IT REASONABLE TO THINK THAT DOW CORNING SHOULD HAVE ACTED DIFFERENTLY?

Dow Corning's decision to hold "close to the chest" the risk information it possessed, or readily could have obtained, created a kind of information vacuum that was gradually filled with a perception of breast implants as an unacceptable risk imposed upon women without their consent. The ultimate consequences of the implant controversy include the possibility of a massive class-action settlement against the company and the loss of most of the sizable North American market for its product.[43]

But are these two happenings necessarily related? Is it reasonable to suppose that a different track record in risk communication by Dow Corning would have affected the outcome of the legal wrangles? To answer this question in the affirmative, we would have to accept the plausibility of the following contention: If the company had informed breast implant patients directly of the known risks of silicone bleed, capsular contracture, malformation, rupture, and so on, and if it had been candid in the reporting of the studies it had undertaken, including the nature of the uncertainties in them, there would have been little basis for the courts' findings of fraudulent or unethical behaviour on the company's part, which were major factors in the award of damages. This is largely because the allegations of systemic health impacts themselves stem at least in part from the fears created by the revelations of the company's suppression of the other risk information it had.

In order to see whether it is reasonable to think that a different risk communication practice might have changed both the course and the ultimate outcomes of this bitter controversy, let us summarize the key points, drawn from the documentary record reviewed in this chapter, on which there is some measure of agreement across the spectrum of positions:

- According to Marcia Angell, a strong critic of the plaintiffs' case, the breast implant manufacturers did not fulfil their responsibility to look hard for evidence of insufficient safety.
- In the very wide range of estimates for rupture rates, for a long time Dow Corning argued for numbers in the extreme low end of the range.
- Dow Corning, consistent with established practice, insisted that communicating about risks with surgeons rather than patients was the correct procedure, but of course the surgeons were deriving revenues from the implantation procedures and were therefore interested parties.
- By any fair and unbiased reading, the internal company memos show what is at best an indifferent attitude toward the developing risk information.
- Dow Corning conceded that the way in which the dog study results were published was "inappropriate."

- Finally, and most critically, there is the act of sealing the files in the settlement of the *Stern* case. At this point (1984) and thereafter, Dow Corning was aware that some of its actions to that point reasonably could be interpreted in a court of law as evidence of bad faith or worse.

We have made an effort to exclude from this list all those matters of fact and interpretations in the record that, in the opinion of Dow Corning officials, do not support either the legal or the ethical finding of fault against the company. To strengthen our case we are even willing, for the sake of argument, to accept Dow Corning's own interpretation of *all* of the contested points in the documentary record as presented in this chapter. And so our list includes only those points which, we surmise, would be found to represent a fair and unbiased reading of the documentary record in the eyes of at least most disinterested parties.

We are well aware that Dow Corning officials believe their company has been the victim of both unscrupulous behaviour by lawyers and some advocacy groups as well as of lack of professionalism by a scientifically naive media. We do not think that this is the whole truth, however. We think that there is also a serious lack of good risk communication practice evident in that list. To be sure, we have the benefit of hindsight in arriving at this judgment: we are not in a position to say whether or not Dow Corning's actions were or were not appropriate to the standards of the time in which they occurred. Our primary interest is in suggesting guidelines for better practices in the future.

The concluding chapter suggests those guidelines in the form of lessons drawn from the full set of case studies in this volume. So far as the implant controversy itself is concerned, the principal conclusions are as follows. First, Dow Corning had early warning (in the *Stern* case) that an interpretation of its risk management and communication actions prejudicial to its interests could be made, and a prudent risk management stance should have impelled the company to be much more forthright about communicating the risks of these products thereafter. Second, its internal memos show at best a cavalier attitude towards the accumulating record of complaints against the product made both by women with implants and by some health professionals.[44] Third, because the appearance of its product on the market predated the newer FDA testing and disclosure rules, Dow Corning did not aggressively pursue of its own accord the full range of scientific studies necessary to characterize the relevant hazards and estimate carefully the risks – and therefore was not in a position to communicate an accurate account of the risks to the end users.

Fourth, for the local complications risks, where the company had good information (rupturing and associated effects), it chose to accept as best estimates the numbers at the very lowest end of the range, which cannot be regarded as the exercise of prudent judgment. Fifth, the company decided not to regard those end users as the legitimate recipients of risk information, despite the fact that both the product itself and the requisite medical procedure might reasonably have been regarded as being particularly sensitive domains in health care. For these and other reasons the company put itself in a situation where others could draw inferences about its behaviour that were prejudicial to its business interests.

Let us even concede that at least some reasonable persons might concur that, while these five items indeed are mistakes in risk communication practice, they are relatively small mistakes. Fine. In this case the lesson to be drawn from them is even clearer: where incipient risk controversies are concerned, if small mistakes are not counteracted promptly, the process of risk amplification, fed by both the scientific uncertainties and the mistrust of institutions that are endemic in those controversies, can turn small mistakes into big problems indeed.

THE *HOLLIS* CASE

Hollis v. Dow Corning Corp. involved damages sought for the rupturing of an implant *in situ* and the question as to whether the woman receiving an implant had been adequately warned of such risks through her doctors or surgeons. In a decision handed down by the Supreme Court of Canada in December 1995, the majority held that the duty to warn had been breached by Dow Corning, because the company had not communicated its awareness about rupturings in a timely fashion to medical practitioners, and it upheld the award of damages made by a lower court. The court held that the "duty to warn" is especially severe for products that are to be ingested or placed into the body, and the *Hollis* decision confirmed that the duty can arise even where the risk is statistically small, provided that the potential harm is serious. Nevertheless, it is important to realize, in terms of the foregoing discussion, that the case dealt only with the "local complications" risks; there was no mention at all of systemic risks in this litigation.

In *Hollis* the Canadian Supreme Court adopted for the first time the so-called "learned intermediary" rule fashioned by u.s. courts. This rule holds that, where products are of a highly technical nature and are not sold directly to the non-expert public (such as breast implants, which are sold to surgeons), the company's duty to warn the public is discharged if it discloses all information in its possession about relevant risks to the intermediary. (This includes what the company reasonably ought to have known, as well as what it did in fact know.) In a public commentary on that decision, one of the members of the Supreme Court, Mr Justice J.C. Major, explained the court's reasoning as follows:[45]

The *Hollis* case imported the "learned intermediary" rule into Canadian law. This rule relieves the manufacturer of the obligation to warn the consumer directly if the product is technical and an expert will be advising the consumer … The learned intermediary rule is seen as a sensible development in that it saves the manufacturer from having to attempt to translate complex and technical matters into information that could be understood by a lay person. This applies in situations where direct communication would be difficult, expensive, and ineffective and where there is present a learned intermediary.

Thus the legal resolution of the breast-implant lawsuits to date in Canada would not support any conclusion from the preceding analysis suggesting that more risk information should have been provided directly to the product end-users.

Considering these comments from the standpoint of good risk communication practice, we cannot concur with Mr Justice Major in praising the learned intermediary rule for saving "the manufacturer from having to attempt to translate complex and technical matters into information that could be understood by a lay person." We cannot imagine any situation in which it would be prudent for a firm not to disclose information pertinent to health risks directly to those affected, no matter what other supplementary communications (e.g., to health professionals) also are undertaken. The logical fault in the learned intermediary rule, at least insofar as risk matters are concerned, is that it sets up the intermediary (the surgeon and attending physician) as a "neutral" media channel for the simple conveyance of risk information from one party (the manufacturer) to another (the patient). This rule does not even recognize the "encoding" and "decoding" processes for information transfer that is a staple of communications theory.[46] It appears to assume that the reinterpretations (especially the choice of qualitative terminology) which the intermediary might impose on the manufacturer's written information, in the process of chanelling it *orally* from its original source to a patient, will have no impact on the patient's perception of the associated risks or her ultimate decision. As chapter 2 indicates, we now know enough about the different languages of risk to regard this as a most unwise assumption.

In our opinion, if firms were to rely on *Hollis* as the primary guide to their public risk communication responsibilities, they might thereby incur a significant business risk. This is because firms cannot rely on the public to accept the logic of the learned intermediary rule in risk communication matters, even if the Supreme Court justices do so. We think that the public will find it unacceptable not to have direct risk communication from those who have intimate knowledge of the risks (in the foregoing case study, the implant manufacturers). This expectation includes, specifically, evidence of a reasonable attempt to translate technical information into understandable terms for a lay person. Failure to do so, we believe, will erode trust in those parties; and public perception of the trustworthiness of corporate actors, especially where health risks are concerned, is a potent factor in citizen behaviour. Even if legal liability for damages were to be avoided by reliance on the learned intermediary rule, citizens and consumers have other ways to punish corporate actors they hold to be responsible for unethical or irresponsible conduct. The prudent course of action for those whose activities generate risks is, first, to search diligently and continuously for all pertinent risk information, and second, to make full, fair, timely, and clear disclosures of it.

POSTSCRIPT

At the time of writing, the class-action litigation still has not been settled. Dow Corning filed for protection under Chapter 11 of the U.S. Bankruptcy Code in May 1995, proposing a $3 billion reorganization plan to the court. Creditors have filed an alternative plan before the court in the bankruptcy proceedings. Three other manufacturers, Bristol-Myers Squibb, Minnesota Mining and Manufacturing, and Baxter International, have proposed a $2 to $3 billion class-action settlement in an Alabama federal court. The federal judge in Alabama has appointed a scientific panel to advise him about the merits of the evidence, and a final decision is not expected for a year. In December 1996 another federal judge in Oregon on the basis of the information of an independent scientific panel dismissed seventy claims, ruling that plaintiffs cannot introduce evidence of implant-caused disease because such evidence is not scientifically sound. Since then there have been further cases with similar decisions.

Finally, in December 1996 Dow Corning introduced a dramatic new element into this long-running controversy, proposing to the bankruptcy judge that a "megatrial" be held – restricted to the sole issue of resolving the scientific issues associated with implants. In this proceeding no plaintiffs would be present; rather, a jury would hear testimony from a court-appointed panel of medical experts and scientists and be asked to rule on the question of whether the implants cause immune-type diseases.[47]

PART TWO

Waiting for
the Regulators

6 Lost in Regulatory Space: rBST

At 10 A.M. on 23 January 1996, the Chicago-based Cancer Prevention Coalition and the Vermont-based environmental group Food and Water held a news conference at the National Press Club in Washington, D.C., to release a study that concluded that "milk from cows injected with rBGH increases risks of breast and colon cancers in humans."[1]

The study, authored by Dr Samuel Epstein, a professor of environmental medicine at the University of Illinois School of Public Health and chairman of the Cancer Prevention Coalition, was a review of research relating to the carcinogenic potential of insulin-like growth factor-1 (IGF-1) in humans and the possibility that recombinant bovine somatotropin (rBST, sometimes referred to as rBGH, or recombinant bovine growth hormone) increases IGF-1 in milk. It was published in the January 1996 issue of the *International Journal of Health Services*, which, according to its inside cover, specializes in "health and social policy, political economy and sociology, history and philosophy, and ethics and law." Epstein also serves on the journal's editorial board. Said Epstein in a prepared statement, "rBGH poses an even greater risk to human health than ever considered. The entire nation is currently being subjected to a large-scale adulteration of an age-old dietary staple by a poorly characterized and unlabeled biotechnology product which is very different than natural milk."[2]

Besides the study, Canadian journalists received an additional press release one day before the scheduled press conference, from the Council of Canadians (COC), a nationalistic organization which has called for a moratorium on the use of rBST in Canada. The COC release cited the new review and called on then Health Minister Diane Marleau to ensure there was an independent investigation of the impact of rBST on human health. The story was widely reported in the Canadian and American media. However, the basic facts of this new review and the allegations of health risk from rBST had been made at least five years earlier, also by Dr Epstein. So how is it that an old story was recycled as news? With the imprimatur of science, trash can often be recycled; and in the absence of a timely and credible refutation, garbage accumulates, adding to consumer mistrust.

As one of the first products of molecular genetic engineering, recombinant bovine somatotropin and the prospect of its commercial use has generated unprecedented scientific analysis and public discourse in North America. An important theme in the history of resistance to technology is the question of public control over technological decisions, challenging the authority of experts and questioning the motives of public officials,[3] all of which characterize the rBST discussion in North America. In examining the public evolution of risk controversies, such as the use of rBST, Leiss and Chociolko offer the following methodological guidelines:

- have any risk communications occurred?
- are risk assessment assumptions made explicit?
- is the nature of public concern understood?
- did any agency take responsibility and forge consensus?

In examining rBST in Canada, the answer to the latter three questions is no. And what constituted risk communication messages by the various social actors were confusing, inadequate, and failed to recognize the broader social context in which the rBST debate in Canada took place.

THE SCIENCE OF rBST

Over the past two decades more than 1,800 research papers have been published on the subject of BST. Many researchers have stated that BST has been responsible for more dairy science literature than any other topic. Dozens of American medical and scientific groups have publicly concluded that food products from rBST-treated animals are safe for human consumption. Regulatory agencies in at least thirty-one countries, including Canada, have also concluded that food products from rBST-treated animals are safe for human consumption.[4]

Research on bovine somatotropin – and on somatotropins in general – dates back to the 1930s, when scientists first attempted to increase the milk output of cows. Researchers injected fluid from the pituitary gland of dead cows into lactating cows and discovered that the pituitary ingredient responsible for increasing milk yield was somatotropin. In the 1950s scientists attempted to help somatotropin-deficient (dwarf) children grow to normal size by injecting them with BST; they concluded that BST was completely ineffective in humans. In 1959 researchers discovered that injecting monkeys with somatotropin extracted from other monkeys produced effects that BST did not produce, revealing that although all somatotropins perform the same functions, the somatotropins from different animal species are different. It was also discovered that injecting somatotropin-deficient children with somatotropin extracted from human pituitary glands helps these children grow.

In 1979, the gene encoding bovine somatotropin was isolated and cloned in bacteria. This made large amounts of the hormone available for study. The first trial involving the supplementation of cows with rBST was conducted at Cornell University by Dale Bauman in 1982. In 1984 studies of rats fed large amounts of rBST showed that the hormone was not active when consumed.[5] Through the mid-1980s, studies showed that rBST does not compete with human somatotropin (HST) in humans. In 1986 the Bureau of Veterinary Drugs (BVD) in the Health Protection Branch of Health Canada concluded that milk and meat from rBST supplemented cows was safe for human consumption, one year after a similar conclusion was reached by the U.S. Food and Drug Administration.[6]

In the late 1980s studies focused on animal health and milk quality, with researchers concluding that supplemental rBST does not increase the amount of BST in milk, that cows respond to natural BST and synthetic rBST in the same way, and that rBST supplementation does not alter milk composition.[7] University scientists demonstrated that the breed of the cow, stage of lactation, age of the cow, diet consumed, and season of the year have a larger effect on milk composition than does supplementing the cow with rBST.[8]

In 1988 German scientists tested rBST-supplemented cows for insulin-like growth factor-1 (IGF-1) concentrations and found that milk from rBST-supplemented cows had 25 per cent more IGF-1 than milk from untreated cows. The next year additional studies concluded that IGF-1 was not orally active.

In 1990 two of the FDA's scientists explained the methodology used to conclude that milk from rBST-supplemented cows was as safe as –

and not different from – milk from unsupplemented cows, in a paper published in *Science*.[9] Such a move was unprecedented in that FDA decisions were previously confidential. The scientists reviewed more than 120 papers on rBST, including scores of tests the FDA ordered, designed, monitored and analysed.

That same year, various U.S. health authorities began to support the use of rBST. A *Journal of the American Medical Association* article urged members to reassure the public about rBST milk safety. After reviewing the extensive body of research documenting supplemental rBST's safety, the review states: "Based on the scientific evidence, comments from health professionals can play an important role in reassuring the public about the safety of milk and refuting misstatements or misconceptions about rBST."[10] An editorial in the same issue urged people not to play on unfounded rBST health fears. Confirming that milk from rBST-supplemented cows had been shown to be safe, the editorial pointed out that there is "an especially vocal group who are against any form of genetic engineering regardless of ... the potential ... benefits." The editorial continued: "Because milk produced from cows treated with Bovine Somatotropin [sic] is no different than milk from the untreated cow, it is both inappropriate and wrong for special interest groups to play on the health and safety fears of the public to further their own ends."[11] A three-day scientific conference on milk safety hosted by the U.S. National Institutes of Health concluded: "The composition and nutritional value of milk from BST-treated cows is ... the same as milk from untreated cows ... Meat and milk from BST-treated cows are as safe as from untreated cows."[12]

In November 1993 the FDA issued a registration of rBST to the St Louis-based Monsanto Corporation. After a ninety-day moratorium negotiated as part of the Omnibus Budget Reconciliation Act of 1993 to allow Congress time to consider the impact of BST in the United States, rBST went on sale on 2 February 1994. In Canada the BVD had yet to issue a notice of compliance. The BVD grants approval for commercial use of a product only when the bureau is completely satisfied that the product meets key criteria: all food from the animal supplemented with the product is safe for human consumption; the product does not harm the animal; the product is efficacious; and the product satisfies manufacturing requirements.

Despite the lack of a notice of compliance, the Canadian federal Standing Committee on Agriculture held hearings on the impact of rBST in the spring of 1994. In August 1994 a one-year voluntary moratorium on the use of rBST was announced by the minister of Agriculture. The moratorium stated that if rBST received a notice of compliance from Health Canada, the two manufacturers of rBST in

Canada, Monsanto Canada and Eli/Lilly, would refrain from selling the product until 1 July 1995. In the meantime a committee was established to research social and scientific issues surrounding rBST and was ordered to report directly to the minister of Agriculture on 1 May 1995.

SURVEYS

Smith and Warland summarized eleven surveys conducted between 1986 and 1990 and, despite variations in number of topics, role of respondents as shopper, method of survey, primary focus, and the nature of rBST information provided to respondents, the answers were quite consistent.[13] Respondents had general concerns about rBST in the milk supply, supported labelling of milk from cows supplemented with rBST, and predicted that future milk consumption would likely decline after the introduction of rBST into the marketplace.

Most American surveys conducted in the years prior to FDA approval predicted a 10 to 20 per cent drop in milk consumption if rBST was approved. For example, a 1990 study for the u.s. National Dairy Board estimated that 20 per cent of 592 survey participants would reduce or completely eliminate milk and dairy product purchases after hearing anti-rBST messages.[14] But according to dairy consumption statistics collected by the u.s. Department of Agriculture, dairy consumption has either held even or increased (with caveats for certain geographical areas such as Wisconsin and Vermont, as was reflected in the Agriculture and Agri-Food Canada task force report on rBST, 1995) since rBST went on sale in February 1994. Surveys are often poor predictors of consumer behaviour, perhaps because it is easier to say one thing during a telephone interview and another to actually alter purchasing patterns.

Nevertheless, a survey conducted after the approval of rBST in the United States – which did accurately predict American consumer response – reported that of those respondents who said their milk consumption had decreased in the previous two months (9 per cent), only 6 per cent of that group mentioned anything to do with rBST, hormones, or drugs given to cows.[15] The most common reason for reduced milk consumption, cited by 40 per cent of those who indicated a decreased consumption, involved answers related to fat, cholesterol, calories, or diet.

Another study conducted in the late 1980s reported that 67 per cent of the u.s. population said they would pay an average of 22 cents extra per half gallon of milk if the milk was free of rBST. Yet when Land 'O Lakes dairy provided rBST-free milk in Minnesota supermarkets in

February 1994 at a cost of five cents more per half-gallon, it sat on the shelves.[16]

Nevertheless, many Canadian critics of rBST pointed to a 1994 survey conducted by Ottawa-based Optima Consultants, on behalf of Industry Canada, as evidence of public apprehension about rBST. The Optima survey asked: "Let's start with BST, which is a hormone that occurs naturally in cows and stimulates milk production. Scientists have identified the gene that produces BST and it can now be manufactured for use. With good management practices, farmers can increase milk production by injecting the cow with BST prescribed by a vet. If Canada adopts BST, how likely or unlikely are you to continue to buy milk?" Forty-three per cent said it was likely, 34 per cent said it was unlikely, and 23 per cent didn't know or care. This formed the basis for the oft-quoted statement that 34 per cent of Canadians would stop buying milk if rBST was approved for use in Canada.

The next question asked, "Suppose that Canadian dairy producers adopt BST. Milk would then come from treated cows and non-treated cows. Knowing that milk coming from all dairy farms is pooled when collected, how likely or unlikely are you to continue to buy milk?" Forty-seven per cent said it was likely, 29 per cent said it was unlikely and 22 per cent didn't know or care. Again, the relatively high percentages of "neutral" or "don't know" respondents is indicative of the confusing nature of the questions. Further, the Optima survey found that respondents had almost exactly the same range of responses when asked whether they would buy tomatoes genetically engineered to stay riper longer: 43 per cent said they would buy them, 32 per cent said no and 22 per cent were undecided. Yet every other survey conducted on agricultural biotechnology has found much more support for tomatoes that taste fresh year round than for the use of rBST.[17]

There are additional shortcomings of the Optima survey. From a retained sample of 13,575 telephone contact numbers, only 2,068 individuals cooperated in the survey, reflecting a participation rate of 15 per cent. This is a low rate of participation when the average is 40 to 50 per cent for telephone interviews. Further, according to Optima, "a much larger than normal proportion of respondents who agreed to take part discontinued the interview after it had begun (10 per cent)."[18] In other words, the sample may not be representative of the Canadian public.

MEDIA COVERAGE OF DAIRY

When we look at the role of dairy in today's diet, confusion clearly dominates, with concerns about saturated fats, animal welfare, health, and nutritional claims joining rBST in the public discussion. If global warming and cancer have become universal touchstones to condemn unwanted environmental practices, then fat has become the universal touchstone to condemn not only unwanted dietary practices but avarice, gluttony, and moral failings.

According to a 1993 survey of 1,000 Canadians,[19] 94 per cent think fat is a "serious" or "somewhat of a" hazard. When respondents are asked to suggest the greatest nutrition hazard in food, fat tops the list at 37 per cent, up from 31 per cent in 1991. Cholesterol is next, at 15 per cent, but that's down from 22 per cent in 1991. Sugar, chemical additives, and nutritional value round out the top five concerns. Other surveys reveal broad trends towards reduced fat consumption, but this is not borne out at the grocery store.[20] The apparent consumption of fat has remained fairly constant. Other surveys have been matched with actual buying patterns, either through pantry checks or garbage checks, and the results are equally disparate.[21]

Animal welfare advocates routinely target milk and dairy products as killers. For example, Dr Neal Barnard and his u.s.-based Physicians Committee for Responsible Medicine have called for the demotion of meat and dairy products to condiment status on the nation's tables, with ninety-one-year-old Dr Benjamin Spock as spokesperson. According to guidelines issued by the committee, meat and milk should no longer be part of the daily diet. "Death from coronary arteriosclerosis from cancers and from stroke keep increasing," said Dr Spock, "and there is no question these diseases are linked to high-fat diets, particularly animal fats from meat, chicken, fish, eggs and dairy products." While Spock agreed that babies and toddlers should not be deprived of milk and other dairy products, he said he is convinced that "after the age of three or so, they do not need to drink milk and eat dairy products every day."[22] In a recent analysis, Dr Barnard and others estimated the North American costs of a meat-based diet in terms of heath care and lost productivity at $50 billion, the same as cigarette smoking. Other health claims such as the virtues of raw milk, or the taste benefits of cold-filtered milk round out the risk-reporting on milk.[23]

The Internet carries several newsgroups which discuss the follies of dairy products. One newsgroup, sci.med.nutrition, carries an ongoing discussion of the pitfalls of consuming meat and dairy, including lower intelligence, a propensity for aggressive behaviour, and reduced sexual prowess.

BST IN THE UNITED STATES

Genetic engineering has now replaced nuclear energy as the primary example of "science-out-of-control" in popular culture. In books, movies, and science fiction, food biotechnology is often presented as "Frankenfood," a metaphor based in the deep ambivalence many individuals express toward any technology that manipulates deoxyribonucleic acid (DNA), sometimes referred to as the "code of life." At the same time, distrust in government and in technology has reached new heights.

Further, those who promote biotechnology are characteristically creating unrealistic expectations. Kathleen Day of the *Washington Post* described the biotechnology industry over the past two decades as filled "with predictions of miracle cures, big profit and rapid expansion," but "the U.S. biotechnology industry has yet to fulfill those grand expectations. Product delays, outright failures, regulatory hurdles and the sheer complexity of understanding hereditary material have made most biotech companies money-losing operations year after year. Basing a business on the chemical sequences of life, it turns out, is more complicated than anyone had imagined."[24]

The first report of rBST in the *New York Times* occurred on 16 March 1981[25] when Genentech Inc. and Monsanto Corp. said they had produced the bovine hormone that promotes meat and milk growth in cattle using recombinant DNA technology. On 19 October 1985, the *Times* reported on the experiments of Dr Bauman of Cornell University, documenting the initial results of increased milk production from cows given rBST.[26] Even in this early story, the parameters of the public discussion were being laid out, with experts stating that although rBST could mean lower production costs for farmers and possibly lower milk prices for consumers, milk supply already exceeded demand.

Over the past ten years coverage of rBST in the *New York Times* has been intertwined with general criticism of the U.S. system of price supports for fluid milk. On 28 October 1985, a *Times* editorial lauded the science behind rBST but noted that consumers won't see the benefits because of government intervention at the behest of a powerful dairy lobby that sets milk prices and surplus-purchase policies.[27] By 1989 coverage had shifted to focus on the social implications of rBST use, particularly at the level of the family farm.[28] A subsequent editorial said that farmers would do better to address the need for a safety net for the estimated fifteen thousand dairy farmers who might be forced out of business by rBST rather than trying to hamper the introduction of the technology.[29]

On 25 March 1990 the *New York Times* reported FDA approval of the first genetically engineered food product, chymosin, a form of rennin used in cheese production. In terms of media coverage, this product generated almost no public opposition, especially when contrasted with the response to rBST.[30]

at her cereal bowl. The text lead with, "Caving in to pressure from giant drug and chemical companies, the FDA has approved use of genetically-engineered 'bovine growth hormone.'" It provided a list of dairy processors and their 1-800 telephone numbers, urging consumers to call and complain. By 1995 the Pure Food Campaign admitted the battle over rBST had been lost and turned its attention to genetically engineered crops – at least in the United States. A receptive audience was still at hand in Canada.[40]

While dairy farmers were divided over the use of rBST, dairy processors put up a united front, through the International Dairy Foods Association (IDFA) and the National Milk Board. E. Linwood Tipton, president of IDFA, outlined the processors' position in a November 1993 interview with the trade magazine *World of Ingredients*:

Our association has the position that we are neither for nor against the approval and use of BST. Its safety is something the scientific community has decided and its use is something individual dairy farmers will determine. We have only dealt with negative publicity generated by radical groups who are opposed to biotechnology. We have spent a lot of energy and effort on two fronts. We had to counter negative publicity generated by people whose primary agenda is to raise funds to oppose biotechnology. The same people have also energized animal rights people in opposition to BST. The negative publicity has influenced people's attitudes about drinking milk. Our role is to educate with information and facts and to ensure that the safety of milk is not impugned.[41]

The position was significantly different from that pursued by dairy processors in Canada.

Shortly after rBST went on sale on 4 February 1994, the FDA published draft guidelines which said that labels for cheese, milk, ice cream, and other dairy products could state that they came from "cows not treated with" the hormone, but the label must also carry a statement like, "No significant difference has been shown between milk derived from rBST-treated and non-rBST-treated cows."[42] Labels could not carry the claim that milk is "BST-free" because the hormone occurs naturally in milk, and labels also could not say the milk is "rBST-free" because that would imply the milk is different. In response the *New York Times* wrote in an editorial that FDA labelling guidelines gave "apprehensive consumers the information they need – without implying a risk that regulators insist is not there."[43] Nevertheless, some firms stretched the limits of the guidelines. Marian Burros of the *New York Times* wrote that a newspaper ad for the Elfco Food Co-op of East Lansing, Michigan, said, "Concerned about the use of synthetic bovine growth hormone? Elfco offers milk, yogurt, cheeses and butter from farmers committed to dairy production without the use of rBGH." The statement did not include the suggested caveat about milk from supplemented and non-supplemented cows being the same.[44]

Through 1994, American media coverage of rBST became more supportive of the product. Keith Schneider of the *New York Times* reported that "despite consumer wariness about milk produced with a genetically engineered hormone, thousands of dairy farmers across the country are adopting the new drug to increase production in their cows." "More and more farmers around here are using it," said Jim Winkel, a thirty-one-year-old dairy farmer from Vogel Center, Michigan. "They just aren't talking about it. You just are never sure where a person stands on the thing."[45]

As the first anniversary of rBST use approached, the u.s. National Milk Producers Federation issued a release stating that – according to USDA statistics – consumption of fluid milk and dairy products increased 0.8 per cent from October 1993 to October 1994 ("Year after Gene Controversy – US Milk Consumption Up"). Also, after one year of rBST use, the FDA had received 806 "adverse-reaction" reports from thirteen thousand farmers.[46] After investigating the complaints the FDA was unable to detect any unusual problems with rBST. After this, the story largely dropped off the national scene in the United States.

BST IN CANADA

The first story in the *Globe and Mail* mentioning rBST was published 7 April 1981,[47] a reprint from the *New York Times* detailing the financial prospects for Genentech, which had announced its rBST cloning with Monsanto on 13 March 1981. On 25 February 1985 the *Globe* ran a reprint from the *New York Times* quoting Robert Kalter, chairman of Cornell University's department of agricultural economics and director of a study on the impact of rBST, who said a 15 to 25 per cent increase in milk production would mean lower production costs for farmers and could mean lower milk prices to consumers. "It's going to be an awesome production increase," said Kalter.[48]

Later that year, *Globe and Mail* science writer Stephen Strauss journeyed to Cornell to see for himself the "birthplace of the milk revolution."[49] Already, noted Strauss, the FDA and Agriculture Canada (although he probably meant Health Canada) had cleared the milk as suitable for human consumption. Nevertheless, rhetorical battle lines were clearly drawn. Strauss quoted John Carr, a farmer with the Wisconsin Family Defense Fund, as saying, "Our universities have turned against us ... They are producing technology which is going out to the farmer in an unfair and unequal way. Only those with large capital can use it. The researchers are part of the system which is killing the family farm and the family farmers." In the same story Jeremy Rifkin predicted rBST would "create the single most devastating dislocation in u.s. farm history."

A *Globe and Mail* editorial of 8 May 1989 forecast the public debate to come and the rhetorical tactic of using scientific language to mask socio-economic, cultural, and value concerns.[50] After noting there had been little in the way of a direct attack on milk safety, the *Globe* predicted that "it seems likely that those who have a strong financial interest in fighting any slippage in milk price or quotas will become extremely interested in genetics, given that the main feature of this new development is a genetically altered hormone."

In the fall of 1989 public discussion of rBST escalated in Canada after it was revealed by several local newspapers that milk from rBST test herds in Ontario, Alberta, and British Columbia was being added to the general milk supply. Even though previous stories had noted that milk from rBST-supplemented cows was cleared by Health Canada for human consumption, it was consumer outrage – noted here in the form of quotes – at the perception of underhanded activity that propelled the story to prominence.[51] (The exact pattern of consumer outrage in response to not being explicitly told a product was in the food supply would be repeated six years later after field-test crops of Monsanto's New Leaf potato, genetically engineered with the Bt-gene to be resistant to the Colorado potato beetle, was released without notice). As recounted by Burton and McBride, it was decided at a meeting held by the Ontario Federation of Agriculture on 23 November 1989 in Toronto to take milk from rBST-treated cows off the Canadian market so that "producers and consumers would be quieted."[52] This move "was prompted by hysteria over rBST resulting from public confusion of the rBST hormone with steroid hormones. The quenching of the protesters by the banning of milk sales only added to the public confusion over what rBST was really all about." Burton and McBride completely disregard the notion of informed consent or consumer right-to-know, the lack of which fueled the notion of consumer (and journalistic) outrage.

On 27 March 1990 the *Globe and Mail's* u.s. correspondent, Colin MacKenzie, reported that the first genetically engineered foodstuff, chymosin, the purer form of rennet's active ingredient, had been approved for cheese production in the United States.[53] MacKenzie contrasted the lack of controversy surrounding chymosin with the "ruckus over rBST" and introduced the notion that "in Canada, where family farms are better insulated by marketing boards ... the major concern is that consumers will object to its introduction."

With rumours of a pending rBST approval in the United States, a coalition of groups campaigning to reduce the consumption of beef announced plans to picket four hundred McDonald's restaurants in Canada and two thousand in the United States, demanding a pledge that food and beverages would be free of rBST.[54] The story said that opponents of the hormone used public opinion surveys to show that consumers want products with rBGH to be labelled as such and predict that demand for milk will drop dramatically if the hormone is approved. Spokesperson Keith Ashdown said his coalition was trying to educate people about the environmental and health problems associated with cows and the issue of BGH, and that McDonald's should offer a vegetarian entree. Subsequently, the planned event fizzled, with more reporters than protesters showing up at the designated McDonald's in Toronto. This fact was not reported.[55]

On 3 May 1993, agriculture reporter Jim Romahn of the *Kitchener-Waterloo Record* reported that the Dairy Farmers of Canada had decided to stay on the fence with rBST, neither opposing nor supporting the licensing or use of the product, but that the group would prepare educational material.[56]

Although media coverage in Canada mirrored that in the United States in quantitative terms, qualitatively the coverage became significantly different. Coverage increased after FDA approval in November 1993, as it did in the United States, but then took on a different flavour, fueled by very Canadian concerns. Predominant in the rhetoric used by the leaders of several dairy organizations was the need to educate consumers. The president of the Dairy Farmers of Canada complained that there had been no comprehensive discussion, no education or information programs or an examination of consumer attitudes with respect to rBST (he made no suggestions of what type of educational or informational programs should be undertaken). The president of the National Dairy Council, which represents dairy processors, issued a call for a one-year moratorium on rBST use (if and when Health Canada issued a notice of compliance) "to allow manufacturers of BST to educate consumers about the product. Early response to the use [of BST] has been very negative and resulted in adverse publicity for the dairy industry."[57] No evidence of this adverse publicity was offered.

The next week another executive with the National Dairy Council said a two-year moratorium would give Canadians a chance to learn about rBST and to watch developments in the United States: "We feel the consumer is confused about this."[58] Another two weeks and once again the same message was hammered home by the NDC, requesting a two-year delay because it wanted "time to educate consumers" and noting that the American backlash to the approval of rBST was immediate.[59] The problem here is that any "backlash" was hypothetical because the product was not even on sale in the United States in December 1993 due to the ninety-day moratorium. Consumers had not yet had an opportunity to vote on rBST at the grocery store, and when they did, consumption of milk was unaffected. There was little or no backlash. Further, requesting a moratorium in Canada to "allow manufacturers of BST to educate consumers" was disingenuous. Under the Food and Drug Act, manufacturers are forbidden by law to enter into any promotional discussion of a product under review by Health Canada, something the NDC and Dairy Farmers of Canada both knew.[60]

Two other characteristics of the rBST coverage became cemented in this time period. First was the frequency with which consumer groups and citizens spoke on behalf of all Canadians, with generalizations like "consumers don't want this product."[61] The evidence supporting such a claim was never presented. Second, Health Canada was often asked by reporters when a decision on rBST would be made in Canada.[62] In a fall 1993 radio interview, the head of BVD said he expected a decision in "a few weeks." In a 14 February 1994 *Globe and Mail* story, the director-general of the food directorate in the health protection branch of Health Canada told Mary Gooderham that his department was still reviewing scientific data on the safety and efficacy of rBST for humans and cows: "He expects a decision to be made on registering the product within the next couple of months." Yet Health Canada had already approved the safety of rBST for human consumption in 1986, as was confirmed by the former director of BVD in a *Globe* story on 17 April 1993. Battle lines were drawn over bovine hormone as he was paraphrased to state "the product has already been declared safe for human consumption ... but tests for animal safety and efficacy are still being conducted and analyzed."

 A decision on rBST was always portrayed by Health Canada officials as "coming soon."

After rBST went on sale in the United States on 5 February 1994, coverage again increased in Canada. It was increasingly negative. "Do you know what happens when you put a growth hormone into people. What happens if you elevate growth hormones? Nobody knows. Until we know what it does I wouldn't want to drink the stuff," said Toronto Board of Health Chairman Peter Tabuns. Apparently the 1990 editorial in *Journal of the American Medical Association* which urged people not to play on unfounded rBST health fears had little effect on the Toronto

Board of Health. Statements that "a furor erupted anyway in the U.S. after the hormone was introduced last month" became common.[63]

Eventually the Toronto Board of Health passed the recommendations of the Toronto Food Policy Council (TFPC) at its 28 March 1994 meeting. These included:

- that there be mandatory labelling of all foods produced by genetic engineering, defined as "the deliberate short-circuiting (forced foreshortening of time sequence) of natural processes;"
- that a mandatory socio-economic impact analysis of new technologies be carried out;
- that the TFPC report on rBST be forwarded to all school boards in Ontario requesting that, in the event of licensing of rBGH, they consider passing a resolution requesting that BGH (or foods containing it) be labelled;
- that dairy suppliers indicate whether rBGH-produced milk is being sold to the schools; and,
- that parents be advised by the school boards.

In arguing that rBST may impact on consumer acceptance of dairy products – ultimately impacting on human health – the Toronto Board of Health cited as evidence an *Ontario Farmer* story quoting the NDC, which "has asked for a two-year moratorium on the use of rBGH because it fears negative consumer reaction."[64] A cyclical argument about negative consumer reaction was becoming established, even in the absence of such evidence from the United States.

In March 1994 the Canadian federal agriculture committee held public hearings on rBST and subsequently passed a resolution asking Cabinet to delay the use of rBST, "to allow public fears about the hormone to be addressed."[65] On 14 April 1994, the chair of the Commons agriculture committee reiterated the claim there was not enough information in the public domain and called for public education. Who would educate, where, when and how, was not discussed.

Based on the committee's report, Agriculture and Agri-Food Canada negotiated a one-year moratorium on the use of rBST with Monsanto Canada and Eli/Lilly Canada. This was announced in August 1994 and included the creation of a task force to investigate rBST and report to the minister of Agriculture by 1 May 1995. However, in covering the moratorium announcement, *Canadian Press* managed to initiate the idea that rBST would be available for sale after the moratorium expired on 1 July 1995, even in the absence of approval from Health Canada; this was simply not true. "Manufacturers can still set up marketing and distribution networks to sell rBST a year from now, which they could not have done if the government had legislated a moratorium," said Alex Boston of the Council of Canadians. "After all the momentum is built up, it will be impossible for this task force to turn around and say no."[66]

On 29 November 1994, CBC Television's *Fifth Estate* ran a documentary about rBST that largely ignored available scientific evidence on rBST and focused instead on the corporate behaviour of Monsanto in both the United States and Canada (journalistically, this made a much better story). Near the end of the segment, in an interview with a Health Canada official, it was alleged that Monsanto Canada attempted to bribe Health Canada officials in 1990 with $1–2 million in new research funding in exchange for rBST approval. Monsanto Canada refused to comment on air, deferring to Monsanto headquarters in St Louis.

A letter to employees from the president of Monsanto Canada dated 30 November 1994 said that, "those of you who watched the 5th estate [sic] last night must have felt as shocked and wronged as I did. The accusation of 'bribing' Health Canada strikes at the very foundation of the integrity and honesty of our people. I believe the 5th estate's program was vindictive with the intent to damage the reputation of our company's image, not to mention each one of our people. For that I am deeply sorry, for the employees, the families and friends, as well as those committed to objective and honest journalism."

In a public statement, Monsanto Canada insisted there was "never an offer of money in exchange for product approval ... we proposed to carry out additional meaningful research to complement existing data and to add to the worldwide body of knowledge on BST." Yet the company still failed to explain why such an offer was ever made. Instead, stories repeating the allegation began to appear, including one by the Ottawa bureau of *Canadian Press* (5 December 1994), which stated that "Health Department experts with knowledge of the matter have been ordered not to talk to the media, but a department spokesman confirmed that Monsanto offered money to the department four or five years ago. An official within the Health Department, who spoke on condition of anonymity, said *The Fifth Estate* report was accurate."

According to a Monsanto Canada official who was present at the 1990 meeting, the discussion of additional research was related to recent changes in federal legislation, extending patent protection to pharmaceuticals in Canada, which contained a provision that a small percentage of gross sales had to be reinvested in Canadian-based research and development.[67] The figure of $1–2 million was based on projected Canadian sales of rBST, and Monsanto officials were engaged in discussion with Health Canada officials as to the type of future research that would advance knowledge rather than repeat what had been done in other countries. However, such an explanation was never made public, probably leaving the impression of a bribe in the minds of many viewers and journalists, an impression that would repeatedly surface in subsequent coverage of rBST. According to one Internet posting, the February 1996 issue of *Health Confidential* contained a story about rBST which recounted the *Fifth Estate* broadcast of November 1994 where "Canadian government officials, while debating legalization of BST, received multi-million dollar bribes from Monsanto officials."

Shortly thereafter, rBST became a focus of debate in the House of Commons. Opposition members of Parliament questioned the objectivity of the task force examining rBST (because it included representatives from both Monsanto and Eli/Lilly) and the objectivity of the former head of Health Canada's BVD, Dr Len Ritter, who was identified in a 3 March 1994 *Canadian Press* story – during agriculture committee hearings on rBST – as someone who now teaches at the University of Guelph and "speaks on behalf of the companies that manufacture BST."[68] Dr Ritter refused to talk to the media. The perception of backroom lobbying and inappropriate behaviour on the part of Monsanto was solidified. Further, the Optima Consultants study (1994) predicting a massive decline in milk consumption was released in November and routinely cited by rBST critics. Only one story criticized the survey methodology – "the questions appeared leading and the survey had a response rate of only 15 per cent" – and questioned the results in light of the u.s. response.[69]

Into 1995 the coverage of rBST in Canada became even more negative, picking up extreme aspects of the discussion in the United States and moving them to the mainstream: the alleged link between IGF-1 and breast cancer, even a link between rBST use and mad cow disease (although there was no evidence of BSE in Canada, several groups alleged that cattle using rBST would require a higher-protein diet, and this extra protein would come from rendered animal remains, facilitating the emergence of BSE in Canada). These elements were increasingly mentioned in published stories, with no one to counter the claims publicly.

Three letters in the *Toronto Star* on 5 March 1995 in response to a feature article on rBST were characteristic. One concerned the impact of rBST on breed characterization. One complained, "In all the testing that has been done, have any tests been done on pregnant women? Remember thalidomide? Who would want to volunteer for such testing anyway? How can they know it will not affect fetuses? It has been established that women are seldom used in drug testing." The third stated, "Once again, our federal government appears intent on caving in to big business. On 1 July, it is scheduled to approve the sale of rBST, a new growth hormone, which is injected into cows and increases their milk production. Reputed Canadian associations have expressed serious concerns about associated health problems affecting cows and humans, which are directly related to the use of this drug." The author, Esther Klein, spokesperson for the Animal Defence League of Canada, said that while mastitis is treatable with antibiotics, cows on rBST need three times as much medicine as other cows to clear up the infection; "As a result, the level of antibiotics in this milk is higher." Klein also said the drug gets cows' milk production so revved up that they need high-protein food supplements, and "dead cows are being ground up for this purpose. This increases the danger of cows contracting other diseases such as Mad Cow Disease, which in turn could contaminate our milk supply."

Two other allegations surfaced repeatedly in rBST coverage: the lack of independent scientific research and the lack of long-term health studies. "A big problem in science is that the money for research is coming from industry," said Dr Rod MacRae of the Toronto Food Policy Council. "This is not a matter of a lack of integrity or dishonesty. It is a conspiracy of shared values." No one challenged such statements, defending the integrity of university scientists or asking why taxpayers would fund research into a private sector product. Similarly, no one challenged the difficulties associated with long-term health impact studies (no one suggested how such long-term studies would be conducted, or funded, but every rBST critic was calling for them).

MacRae also said the industry was paying little attention to the broader effects of the technologies on people and the environment. "Bovine growth hormone is, like a lot of biotech stuff, a solution looking for a problem. There's no shortage of milk in this country. In fact, we have more milk than we can use. Why do we have to give hormones to cows to get more milk?" That question was easily answered by several editorials in the United States, which noted increased production efficiencies had environmental and consumer benefits, but apparently stumped Canadian editorial writers.

As the story died down in the United States, it continued to flourish in Canada. Accusations persisted that rBST was being purchased in American border towns and then transported into Canada for use on dairy farms.[70]

The release of the rBST task force report prompted a number of stories concluding that if consumers didn't react negatively, the introduction of rBST could lead to lower milk and dairy product prices, higher consumption, and increased farm income.[71] The report noted that the introduction of rBST in the United States more than a year earlier had little impact on dairy consumption. In fact, dairy consumption rose 0.6 per cent, the first increase since 1992. The report also estimated that sales of rBST-free milk represented less than 2 per cent of total U.S. fluid milk sales; when combined with manufactured milk, less than 1 per cent of sales was represented by milk or milk products specifically identified as rBST free. The states of Wisconsin and Vermont were the exceptions, with rBST-free milk being the overwhelming choice of consumers in Wisconsin and having significant sales in Vermont: "In these areas, however, opposition to rBST seems to have started as much from farmer and rural living concerns as from consumers."[72]

Although Monsanto saw vindication in the report ("I think the milk consumption numbers in the United States speak for themselves," said a Monsanto Canada official: "milk consumption is up") consumer groups dismissed the task force report. A spokesman for the Council of Canadians argued that Canadians "have very different consumer attitudes" (no evidence was forthcoming). "Dairy industry surveys and reaction we have received on the issue suggest there will be a strong demand for BST-free milk." This spokesman also predicted many Canadians would switch to substitutes like soya solutions.[73]

The report also had little effect on the National Dairy Council. On 12 May 1995 the NDC president sent a letter to all members of Parliament, discussing the results of their recent board of directors meeting and stating that the dairy processing industry sees "no benefit whatsoever for itself nor for consumers in the use of rBST in Canada." While the NDC "is not opposed to bio-technology nor advances in the field," it is "opposed to being subjected to an un-needed [sic] and unwanted intrusion into its business which offers no benefit whatsoever to consumers and processors. In this case that intrusion is rBST."

The letter set up a straw person, stating that consumer concerns, whether based on fact or perceptions, cannot be dismissed "as some do, as 'whining from the lunatic fringe.'" There was no reference as to who was actually doing this whining or who made the statement in quotations. The letter went on to shoot down this straw person, saying, "To do so is contemptuous of Canadian consumer concerns." The letter concluded by suggesting that legislators may want to "empower an agency to respond to consumer concerns by refusing the 'right to sell' for rBST or other new controversial products until such time as stated concerns whether economic, administrative, or perceptive have been addressed."

In May 1995 the Angus Reid polling firm released results from its monthly omnibus survey which had included questions on food safety and food biotechnology the previous month. Of the fifteen hundred people surveyed, 46 per cent said they would "definitely" pay 10 per cent extra for milk which was guaranteed to be produced without the use of BST. An additional 28 per cent said they would "probably" pay the additional price.[74] This data was further cited as proof Canadians would reject rBST, even though the exact same prediction failed to materialize in the United States.

Media coverage of rBST once again increased as the 1 July 1995 expiration of the voluntary moratorium approached. The Toronto Food Policy Council sent an open letter to Ontario dairy producers, citing a study it said questioned the safety of increased levels of insulin-like growth factor 1 in milk from rBST-treated cows.[75] A multi-party coalition of rural MPs, consumer-activist groups, and farm-industry organizations asked the federal government to impose a two-year moratorium on the sale of rBST.[76] A story in the *Vancouver Province* about the call for a new moratorium quoted Alan Parker of the Health Action Network: "We're lobbying on this because we think it's an emotional issue. We're talking about milk. You can't trust government any more. You can't trust researchers any more. They only want to sell you crap."

At the same time, the Council of Canadians took out a full-page advertisement in the *Ottawa Citizen* which said, "Do your kids drink milk? They could soon be part of a dangerous experiment." The ad went on to say that "studies show a byproduct in [rBST] milk could cause breast and colon cancers." The ad also equated rBST with other Monsanto products such as the jungle defoliant Agent Orange and polychlorinated biphenyls (PCBs). Monsanto responded by calling the ad "libelous" and then, along with Eli/Lilly, publicly threatened to scale back research and development efforts in Canada if rBST was further delayed.[77] In an editorial, the *Vancouver Province* called the "threat ... nothing more than thuggery."[78]

In an equally bizarre move, an "Open Letter to Agricultural Journalists" was sent to several trade publications in early July 1995, signed by a group of veterinarians and farmers supporting rBST. In the "letter," the rBST supporters state there is a "clear, direct association between several of these influential MPs and the Animal Defence League, the Council of Canadians, and other special-interest groups." This is a common rhetorical tactic, to label those who disagree as "special interest groups."[79] As the *Manitoba Co-operator* correctly pointed out in an editorial, "the irony is that the veterinarians and farmers who wrote this letter are as much or more of a special interest group than any which appeared in front of the parliamentary committee.[80] We know that milk can be produced without BST. It can also be produced, apparently with more profit, with BST. The farmers and vets will receive part of those profits. They are therefore a special interest group."

On 13 July 1995 the *Globe and Mail* published a feature article that picked up where the *Fifth Estate* left off, tracking the corporate misdeeds of Monsanto Canada.[81] In it Doug Saunders wrote that while Monsanto is not permitted to promote rBST until it has been approved by Health Canada, "that hasn't stopped Monsanto from developing a multi-pronged public relations effort that influences public thinking in a more subtle way than advertising and promotions.

"It is quite possible that BST is, in fact, relatively safe – the bulk of scientific research supports this conclusion, and in any case, high levels of BST occur naturally in all modern high-yield dairy cows," wrote Saunders. "But if this is the case, observers ask, why is Monsanto making such an effort to mold public and professional opinion?"

The story wove a thread of conspiracy, implicating governments and scientists who have been bought through Monsanto's largesse, worthy of broadcast on television's conspiracy-minded show, *X-Files*. (A 1994 episode of *X-Files* linked rBST to the injection of alien DNA. After being told by special agent Dana Scully that the FDA approved rBST as safe, agent Fox Muldar responded, "Who trusts the government?") Saunders also recounted the *Fifth Estate* allegations of bribery, but did note that the Royal Canadian Mounted Police investigated the claim and found no evidence to support a criminal investigation.

Opponents of rBST continued to recycle so-called scientific evidence as the basis for rBST risks. For example, a persistent contributor to the Internet newsgroup sci.med.nutrition alleged on 11 August 1995 that, with respect to the functionality of rBST in pasteurized milk, "FDA relied on a published paper written by a graduate student, Paul Groenewegen, from Guelph, Ontario. In a severely flawed experiment Groenewegen pasteurized milk for 30 minutes at a temperature reserved for a 15 second method. After 'cooking' [sic] milk Groenewegen observed only a 19% reduction in levels of BST. When reached at his home[82] Groenewegen was first shocked and then outraged that the FDA had reached an erroneous conclusion from his research. This lie was repeated by every major newspaper and magazine article."

Sounds convincing – except that when Paul Groenewegen was contacted on 22 February 1996 he seemed more outraged by the aforementioned Internet description of his work.[83] Groenewegen recalled that he received a phone call from Robert Cohen "sometime in 1995," inquiring about his Masters research from 1988. Groenewegen said that Cohen kept insinuating that his supervisor at the time, Dr Brian McBride of the University of Guelph, had "set him up" by making

Groenewegen put his name first on the paper describing survivability of rBST under various heating conditions. He recounted that Cohen began citing active levels of IGF-1 in mg/l instead of ng/ml. Paul Groenewegen said, "The only reason you're doing that is to make the numbers sound bigger." Later in the conversation he said he responded, "It's bullshit," in response to Cohen's representation of the data. Apparently this was the source of the shock and outrage mentioned in the previous paragraph.

In a further example, the Internet digest *Rachel's Environment and Health Weekly*, published by the Environmental Research Foundation in Annapolis, Maryland, stated that new scientific studies "suggest that milk from rBGH-treated cows may not be as safe for humans as was previously believed."[84] Included in the charges were the following points:

- some humans suffer from a condition called acromegaly, or gigantism, which is characterized by excessive growth of the head, face, hands, and feet and is caused by excessive natural production of IGF-1;
- two British researchers found IGF-1 induced mitotic activity in human cell cultures;
- IGF-1 promotes the growth of cancer tumours in laboratory animals and in humans by preventing programmed cell death;
- the casein protein in milk prevents IGF-1 from being digested in the stomach;
- milk from rBST-supplemented cows has elevated levels of IGF-1.

According to the FDA, IGF-1 is a natural protein required for normal growth and health maintenance. Structurally and chemically similar to insulin, it is normally present in almost all body tissues and fluids including human breast milk and saliva. The IGF-1 that occurs naturally in human breast milk occurs at about the same concentration as that found in cow's milk. Levels of IGF-1 in cow's milk and meat are very much lower than the levels found naturally in human blood and other body tissues.

The FDA statement goes on to say that IGF-1 is not absorbed intact. Dietary IGF-1 in milk and meat is broken down in the gastrointestinal tract by digestion. Undigested IGF is excreted. In cow's milk IGF levels start high and drop over time. The reported range is from 150 ng/ml in colostrum, to 25 ng/ml for milk from cows one week into their lactation, to as low as 1 ng/ml for cows late in their lactation. If cows are treated with rBST, the treatment doesn't begin until about seventy days into lactation. In cows treated with rBST, IGF-1 levels are higher than in similar cows at the same point in their lactation. Dr Bauman of Cornell University has calculated the daily IGF-1 from saliva and other digestive secretions is equal to that in ninety-five quarts of milk.

Nevertheless, the report in *Rachel's Environment and Health Weekly* formed the basis for a front-page story in the *Victoria Times Colonist* linking rBST use with elevated levels of IGF-1:[85] "Another study shows humans with gigantism, a condition in which the head, face, and feet grow excessively large, also have elevated levels of colon tumors, says *Rachel's Environmental & Health Weekly*. Gigantism is caused by high levels of IGF-1 produced by the body." Such an extraordinary finding must have surely seemed worthy of the front page to the editor at the *Victoria Times Colonist*. No other paper ran the story, which referred to *Rachel's* as "a prestigious report published by the Environmental Research Foundation in Maryland."

Which leads to the press conference on 23 January 1996 hosted by the Cancer Prevention Coalition along with Food and Water, where Dr Epstein proclaimed, "rBST poses an even greater risk to human health than ever considered." Predicting that the hormone would cause cases of breast cancer and colon cancer to soar, he demanded its immediate removal from the market. Shouting "cancer" at the crowded press conference garnered Epstein extensive coverage – including CBS *This Morning*, USA *Today*, CNN and 350 radio and television stations across the United States. Notably, the *New York Times* and *Associated Press* ignored the story. They had heard it before.

In the September/October 1989 issue of the *Ecologist*, Dr Epstein had published an article entitled "BST: The Public Health Hazards," which condemned rBST as unsafe.[86] Since that publication, Jeremy Rifkin has often cited Dr Epstein's research as the basis for new questions about the safety of rBST.[87]

Responding to the Epstein press conference, the U.S. Dairy Coalition stretched Dr Bauman's analogy regarding IGF-1 in milk, stating that "every day, the human body naturally produces the same amount of IGF-1 as can be found in 3,000 quarts of milk."[88]

In Canada, the Epstein press conference received significant attention, beginning with a *Canadian Press* story that stated that the new report "will likely add fuel to the long-running controversy over" rBST.[89] While caveats were added in some newspaper accounts, they disappeared by the time the story reached radio and television: "American cows spiked with growth hormones are a breast cancer risk according to new American research"; "A U.S. study says the cow hormone sanctioned for use in the U.S. and being considered for use in Canada, can increase an individual's chance of getting cancer"; and, "rBGH a hormone injected into cows to boost production has been found to cause breast and colon cancer."[90]

Two weeks later Susan Semenak of the *Montreal Gazette* wrote that "consumer advocates are urging Health Canada to pay close attention to newly published research which links a controversial bovine-growth hormone with increased risk of breast and colon cancer in humans"; the story was reprinted across the country.[91] Semenak also quoted a Health Canada official who, contrary to earlier statements about an imminent rBST decision, said, "They will need to do more work to demonstrate, within cows, its safety and efficacy. We just simply have not made up our minds about this product."

A VACUUM FILLED WITH NONSENSE

As of January 1997, Health Canada had still not made a decision on the rBST application. In September 1995, it had been revealed that Health Canada had asked Monsanto and Eli/Lilly for additional animal health data to support their applications for rBST, a request that was estimated to take well into the fall of 1996 to comply with.[92]

In the summer of 1995, the Canadian press began carrying stories critical of Health Canada's delays over the years. According to two members of a research team that studied rBST at the University of Guelph (they insisted on anonymity because, they said, the current controversy was political and emotional, not scientific), Health Canada's 1995 request for more data was "pure politics."[93] "Both [scientists] said there is lots of data available on both questions Ottawa has raised – efficacy (proof that it works as claimed) and the health of cows – and said the real reason is the regulators want to delay making a decision that is bound to be controversial." Jim Romahn continued his criticism in the *Manitoba Co-operator*: "Health Canada has done an absolutely lousy job of informing the public about what it's doing with BST and why. The bureaucrats and politicians have seldom had a better chance to show and tell the Canadian public why and how they review and regulate these products, but they have consciously, deliberately and persistently stone-walled, even when the federal government set up a special task force to review BST."[94]

An editorial in the *Ottawa Citizen* on 19 June 1995 concluded that Health Canada "will have some explaining to do whatever the decision, because it has taken far too long."[95] Barry Wilson wrote in *Western Producer* that "Health Canada's dithering over rBST represents a cumbersome and unsatisfactory way to make a significant policy decision.[96] A political debate that is undermining public confidence has been allowed to take root and flourish. There are allegations of biased research, bad science, pre-drawn conclusions and a faulty regulatory process ... The debate is making the public suspicious of the product and the process."

All along Health Canada maintained that the review process was based entirely on science. "A favorable decision will only be made if health department experts are convinced that the hormone can be safely used in Canada," said Health Minister Diane Marleau in the Commons. "It is important to keep that in mind."[97] Dr Sol Gunner, director general of Health Canada's foods directorate and the official in charge of reviewing rBST, said: "Health Canada has continually stated that the review process is based on science and that science will be the sole determinant. Other variables such as marketplace, political processes, questions of moratoria are completely not within the realm of how we do business."

Which begs the question: What has been the role of Health Canada in the public discussion of rBST? And how does this compare with the role of the FDA in the United States? In terms of the methodological guidelines of Leiss and Chociolko, Health Canada engaged in no risk communications on rBST, failed to explain risk assessment assumptions (let alone the entire risk assessment process) for evaluating rBST, did not understand the nature of public concerns, and utterly failed to take responsibility on the issue of rBST approval.[98] In terms of the additional evaluative criteria, Health Canada delivered a simple message – rBST would be evaluated by science alone – but failed recognize the variety of socio-economic concerns which would accompany any decision regarding rBST. Why Health Canada has yet to proffer a decision on the rBST submission is unknown. What is known is that this silence helped create a risk information vacuum that was eagerly filled by many others.

In contrast, the FDA understood that there were public concerns about rBST and published a paper in *Science* explaining the risk assessment of rBST. When a decision was reached, the Department of Human Health Services issued a press release announcing the decision. It is Health Canada policy not to issue press releases on any product decisions; it is up to the companies to do so.[99] The FDA hosted several scientific consensus reviews that were at least reported in the press. Health Canada has not.

The reaction of dairy processors in the United States and Canada also differed in response to the introduction of rBST. The U.S. National Dairy Board insisted that rBST was safe, and that it was up to individual producers to decide if rBST made sense in their individual dairy operations. They also countered negative claims about the safety of milk from rBST-supplement cows. In Canada the National Dairy Council backed calls for a moratorium on rBST, even if Health Canada declared rBST safe. "It's not a health issue, it's a marketing issue," said the NDC president.[100] Does this mean the marketing of dairy products becomes a responsibility of Canadian legislators? The NDC also demanded that if rBST were approved, all products should be clearly labelled. Does this mean that all dairy products should be accurately labelled for fat content, considering that a diet high in saturated fats is a well-documented health risk? As Franklin Loew, dean of Tufts University's School of Veterinary Medicine, wrote in a *Boston Globe* opinion piece on 10 October 1989, "Premium ice creams (like Ben and Jerry's, which actively lobbied against rBST approval in the U.S.) contain nearly 24 grams of fat and 349 calories per cup.[101] Highly saturated, cholesterol-laden butterfat supplying 62 per cent of the calories is a serious threat to sensible dietary practice, with or without BST."

Another possible explanation for the stance of the National Dairy Council is that, yes, they were concerned about the marketing of dairy products, not because of public perceptions of rBST but rather because of a challenge to Canada's supply management system for dairy products and the possibility of increased U.S. imports under the North American Free Trade deal. The United States launched a challenge to Canada's dairy and poultry marketing system in July 1995, and the matter has gone to an arbitration panel.[102] If the Canadian border were opened to American dairy products, this would represent a significant threat to the markets of Canadian producers and processors. But if rBST were not in use in Canada because of a moratorium, American dairy products could conceivably be denied market access because they might have been created with the aid of rBST. The U.S. Executive Branch of the Federal Government warned of such a scenario in its 1994 report, noting that "several countries appear content to observe the U.S. experience before acting on rBST approval." The report goes on to state that "the exhaustive study of the safety, quality and efficacy of BST under standard FDA procedures lends credibility to the product. A country wishing to ban imports of dairy products originating in the U.S. or another country that uses BST would incur the risk of a trade dispute because the ban would be seen as a non-tariff trade barrier." The language of the NDC is quite similar to the language used by officials of the European Union to bar North American beef imports. Although international regulatory bodies have declared that growth hormones used in beef production are safe, the E.U. has banned imports of American beef because, the E.U. argues, there is a consumer perception that growth hormones are a risk.

Surveys suggest that consumers would reduce beef consumption if American beef, possibly raised with growth promoters, was imported; therefore, American beef must be banned to retain consumption levels. The United States recently filed a complaint with the World Trade Organization, saying that the E.U.'s position on growth hormones in beef was nothing more than a non-tariff trade barrier.

American dairy farmers remain divided on the use of rBST, with strong opposition in Wisconsin and Vermont. But their concerns are largely economic and political, which are traditionally matters of social policy. The report by the U.S. Executive Branch of the Federal Government (1994) found that rBST was likely to reinforce productivity changes, such as larger, more productive farms with lower employment, that have been occurring for decades in the American dairy industry. Science is a poor conduit to air social concerns because it creates mistrust in the entire scientific approval system. An editorial in the *Wisconsin State Journal*, about a report from the Office of Technology Assessment which found rBST posed no threat to humans, noted as much, concluding that "many farmers may reject this new technology ... but it ought to be their choice, not the choice of legislators who can't back up their case with hard science."[103]

The primary concern for dairy farmers seems to be that of individual choice. As a management tool, rBST favours good herd management rather than small or large farms, and its adoption pattern to date in the United States suggests that it has a specific niche role to play in managing a dairy farm. Of nine technologies introduced in the U.S. dairy industry over the past several decades – scientific feeding, Dairy Herd Improvement (DHI) testing, mechanical milking, artificial insemination, electronic farm records, milking parlours, bulk tanks, freestall housing, and embryo transfer – only two (mechanical milking and bulk tanks) were used by 100 per cent of American dairy farmers in 1985. The other technologies in the list ranged from 0.5 to 70 per cent adoption.[104]

Officials at Monsanto Canada have expended considerable resources on communication about rBST, hosting workshops on risk communication and attempting to balance the legal requirement not to promote rBST while it was being considered for approval by Health Canada with a need to provide what Monsanto officials called balanced, factual information: to present their side of the story. Yet despite this investment, Monsanto Canada refused to be interviewed by the *Fifth Estate*, deferring to company headquarters in St Louis, even though there was clearly a Canadian angle to the story. Further, despite extensive training in risk communication, some company officials resorted to the Luddite-allegation: "The people who oppose the technology do it on emotion and scare tactics but not on scientific grounds," said Bob Toth, director of animal sciences for Monsanto.[105]

Monsanto officials, when quoted in the press, would consistently stress that rBST was safe, that rBST had been reviewed and endorsed by every major medical and regulatory body, and that rBST had received more scrutiny than any other animal health product. Monsanto officials were talking about scientific risk, whereas many consumers have a much broader definition of risk. Nelkin suggests that efforts to convince the public about the safety and benefits of new technologies like genetically engineered food, rather than enhancing public confidence, may actually amplify anxieties and mistrust by denying the legitimacy of fundamental social concerns.[106] Certainly this is evident in the Canadian discussion of rBST, where attempts to reassure citizens on the basis of safety have been utterly futile.

Journalistic support for rBST appeared stronger in the United States than in Canada, at least on a relative basis. This may be partly explained by the availability of scientists and others knowledgeable about rBST to comment publicly. In Canada, supporters of rBST were overwhelmingly silent. With a few notable exceptions, many of the researchers who conducted field trials of rBST in the 1980s simply refused to talk to the media, citing the 1989 incident when milk from test herds was pulled from the general milk supply.

Burton and McBride, exploring the broader implications of rBST, argue that "the affiliation of rBST researchers with manufacturers of the product is of necessity a strong one. This leads to further public mistrust and skepticism regarding published scientific results. As a result, misinformation from unqualified (and often unidentified) sources pours into the media. This misinformation causes undue hysteria among dairy producers and consumers."[107] Yet these authors fail to offer solutions – such as always disclosing the source of research funds when talking about research – and utterly fail to appreciate the practice of journalism. Media accounts rely on interviews with individuals; if scientists refuse to talk to the media, what is a journalist supposed to write? Further, the sources in the stories examined here were almost always identified, and the link between misinformation and hysteria sounds more like a rhetorical twist than the results of a research program. The outright refusal publicly to discuss rBST by many Canadian scientists – even when they were obviously what would be considered the Canadian experts on the topic – also contributed to the risk information vacuum and the general perception that rBST was simply bad stuff.

In the absence of credible scientific evidence in the Canadian discussion of rBST, the negative perception that is thereby created can be extremely profound. During a recent seminar about forty members of a local health unit, almost all trained in science, were asked, "Would you drink milk from cows treated with rBST?" One person raised a hand. When asked why they would not drink such milk, several said, "The human health impacts are unclear," or "The animal health impacts are unclear." The health practioners were then asked what scientific information they knew about that the FDA, World Health Organization, and dozens of other professional health bodies that had endorsed rBST were apparently unaware of. They were asked what experiments could be conducted to demonstrate safety and efficacy that had not been conducted to date. Silence followed.[108] The implications of arguing that health regulatory authorities are involved in some sort of conspiracy or that they are ignorant would therefore need to be applied to literally thousands of medical devices, procedures, and pharmaceuticals that are reviewed and regulated each year.

In examining the public discussion of rBST in Canada, traits that are common to the introduction of other new, revolutionary technologies can be identified in the public response: confusion, unrealistic expectation, and finding a way to cope.[109] The United States has found a way to cope. Canada has not.

7 Gene Escape,
or the Pall of Silence
over Plant Biotechnology Risk

WITH ANGELA GRIFFITHS AND
KATHERINE BARRETT

The use of chemical inputs into agricultural food production has a lengthy history. As early as 1000 B.C. the Chinese used sulphur as a fumigant. In the sixteenth century arsenic-containing compounds were utilized as insecticides. By the 1930s the production of modern synthetic chemicals commenced. With the onset of World War II there was a rapid increase in the production and use of chemical substances such as DDT, used for control of insect-transmitting malaria. The post-war era marked the start of the modern agrochemical industry, and as a direct result of technical advancements in chemical production during this period, various insecticides, fungicides, and fumigants found their place in agriculture and food production.[1]

Today, rather than spraying chemicals in fields to bolster crop production, genes from naturally occurring organisms with pesticidal properties are being genetically engineered into plants. And, just as in the earlier period of chemical pesticides use, the public discussion of agricultural biotechnology is being framed narrowly in terms of risks versus benefits rather than in a more complete outlook where the objectives are to maximize benefits while minimizing risks.

BIOTECHNOLOGY IN CANADA:
DEFINITION AND REGULATION

Biotechnology is defined in the Canadian Environmental Protection Act as "the application of science and engineering in the direct or indirect use of living organisms, or parts or products of living organisms in their natural or modified forms."[2] This definition is used by all government departments. Such general definitions are controversial because they can be used to describe processes and products as diverse as the use of yeast to make bread and beer at one end of the spectrum to gene replacement in humans on the other.

Defining biotechnology so broadly allows the government to support its position that biotechnology is nothing new and can therefore be regulated on a product-by-product basis under existing legislation, some of which dates back to the early part of this century. John Durant has noted that attempts to characterize biotechnology as merely trivial extensions of the familiar techniques of baking, viniculture, and breeding are "pedantic" at best: "The technologies employed are completely different and it is the power and precision of the new molecular biology that drives both industrial growth and public concern."[3] The notion that, for example, human gene therapy is "just like" making beer offends common sense. So already in the basic conception of this technological domain itself Canadian government regulators have assumed a stance that has the potential to arouse controversy.

The term "biotechnology" actually describes many different techniques. Recently it has become synonymous with genetic engineering, which involves the transfer of a specific piece of genetic information from one organism to another. For example, genes from viruses can be inserted into plants, and genes from humans can be inserted into pigs. These processes result in what are called "transgenics" or genetically engineered organisms, also called genetically modified organisms, or GMOs. Genetic exchange between different species also occurs in nature, usually via bacterial species and viruses; the extent to which genetic engineering accelerates such natural processes is controversial.

The European Economic Community (EEC) differentiates natural genetic exchanges from genetic engineering by defining a genetically engineered organism as "an organism in which the genetic material has been altered in a way that does not occur naturally by mating and/or natural recombination."[4] The EEC does not consider traditional breeding programs, mutagenesis, cell fusion, in vitro fertilization, or polyploidy induction as techniques that lead to the production of genetically modified organisms because these techniques do not result in the introduction of foreign DNA into an organism.

The structure and nature of deoxyribonucleic acid was elucidated in the decades between 1940 and 1960, and geneticists Cohen and Boyer created the first genetically engineered organism in 1975.[5] About the same time a self-imposed moratorium on genetic engineering experiments by the scientific community was championed by Paul Berg in 1974, and the subsequent Asilomar conference in California in 1975 then took up the risks associated with genetic engineering in terms of laboratory safety and accidental escape. The result was widespread public debate. Whether such actions were actual concern or public relations, they have served the biological community in a way the nuclear industry can only dream about: regardless of the actual outcome (and many believe the debate led to positive guidelines), the perception was of a community that cared enough to debate the issues in a very public way. The moratorium was lifted the following year, when the U.S. National Institutes of Health issued guidelines for experimentation with genetically engineered organisms.[6]

In Canada most biotechnology research has focused on agricultural biotechnology and the production of pharmaceuticals. Over three thousand field trials of genetically engineered plant material have been conducted in Canada since 1988.[7] There are also fifty current applications for field trials for microbes that act as fertilizers. Dozens of genetically engineered food products have been approved for commercial use, including canola, soybean, potato, corn, and tomatoes. The regulation of biotechnology is complex, and jurisdiction is spread over several government departments with different mandates. In general, regulation is based on end products as opposed to the process by which the products were made, as is shown in table 7.1.

This chapter provides an overview of risk communication activities related to a specific group of plant biotechnology techniques, namely, the creation of what are called "plants with novel traits" (PNTs). PNTs are regulated by the Plant Biotechnology Office in the Food Production and Inspection Branch of Agriculture and Agri-Food Canada (AAFC). All plants with novel traits are required to undergo an environmental safety or risk assessment, based on information provided by industry applicants to the Plant Biotechnology Office, before they can be field-tested or offered for sale. None of this information is freely available to the public, unless the company or agency chooses to release it; the Plant Biotechnology Office publishes "decision documents" after a PNT has been approved. The decision document as a communication tool will be discussed later in this chapter.

EXPECTED RISKS AND BENEFITS OF BIOTECHNOLOGY

Many applications of biotechnology, including genetic engineering in particular, have raised public concerns. These centre around environmental, health, and ethical issues and are outlined in table 7.2.

Common to all of the concerns outlined above are four broad issues:

Table 7.1
Regulation of products of biotechnology

Type of Product	Function of Product	Regulating Acts and Departments
Plants	Agricultural crops (including pesticidal plants) Forestry species Plants for bioremediation	Seeds Act and Plant Protection Act Agriculture and Agri-Food Canada
	Plants or plant parts which are for human consumption	Food and Drugs Act Health Canada
	Plants or plant parts which are for animal consumption	Feeds Act Agriculture and Agri-Food Canada
Microbes	Biofertilizers	Fertilizers Act Agriculture and Agri-Food Canada
	Bioremediation	Canadian Environmental Protection Act Environment Canada
	Microbial pesticides	Pest Control Products Act Pest Management Regulatory Agency Health Canada
Animals	Animals for human consumption and for the production of pharmaceuticals	Health of Animals Act Agriculture and Agri-Food Canada Food and Drugs Act Health Canada
Fish	Fish (for human consumption)	Food and Drugs Act Health Canada Fisheries Act Department of Fisheries and Oceans
Pharmaceuticals	Human treatments	Food and Drugs Act Health Canada
	Animal treatments	Health of Animals Act Agriculture and Agri-Food Canada Food and Drugs Act Health Canada

1 The levels of uncertainty inherent in the release of genetically modified organisms into the environment

Current knowledge of ecological systems, particularly microbial systems, is limited, making it difficult to predict interactions and impacts.[8] The use of living organisms also imparts a high level of uncertainty, since they continuously reproduce and mutate. Recombination between viral DNA and wild viruses to create new pathogens is of particular concern.

A related concern is the commodification of life. Much biotechnology research and development is carried out by corporations or by public research institutions in partnership with industry.[9] Therefore, the products and processes developed are proprietary. One of the most controversial issues that has arisen as a result of ubiquitous industry involvement in biotechnology research is the patenting of life forms. A patent gives the holder exclusive ownership of that organism and all its offspring. In the case of a cell line, the patent holder would have rights to any product developed from that cell line.

2 Ensuring adequate consent from all persons directly or indirectly affected by biotechnology

Issues of obtaining adequate consent are most often associated with the collection of DNA from indigenous peoples and with the patenting of human cell lines. John Moore, whose doctor was granted a patent on his spleen cells, argued in a court case that he did not give consent for his cells to be patented and that he should at least be entitled to a share of any revenues generated by the cell line.[10] He lost the court case on both counts. This decision implies that one does not "own" the cells in one's body and DNA and therefore that one's consent for others to appropriate them is not required.

3 Communicating adequately the risks and benefits of biotechnologies to the public

Communication with the public about the possible risks of new technologies is very important, especially when specific individuals or groups will be exposed to those risks. The regulators' pretensions to the contrary, to the majority of citizens these are novel technologies with characteristics that are most unfamiliar. Indeed, they are capable of arousing apprehensions, such as the fear that there may be unintended consequences of releasing an engineered organism into the environment, unforeseen to its developers, which adversely affect the health of humans or other species, and which cannot then be undone or mitigated adequately. The greater part of this chapter will focus on the provision of information to those directly and indirectly affected by biotechnology.

4 The fair distribution of risks and benefits among all parties

This concern is common to many risky technologies. For example, benefits of nuclear power may be enjoyed by thousands in the form

Table 7.2
Public concerns about biotechnology

Issue	Specific concerns/risks
Environmental	Increased weediness and/or invasiveness of plants
	Escape of gene to other organisms
	Competition of transgenic organisms with indigenous organisms
	Development of target species resistance
	Effects on biodiversity and sustainability
	Unforeseen impact on ecosystems
	Development of new plant pathogens
Health	Creation of new pathogens, allergens and/or irritants
	Increased antibiotic resistance in pathogens
	Unknown hazards of recombinant vaccines
	Occupational safety
Ethical	Patenting of life forms and traditional knowledge
	Eugenics
	Animal welfare
	"Playing God"
	Labelling and consumer choice
	Implications of genetic screening (privacy, discrimination, anxiety)
	Abuse and/or loss of control over reproductive technologies
	Effects of biotechnology on developing countries
	Targeting specific groups of people as sources of genetic information (e.g. human genome and diversity projects)

of cheap energy, but the bulk of the risk is borne by those living in the proximity of a nuclear power plant. Such public concerns have been reflected in media coverage of plant biotechnology. For instance, Dan Westell wrote in a *Globe and Mail* story, "Canada's first gene-modified commercial crop is ready for planting next month in Saskatchewan, primarily in the interests of selling a herbicide." The story mentions that the canolas have been deemed safe for people, animals, and the environment by the federal departments of Health, Agriculture, and Environment, and that "it is multinational chemical companies that are carrying out the research to increase resistance to herbicides. A seed that can tolerate a specific herbicide potentially means more sales for the herbicide manufacturer."[11]

Steve Meister, communications manager for AgrEvo Canada Inc. of Regina, the developer of one of the approved genetically engineered canolas, is quoted as saying that selling herbicides "is really our interest in it":

Possible benefits of biotechnology include improved tools for treating disease, improved bioremediation technologies and increased productivity in agriculture. The introduction of herbicide tolerant canolas may result in a shift towards the use of more "environmentally friendly" herbicides like glyphosate, thus reducing the environmental impact of agriculture. Traits like stress tolerance, insect and virus resistance may reduce the need for some pesticides and extend the geographical range that some crops can be grown in, thus increasing production and productivity. Genetically modified microbes may also be enhanced to improve their ability to clean up degraded lands and toxic waste dumps. These have the potential to become significant, beneficial technologies. The goal, again, is to maximize the benefits this new technology can bring, while minimizing risks; and to do so in a socially responsible manner.

Agricultural biotechnology has been represented as the next "green revolution" and is predicted to have a significant impact on the future of agriculture, by groups as diverse as the United Nations Conference on Environment and Development, the Organization for Economic Co-operation and Development (OECD), the biotechnology industry, Agriculture and Agri-Food Canada, agricultural researchers, and environmental groups.[12] Agriculture is an extremely important source of trade revenue for Canada. In 1994 agricultural production accounted for 8 per cent of Canada's GDP and 15 per cent of Canadian jobs.

Nevertheless, given the number and range of the troublesome issues that have been raised about biotechnology (summarized in table 7.2 above), concerns have been raised about the strong promotional culture in favour of genetic-engineering technologies in Agriculture and Agri-Food Canada, to the exclusion of alternative technologies.[13] For example, a handout from the Research Branch supplied to the public bears the heading "Research Branch: Where Biotechnology Is a Way of Life." The combination of promotional and regulatory activities within a department may represent a conflict of interest and certainly calls the credibility and independence of the department as a regulator into question.[14] The transfer of the Biotechnology Strategies and Co-ordination Office to the newly created Canadian Food Inspection Agency (effective 1 April 1997) may alleviate some of these concerns by, theoretically, separating the promotional and regulatory functions.

In the sections that follow we focus on two products of agricultural biotechnology that have been commercialized in Canada: first, canola engineered to contain a gene that makes this plant tolerant of particular herbicides; and second, genetically engineered potatoes incorporating a gene that produces an insecticide (Bt) that confers resistance to an insect pest (the Colorado Potato Beetle).[15]

HERBICIDE-TOLERANT CANOLA AND THE RISK OF GENE ESCAPE

1 The Problem – and the Biotechnology Solution

Weed control is a major problem in canola because the plant closely resembles many weedy species, and thus it is difficult to kill the weeds without also harming the canola. As canola is an important cash crop in Canada, second only to wheat in terms of acreage,[16] maximum yield and cost-effective use of herbicides and insecticides is of great interest to many commercial growers and to Canada's balance of trade.

Weed management in canola currently requires the application of several expensive herbicides in order to obtain adequate weed control.[17] However, through genetic engineering, crops such as canola can be designed to tolerate broad spectrum herbicides – which would normally kill the crop – by introducing genes that detoxify the herbicide, or by replacing the plant gene product that is sensitive to the herbicide. The broad-spectrum herbicides currently available are more environmentally benign, at least in a range of impacts on non-target organisms, than were their crop-specific predecessors. As a result, projected benefits of herbicide-tolerant plants include reduced overall herbicide use, resulting in reduced input costs, and some lower environmental impacts than other current options. Four transgenic canola varieties were approved by AAFC in 1995, and three more were added in 1996. These canola varieties are tolerant to several different chemicals, including glyphosate, glufosinate, and imidazolinone.

2 Risks Identified in the Scientific Literature

In agricultural settings existing management practices may become ineffective in controlling weeds. In natural ecosystems new, persistent, or invasive plants may change population dynamics and alter interactions among many organisms, with unknown long-term effects. Most of these environmental risks turn on the concepts of "weediness" or "invasiveness." Two specific questions about risks are usually posed: First, will the transgenic plant itself become a weed through the presence of the new gene? Second, will the new gene spread from the original transgenic entity to other organisms in the environment?

This risk of a plant becoming a weed is termed "increased weediness." However, the phrasing is sometimes misleading because canola already displays several weedy characteristics. For example, canola flowers produce a tremendous amount of pollen, a trait which may promote outcrossing if this pollen is widely dispersed. Furthermore, once seeds are formed in the plant, the seed heads readily shatter, efficiently spreading the seeds to new ground.

The risk of a gene spreading from the transgenic organism to other organisms in the environment is termed "gene escape." This can occur in several ways. The most common "escape route" is through hybrid-ization (sexual reproduction), where pollen from the transgenic plant is carried by wind or insects to a non-transgenic, wild plant. If the pollen fertilizes the wild plant, the resulting hybrid will contain the transgene. This process is also referred to as cross-pollination or out-crossing. If the new hybrid plants survive and reproduce with other wild plants of the same species, the transgene may become firmly established in the wild plant population. These processes have likely occurred with crop plants since the beginning of agriculture; however, the introduction of completely new genes adds new risks.

Gene escape can also occur through means such as accidental spreading of seeds during transportation (seeds often fall off trucks, resulting in familiar roadside growth); transfer of genes through micro-organisms or viruses; and spread of the transgenic plant through vegetative growth, such as tuber production in potatoes. The consequences of gene escape are manifold and difficult to predict, and thus the whole issue of gene escape from herbicide-tolerant crops is beset with controversy and ambiguity.

Brassica napus, the canola species currently released as a transgenic variety, is a primarily self-fertilizing plant, whereas *Brassica rapa*, the other commonly grown canola species, is primarily cross-fertilizing. No transgenic *B. rapa* varieties have been released as yet, but field trials are underway. In self-fertilizing plants, pollen (male) and egg (female) from a single plant can combine to produce seed, and cross-pollination from another plant is not necessary for reproduction. However, as discussed earlier, canola produces a vast amount of pollen, and it has been known for decades that this pollen can be carried long distances by wind and insects. Trapping experiments for wind-borne pollen carried out at least since 1955 have detected canola pollen in the air 70 km from the plants. The major insect pollinators of canola are honeybees and bumblebees, and both species are capable of carrying pollen for several kilometres.[18] Many of these early studies of pollen dispersal were aimed at controlling the inflow of pollen to canola fields because farmers were interested in keeping "pure line" crops unaffected by outside pollen sources. The outflow of pollen from fields – gene escape – only became a seriously studied problem after the development of transgenic plants.

Given that pollen dispersal from transgenic canola certainly will occur, two possible scenarios arise: one, transgenic canola pollen will fertilize non-transgenic canola plants; or two, transgenic canola pollen will fertilize non-transgenic wild plants: that is, the transgenic variety will form hybrid plants with different plant species.

Theoretical arguments for the escape of transgenes in particular have been expressed in scientific literature at least since 1988.[19] Although there is no well-argued reason why transgenic canola cannot hybridize with wild species, and no reason why such hybrids cannot express and pass on the transgenic characteristic, experiments that clearly demonstrated this phenomenon were not published until March 1996. In a research paper published in *Nature*, Mikkelson *et al.* report that transgenic herbicide-tolerant canola readily hybridizes with the wild species *B. rapa*. The resulting plants retain many wild, weedy characteristics but are also herbicide-tolerant. Furthermore, the new hybrid variety could "backcross" with other wild plants, thus establishing the herbicide-tolerant gene in the wild population. The authors therefore predict "a possible rapid spread of genes from oilseed rape to the weedy relative B. campestris [rapa]."[20]

It is generally accepted among the scientific community that gene escape from transgenic canola plants will occur, and in this light many researchers are calling for studies on the possible environmental effects. Specific research questions that should be addressed are: Will the transgene be maintained in the new hybrid? Will the hybrids be weedy or invasive? What will be the impact of the new hybrids? Some researchers claim that herbicide-tolerant crops will not have a significant impact on the environment because the herbicide tolerance trait will be lost in plant populations which are not subjected to the selective pressure of the agricultural fields on which herbicides are applied. However, other researchers dispute this claim, pointing out that herbicides are frequently sprayed on field margins and roadsides. This is important because an exacerbated weed problem within the agricultural ecosystem as a result of increased herbicide usage may still have a significant environmental impact, not to mention effects on yields and farm income. As well, this argument cannot be used for insect-tolerant and stress-tolerant plants, which may also have a selective advantage in natural settings.

As mentioned above, evidence for the environmental impact of herbicide-resistant crops is fraught with uncertainty and controversy. Although it has been clearly established that gene escape will occur, there is no scientific consensus on the significance this will have for the environment. Much of the difficulty in predicting impact lies in the inherent complexity of ecosystems. Ultimately, environmental impact depends on the genetic characteristic expressed in the plant, and the effect that the transgene has on the plant's survival in relation to other organisms in the environment.

3 Public Dialogue about Risks Associated with Herbicide Tolerant Canola

Few government documents have been published which are specifically intended to communicate with the public about possible risks associated with biotechnology. However, theoretical risks and concerns have been identified in several government publications and workshops since 1980.[21] The only documents that AAFC has published that are specifically aimed at public communication are *Biotechnology: Science for Better Living* and the pamphlet series *Biotechnology in Agriculture and Food*. Both of these documents were produced by the Biotechnology Strategies and Coordination Office (BSCO), whose mandate is primarily to promote inter-departmental communication about biotechnology regulation. In an interview conducted with one of the authors in September 1996, representatives of both the Plant Biotechnology Office and the BSCO were adamant that their mandate is not to promote biotechnology.[22]

The title of the first document, *Biotechnology: Science for Better Living*, clearly implies a positive attitude towards biotechnology, an impression reinforced in a section entitled "Questions about the new technology." The pamphlet assures the reader, "Before anyone releases these new products into the environment, it is important for research to be carried out to demonstrate that the organism does not turn into a future pest or weed, the organism does not exhibit unexpected characteristics outside the laboratory, which could affect other useful plants or organisms, and unintended characteristics do not spread to related species." The statement implies that this research has already been conducted (much of it has not) and certainly does not reflect the level of scientific disagreement over issues like gene escape and good management practices. What is worse, it can easily be read as suggesting or implying that the department would not approve for release or sale any transgenic plant that could increase weediness or spread any of its novel traits to other species. This ambiguity makes the statement quoted above at least potentially misleading; if the construction of this ambiguity were intentional, it would be a serious matter indeed.

The second BSCO publication consists of a series of pamphlets, only two of which make reference to risks or concerns. In one of them we read: "Some people have expressed concern about the safety of these new technologies, especially the possibility of genetically modified organisms adversely affecting plants and other organisms outside the lab. To deal with these concerns, scientists and government regulators have taken steps to carefully assess all new products of biotechnology. Before a product can be released into the environment, it must be evaluated for safety and effectiveness, based on data collected from extensive testing." Concerns are attributed to unidentified "people," whereas "scientists and government regulators" are the ones who are said to have assessed the risks. The statement implies that no scientists have expressed concern about the release of transgenics. This implication is misleading.

The following government documents and workshops also constitute an indirect form of public communications. In 1980 the Science Council sponsored a workshop on biotechnology involving academics, government, and industry. In general the workshop report is positive towards biotechnology, and most of its recommendations relate to how biotechnology can be supported financially and structurally in Canada. Industry, Science and Technology Canada conducted a workshop in 1993 entitled "Biotechnology and Public Awareness" for government, industry, and the public. At the workshop Joyce Byrne, then head of the Biotechnology Strategies Office of AAFC, gave an overview of Agriculture Canada's communication strategy on biotechnology:[23] "The communication strategy identifies a number of specific measures for promoting biotechnology, including a glossy brochure aimed at building public awareness. The brochure is designed to be eye-catching and is intended to leave readers with a positive feeling about biotechnology and its potential." Note that risk communication is not listed as one of the objectives.[24]

Finally, a consultation program by AAFC on biotechnology regulation was also held in 1993, in which three major issues were suggested for discussion: food labelling, plants with novel herbicide tolerance, and insect-resistant plants. Although risks of transgene escape were brought up in the discussions conducted by AAFC, no specific research program or follow-up monitoring of the issue was implemented.

AAFC issues two types of documents dealing with specific crop types: "information documents" on the biology of crops and "decision documents" on the transgenic variety. The biology document for *B. napus* indicates that outcrossing rates can be up to 20 to 30 per cent, and that pollen is transferred primarily through insects rather than wind. The document also comments that *B. napus* can be quite problematic as a volunteer weed and can occur in large numbers in subsequent crops, due to small seed size and shattering. It goes on to state that in disturbed areas, these species can be persistent because of their "primary colonizing nature." That said, the document concludes that since these species are not listed in the Weed Seed Order nor recorded as being invasive of natural systems, "there is no evidence that in Canada B. napus has weed or pest characteristics."[25] *Weeds of Canada* defines a weed as "a plant that grows where man does not want it to grow, in grainfields, row crops, pastures, hay fields, lawns and other disturbed areas."[26] According to this definition, canola definitely can be a weed.

This point is a key one, because the assertion that canola is not weedy is one of the main rationales used in the decision document to prove the environmental safety of the herbicide-tolerant plants. In fact the definition of a "weed" is surprisingly controversial among agronomists, ecologists, and weed scientists. Furthermore, a paucity of information on invasive and weedy species frequently renders the "no evidence" argument untenable at best. Planned studies to determine if natural outcrossing under field conditions occurs are also mentioned in the biology document. However, this document was issued in December 1994, and the first herbicide-tolerant canola varieties were approved for commercial release in spring 1995; one can only conclude that the studies were not done before commercial release was approved.

Decision documents are made available to the public after a transgenic plant has been approved for field trials or commercial release. In the canola decision documents, transgene escape is linked to increased invasiveness of the recipient plant. In other words, the possibility of transgene escape is acknowledged but is only deemed important if invasiveness is increased thereby. The document does not specify under what conditions invasiveness was studied by the applicant, if at all. For all the herbicide-tolerant canolas, AAFC concludes that there is no reason to believe that the transgenic lines would behave differently from parent lines in their interactions with the environment. However, a note is added in all of the herbicide-tolerant canola decision documents:

A longer term concern, if there is general adoption of several different crop and specific weed management systems, is the potential development of crop volunteers with a combination of novel resistance to different herbicides. This could result in the loss of the use of these herbicides and any of their potential benefits. Therefore, agricultural extension personnel in both the private and public sectors, should promote careful management practices for growers who use these herbicide tolerant crops to minimize the development of multiple resistance.

No specific recommendations are made as to what constitutes careful management practices. It is well documented that farmers frequently do not follow recommended practices and have a strong mistrust of government information sources.[27] Therefore, relying on good management practices at the farm level does little to minimize or communicate risk.

AAFC's handling of the risk of transgene escape is inconsistent. In the biology documents and the decision documents, the department acknowledges the possibility of transgene escape, but in its more general public documents, the public is assured that risk is negligible. In addition, there has been no attempt to gauge the impact of transgene escape or to communicate risk information to the users of the product.

ENGINEERED POTATOES AND THE RISK OF INCREASING INSECT RESISTANCE

1 The Problem – and the Biotechnology Solution

Potatoes are the most valuable vegetable crop in Canada, worth about $293 million in 1994, and they are grown in all Canadian provinces. A primary concern of potato growers is the effective control of insect pests, especially the Colorado Potato Beetle (CPB), the most significant pest of potatoes across Canada and in many growing areas of the United States.[28]

By using the techniques of genetic engineering, it is now possible to produce crops that contain an active pesticide in each cell of the plant. Topical application of that particular pesticide can therefore be reduced or eliminated, since pests are killed when they ingest a small part of the transgenic plant. A gene that expresses a protein toxic to CPB has been inserted into Russet Burbank potatoes, and the resultant transgenic variety has been shown to effectively control CPB damage in field trials. The gene used in creating these potatoes was isolated from the bacterium *Bacillus thuringiensis*, and the plants have been nicknamed "Bt potatoes." To understand this technology, and the resulting risks and benefits, it is necessary to review some of the bacterium's biology.

Bacillus thuringiensis (Bt) is a common soil bacterium first identified in Germany in 1911 and named after the German province of Thuringia. Although its ecological significance is poorly understood, Bt has played a vital role in agricultural and forestry pest control for over fifty years. It was first used as a commercial insecticide in France in 1938. Since then, preparations of Bt have been used against serious pests including gypsy moth, spruce budworm, and the European corn borer.[29] Bt's insecticidal properties have provided several important advantages over chemical sprays. Bt toxins are very specific, and so there is little or no effect on non-target insects or other animals, including humans. The toxic Bt proteins are readily degraded by ultraviolet light, and there are no known long-term environmental effects.[30] This lack of persistence is particularly important for delaying development of insect resistance to Bt. Since Bt toxin is derived from a naturally occurring organism in the environment, the short-term effects of application may be more predictable and less harmful than for synthetic chemicals. For these reasons, Bt has become an extremely valuable, low-impact method of insect control. It has been widely used in industrial agriculture and organic farming alike, as well as in forest pest management for spruce budworm control.

The secret to Bt's insect-killing success lies in protein crystals formed when the bacterium enters the spore-producing stage of its life cycle. The proteins that make up these crystals are called "delta endotoxins," and they are toxic to particular insect species. To be effective the endotoxin must be ingested by the target insect. Ingestion results in gut paralysis, and the insect stops feeding and dies after consuming very little foliage. Many different delta endotoxins have been characterized in terms of their toxic properties, and the genes that encode for the different proteins have been isolated. Known as "Cry," these genes are categorized according to the family of insects susceptible to the encoded protein toxin: Lepidoptera (including gypsy moth and spruce budworm); Diptera (including mosquitoes and black flies); and Coleoptera (including CPB, elm leaf beetle, and yellow meal worm).[31]

The isolation and characterization of the Cry genes made the development of Bt-producing plants possible. Transgenic crops (including potatoes, corn, cotton, and soybeans) have subsequently been developed which incorporate different Cry genes, rendering them resistant to different insects. The Cry-3 gene was isolated from the *Bacillus thuringiensis* subspecies *tenenbrionsis* and is known as Btt. The Cry-3 gene product is specific to some Coleoptera, including CPB. Nature-Mark Potatoes, a business arm of Monsanto, developed potato plants that contain the Cry-3 gene and resist CPB attack. Confined field trials of Bt potatoes have been conducted in Canada since 1992, in seven different provinces to date. In 1995 Health Canada concluded that the transgenic variety and currently commercialized varieties of potatoes were "substantially equivalent" in terms of human health and safety.[32] The United States approved Bt potatoes for commercialization in 1995. In January 1996 AAFC released the decision document stating that "AAFC has determined that these plants with novel traits should not pose concern to environmental safety" and authorized unconfined release of Bt potatoes under the trade name "NewLeaf."

2 Risks Identified in the Scientific Literature

Ironically, the arguments for replacing Bt-based sprays with transgenic Bt crops often rest on regarding the very advantages of Bt foliar sprays – discussed above – as problems that could be overcome by genetically engineering the toxin into the plant cells. The promised advantages of transgenic crops include a broader host range (since several genes can be engineered into the same plant) and continuous presence in the field (since the toxin would not be washed away by rain, or degraded by UV light). However, these same "advantages," especially persistence of the toxin in the field, may increase the risk of adverse environmental effects and the development of resistance in insects.

Although several risks have been associated with the release of Bt crops, here we focus on the development of insects that are resistant to the Bt toxin. Constant exposure to the pesticide, as in the case of transgenic crops, selects for those few individuals that can survive the dose. In a typical "survival of the reproductively fittest" scenario, the resistance mutation is passed on to subsequent generations, potentially resulting in a completely resistant population of insects. If insects develop resistance to Bt, this valuable method of pest control is rendered useless.

Prior to 1985 "all efforts to select strains of insects resistant to the delta endotoxins had failed," and it was therefore generally concluded among scientists that resistance could not occur.[33] However, the theoretical possibility of resistance development had been recognized since at least 1971,[34] and in fact resistance in CPB is a particularly logical prediction for several reasons:

- By 1993 CPB had developed resistance to all registered chemical insecticides and had been shown to develop resistance to these chemicals in as little as one season.
- Coleopteran species are particularly likely to develop resistance to pesticides because, unlike other families, both the larval and the adult stages feed on the host plant. This activity increases selective pressure by increasing exposure to the pesticide. According to Ferro, "Few other agricultural pests have been as successful as Colorado potato beetle in developing resistance to insecticides."[35]

Resistance of several insect species to the Bt toxin has been described for at least thirty years. The first report of resistance in an agricultural pest, however, was made in 1985.[36] In this case moths trapped in storage bins of Bt-treated grain developed resistance to Bt within a few generations. Significantly, the researcher commented that such conditions are ideal for selection of resistant insects: the Bt toxin is stable, and successive generations of insects are exposed to high doses. Note that these are precisely the conditions created by the use of transgenic Bt crops.

Bt resistance in CPB was first detected in the laboratory in 1990.[37] Further experiments in 1993 demonstrated that CPB could develop resistance to the Cry-3 gene product in as little as three generations; after twelve generations the selected strains of insects were fifty-nine times more resistant to Bt than were the unselected strains.[38] The researchers predicted that resistance in CPB populations could develop within three to five years, especially under the high exposures supplied by transgenic plants. Similar predictions of resistance and experiments showing resistance development were published by entomologists and ecologists in 1992, 1993, 1994, and 1995, right up to the time that Bt potatoes were approved by AAFC and the U.S. Environmental Protection Agency (EPA).[39] It is now well recognized among scientists and government regulatory agencies alike that CPB will eventually develop resistance to the Bt toxin, both to the transgenic crops and, as a result, to the valuable Bt-based foliar sprays.

The key question now is: Can the development of Bt-resistance be managed or at least delayed? The most frequently recommended management strategy is the use of "refugia." This means that when Bt crops are planted, a small section of the field is sown with non-transgenic crops. The idea is that this small area would provide a "refuge" in which insects could breed which would not be in contact with the toxin and therefore would have no need to acquire resistance. The constant supply of non-resistant insects would then interbreed with the resistant ones flying amongst the transgenic crops, thereby diluting the number of resistant individuals in the population. The refugia strategy is often combined with a "high dose" strategy, yielding the much discussed "high-dose-plus-refugia" management scheme. The dose refers to the level of expression of Bt in the plants: a high dose will kill most insects, and a mid-range or low dose will only kill some insects, thereby selecting for those which are resistant. The trick is to combine just the right-sized refuge with the right dose of Bt.

Other management strategies have been proposed. Among them are: rotation of plantings between transgenic and non-transgenic crops (in the years when non-transgenic crops are planted, use of other insecticides would be required); mixing seeds so that each field contains a variety of crops, each carrying different toxin genes; engineering two or more toxin genes into a single plant (the latter two schemes assume other toxin genes have been identified and are effective); and finally, modifying the transgene so that the toxin is only produced in certain plant parts, or at certain times during plant development. There is no lack of theories. What is lacking, however, is experimental evidence showing any one of these strategies is actually effective. Although computer simulation models have shown that management strategies should work, at the time of writing (and certainly at the time AAFC approved Bt potatoes) no experimental results were published showing that "sound management practices" would prevent or even delay resistance development in CPB. Part of the problem is that such data are difficult to collect without first releasing the crops on a large scale and then conducting extensive monitoring.

3 Public Dialogue about Risks Associated with Bt Potatoes

The decision document on the environmental safety of NewLeaf potatoes (January, 1996) fully acknowledges that "resistance to the Btt protein could ... develop following continued exposure to the NewLeaf potatoes" and that "development of such a resistance would result in the loss of these valuable Btt tools." It also comments that target insects are exposed to significantly higher levels of Btt when feeding on the potatoes than they would be with a foliar spray, leading to high selection pressures for Btt-resistant insects. The document therefore recommends use of refugia as a "major component of the resistance management plan." At the same time it acknowledges that "even though the majority of the scientific community agrees that this approach sounds effective in theory, it is very difficult at this point to predict the extent and rapidity of resistance development without field validation of the proposed strategy."

Although AAFC's decision documents contain a discussion of possible risks, AAFC does not have a policy to ensure that these documents are widely distributed. Interested parties have to request them from the Plant Biotechnology Office, or obtain them from provincial extension agents who are not explicitly informed about the risks. Electronic distribution and the World Wide Web could facilitate a greater discussion of risks and benefits.

AAFC granted approval for NewLeaf potatoes based on an agreement that the manufacturer, Monsanto Canada, would devise an adequate management strategy. Furthermore, AAFC gave Monsanto the responsibility for communicating this strategy, its related risks, and any observed operational shortcomings to farmers, field managers, and AAFC itself. To analyse AAFC's proxy risk communication effort, therefore, we must examine the actual risk communication practices of private companies such as Monsanto. An eagerness to get Bt crops into the field is reflected in Monsanto's recent advertisement in *Ontario Farmer* magazine. The ad, for corn carrying Monsanto's "Yield-Guard" (Bt) gene, gives a clear message to farmers about using this product: "You don't change the way you do things, such as adjusting your planting schedules, crop management or herbicide program." There is no mention whatsoever of risks or refugia. Based on the scientific evidence outlined above, we can confidently say that this advertisement constitutes neither "sound management practices" nor adequate risk communication of any kind.

NatureMark, the developers of the Bt potato, have issued several technical documents aimed at farmers growing Bt potatoes. In one of them the following comment is made: "Studies have shown that high expression [of Bt], in combination with an adequate refuge, can delay resistance development for many years." For the recommended size of refugia the technical information says: "Entomologists recommend that at least 20 per cent of your acreage should be unimproved potatoes." But these documents never mention specific monitoring plans for resistant insects, which is stipulated as a requirement in the decision document for commercializing these crops. In general, the technical information supplied by the company infers a scientific consensus on the effectiveness of refugia for delaying the development of resistance and on the proportion of refugia in the planted fields as a whole. As we have seen, such a consensus does not exist.

Several stories in both the farm and general press have discussed the propensity for genetically engineered Bt-containing potatoes to accelerate the development of resistance in CPB.[40] During the summer of 1996, a debate raged in American newspapers and journals over the effectiveness of Bt-engineered cotton after potentially damaging bollworms cropped up in high numbers that year throughout the Cotton Belt, even on plants grown from Monsanto's genetically engineered Bollgard seeds – advertised as all but bollworm-proof.[41] Nevertheless, many agricultural scientists said it was far too early to assess whether the Bt-containing crops were a success or not. What did become apparent is that, regardless of the resistance management strategies suggested by science, no one knows what margin of error is needed to compensate for farmers who will not observe the recommended refuge practices.[42]

Several stories in the United States have described the major scientific effort now underway designed to come up with adequate Bt resistance-management strategies. Organizations such as the international Insecticide Resistance Action Committee – a group of about twenty companies – are working together to make sure their products are effective over time, and the EPA and USDA have organized major conferences on this theme, such as the National Forum on Insect Resistance to *Bacillus thuringiensis*, held in April 1996.[43]

4 Public Opinion and Discussion of Biotechnology

There have been many public opinion surveys of biotechnology in general and agricultural biotechnology in particular. In his comprehensive history of biotechnology, Bud begins by asking: "What other single word is itself the subject of worldwide polling?"[44]

Public perceptions of biotechnology have received extensive attention in recent years in most western countries, including articles, book chapters, conferences, a public perception bibliography series, studies of social implications and public concerns about biotechnology, and entire books.[45] There have been many general surveys of public perception of biotechnology.[46] One U.K. survey specifically related to public perceptions of food production and consumption has been completed and analysed using the psychometric approach developed to understand public risk perceptions.[47] Kelley recently completed a survey of public perceptions of genetic engineering in Australia; several such surveys have also been conducted in Canada. Other regular surveys are now also including questions about biotechnology.[48]

Although relatively few Canadians had heard or read much about biotechnology, opinions regarding specific biotechnology applications appeared strong. Kelley also concluded that Australian voters had firm opinions about biotechnology, and noted that in a democracy voters routinely make decisions about policies about which they have no detailed academic understanding. Consumers will continue to make decisions about biotechnology, whether they are "better educated" or not.

Although those who said they were more aware about biotechnology thought it would offer more benefits than did those who said they were less aware, these same people also thought biotechnology would give rise to more dangers. The notion that enhanced education would automatically increase acceptance of biotechnology is not borne out by these results. An alternative suggestion is that those with more education may be better able to assess critically both the risks and benefits of a new technology such as biotechnology. Kelley made a similar observation and suggested that increases in knowledge lead some people to be more supportive of genetic engineering but lead other people to be less supportive, so that the two effects cancel each other out.

Hagedorn and Allender-Hagedorn concluded the public has expressed a strong perception of being omitted from the process.[49] This is the case even though this same public has been the focus of many different biotechnology educational initiatives that call for including the public as a legitimate partner, using the media to develop public awareness, instituting nationwide public school programs, and developing a special infrastructure to meet legitimate public concerns.[50] These initiatives have shown varying degrees of success or acceptance.[51]

The relatively low levels of public support for a variety of gene transfers change dramatically when a gene transfer is tied to achieving a specific goal that is deemed worthy, such as increasing nutritional content in a food crop. Kelley made this observation and went on to argue that most Australians approve of genetic engineering because they see it as serving goals that they value, not because they understand much about it. Such results can inform risk communication efforts; one interpretation is that risk messages regarding agricultural biotechnology must contain a rationale for engaging in such activity. While many respondents suggested medical or agricultural applications when asked about benefits from biotechnology, these same respondents were concerned about the lack of oversight or felt that the science was "out of control." Risk messages should therefore be designed to address this underlying concern. A related perception on the part of respondents was that experts were not involving citizens in decision-making. Taken together, these results suggest that current regulatory procedures may be perceived to be inadequate.

Media coverage of genetically engineered food, and biotechnology in general, is often polarized: safety versus risk, science moving forward versus science out of control, and competitiveness versus safety. Several opinion pieces were published by all of the dailies surveyed, again emphasizing the polarized aspects of the debate. In "Genetic Engineering: Cause for Caution," Lippman and Bereano contend that the credibility of those promoting the technology is undermined: "Substantial conflicts of interest exist in which the development of science and technology is increasingly bent to the service of private and government interests ... Thus, agricultural plants are genetically engineered to make them tolerant to herbicides so that corporations can continue to sell pesticides along with the new seeds."[52] Compare this with Dennis, who cites the need for biotechnology as the basis for a new, clean, economic engine: "biotechnology will transform the way we live."[53]

Films and novels have a long history of feeding the public an image of science out of control, and when this is coupled with western society's tendency to attach unrealistic expectations to technology, an ideal environment for public apprehension is created.[54] Many print media reports raised the spectre of science out of control, as best exemplified in the 1993 movie Jurassic Park, where recombinant DNA technology replaced nuclear energy as the latest science to fail society. Stories with titles such as "Research Skewed: Bioengineered Food Serves Corporate, Not Public, Needs," "Science Is Playing with Our Food," "Invasion of the Mutant Tomatoes," and "Genetics Expert Fears Mutant Monsters" provide ample fodder for editorial cartoonists, who almost invariably draw upon the Frankenstein ("Frankenfood") metaphor.[55]

Some food writers routinely cite the general dangers of biotechnology. For example, Marion Kane of the Toronto Star calls biotechnology the "most worrisome food trend" and continues: "The genes of animals and plants are sliced and spliced, usually with the object of making more food more cheaply without due regard for the potential harm to human health and the environment."[56] Interspersed with such stories are articles and letters to the editor about business consolidation within the agricultural biotechnology sector, ongoing protests spearheaded by Greenpeace in the European Union about the importation of genetically engineered foodstuffs, and the need for labelling of genetically engineered foods.[57] Late in 1996 the Natural Law Party mounted a cross-Canada book tour featuring Dr John Fagan, which received extensive coverage. Among the exaggerated or erroneous claims promulgated by Fagan and others, and one that deserves specific attention, is the statement that "40 people were killed and thousands were crippled by exposure to gene-tinkered food."[58]

In 1989 there was an outbreak in the United States of a newly recognized fatal blood disease called eosinophilia-myalgia syndrome (EMS). At least twenty-seven people were killed and another fifteen hundred sickened, and the cause finally was traced to certain batches of the amino acid L-tryptophan, manufactured in Japan by Showa Denko and widely available in the United States as a nutritional supplement. It has been estimated that, prior to this outbreak, up to 2 per cent of the U.S. population took L-tryptophan in the belief it helped manage sleeping difficulties, premenstrual syndrome, stress, and depression – this in the absence of any medical data supporting the supplement's effectiveness.

L-tryptophan is manufactured in a fermentation process using a bacterium, Bacillus amyloliquefaciens, in the same way that yeast ferments the sugars in barley into ethanol in beer. Subsequent investigations by American health authorities revealed that Showa Denko made two changes to its L-tryptophan manufacturing process in 1989 which allowed the supplement's contamination. First, the company began using a strain of *B. amyloliquefaciens* that had been genetically engineered to produce larger amounts of L-tryptophan. Second, the company reduced the amount of carbon used to filter out impurities from the final product. Studies have shown that the disease-causing molecule only appears during purification and that cases of EMS have been linked to L-tryptophan produced by Showa Denko as early as 1983, long before the company used a genetically engineered bacterium. The risk information vacuum for biotechnology allows such alarmist and erroneous versions of events to take root and flourish.

5 Maximizing Benefits and Minimizing Risks

Risk communication should be an active, ongoing process between the decision makers and would-be communicators, the scientific community, and the public.

AAFC, for example, should be actively collecting and generating information about biotechnology risks. This includes keeping up to date on published scientific literature, industry information (submitted with environmental assessments), and information from interest groups – such as the major studies published in draft form in the United States by the Edmonds Institute and Public Employees for Enviromental Responsibility (PEER) – and public consultations.[59] Active collection of information is necessary to avoid biases which may arise if AAFC collects only industry information. AAFC – or the plant biotechnology industry acting on its behalf – should also be actively and directly collecting information from farmers who are using the technologies and monitoring for problems that might arise in the field. Databases on particular technologies should be formally maintained, and the public should be allowed reasonable access to them.

AAFC should ensure that up-to-date information is communicated to the public and to users affected by the technologies. At present AAFC's Plant Biotechnology Office does not have a mandate to communicate with farmers directly; instead, they rely on indirect communication through the provincial government and industry. However, at least one branch in the department, the Prairie Farm Rehabilitation Association (PFRA), has a long history of interacting and communicating directly with farmers on conservation issues. In biotechnology matters AAFC should also communicate directly with users, especially about risks, for example in a pamphlet on risks that must accompany seed purchases (which is now done only by industry).

Intra-departmental communication within AAFC is necessary to ensure that research is done to support regulatory needs. The Research Branch has committed itself to biotechnology research. However, searches of the Canadian public research databases (Inventory of Canadian Agricultural Research) failed to reveal any work done by Canadian researchers in addressing ecological or economic risks associated with the commercial release of biotechnology. Better coordination among branches of AAFC might ensure that research and policy considerations (including regulatory policy) are integrated. In particular, steps should be taken to ensure that gaps in the scientific literature surrounding risks of biotechnology should be specifically targeted for research support. USDA's Biotechnology Risk Assessment Research Grants Program funds several projects aimed at quantifying the risks posed by agricultural biotechnology.[60]

Labelling of genetically engineered foodstuffs remains a troublesome area.[61] Choice is a fundamental value for Canadian consumers, as are honesty, balanced budgets, and an inexpensive food supply. The question is not whether to label genetically engineered foods but how to do it in a cost-effective manner that provides the information shoppers actually want. The Flavr Savr tomato, engineered to stay riper longer using the mirror image of a regular tomato gene, is a whole food that is voluntarily labelled by the company. However, when that same tomato is used in a sauce – the Flavr Savr has a higher concentration of solids, valued by tomato processors – which is then used in frozen pizza, the label disappears.

And what of the humble potato? Should the French fries sold at the local ice-rink, ballpark, and soccer-field – possibly derived from Bt-containing potatoes and cooked in oil derived from genetically engineered canola – carry a sticker proclaiming the involvement of biotechnology? If there is no health risk, as Health Canada has decided in the case of both of these products, the answer is no. Should consumers be able to determine the origins of the fries? Absolutely, yes: and then they can decide for themselves if they want to have further information about how they originated.

Mandatory labelling is expensive and, in a society that values convenience over cooking skills, impractical as well. Instead, consumers can be informed about the products they purchase through 1-800 numbers or point-of-purchase information. (Those who desire organic produce – whatever that means – can make that choice today, yet supermarkets still carry regular produce.) Those who desire "biotech-free" products – whatever that means – should also be able to make that choice. But this does not necessitate imposing on us all a huge amount of technical information we may not want or need.

In the United States many grocery food packages scream "fat-free," "salt-free," and "cholesterol-free" at the hapless shopper, reminding one of a food science professor who once said that processing was all about selling air and water for higher prices. Researchers at Purdue University and Pennsylvania State University have found in separate studies that people who were told they were eating low-fat foods (when, in fact, they weren't) would subsequently consume more food at the next meal. In other words, people who made low-fat choices some of the time overcompensated by eating too much food at other times. Labelling carries risks as well as benefits.

Canada's farmers also value choice. If a product is deemed to be safe by capable regulators, then let the country's producers choose whether something like the Bt-containing potato, which may require fewer sprayed chemicals, is worth the extra cost. They know how to best manage their farms.

Most worrisome is that the public discussion of agricultural biotechnology seems to be following the path laid out by the widespread adoption of agricultural chemicals in the post–World War II period, with proponents urging better education and critics deriding the value of high-yield agricultural production. A 1961 editorial by the *New York Times* urged "discriminate use of pesticides, and education on the hazards of misuse,"[62] a strategy that resonates in many of today's pesticide reduction strategies such as Ontario's Food Systems 2002. Strangely enough, much of today's newspaper coverage of agricultural biotechnology in North America cites economic benefits but rarely mentions the "hazards of misuse" such as, in the case of genetically engineered Bt-containing crops, the accelerated development of resistance.[63]

In general, AAFC seems reluctant to acknowledge the risks associated with plant biotechnology and therefore does not feel the need to communicate about them or to devise monitoring or management plans for environmental impacts. Communications aimed at the general public emphasize the supposed benefits of biotechnology while minimizing or ignoring possible risks.[64] Although some risks are acknowledged in more specific documents, AAFC makes no attempt to initiate research to quantify impacts or to ensure that these documents reach users of the technologies or the general public.

In response to our questions Plant Biotechnology Office staff stated that they do follow the scientific literature regarding risks and attend conferences but that they maintain no formal database for this information.[65] The federal regulators also stated that they rely on the provincial governments to monitor for problems at the farm level and to communicate this information to companies, who will then (presumably) inform AAFC. In some cases companies are relied upon to both develop and administer risk management plans as well as to communicate risks. We submit that such an indirect, haphazard approach to risk communication is insufficient and irresponsible. At the very least, government should have a set of criteria for evaluating industry's risk management and communication plans and making this information freely available to the public. It is difficult to assess the adequacy of AAFC's risk assessments for transgenic plants, since none of the information submitted by companies is freely available.

Why industry and regulators involved in the public coversation about agricultural biotechnology in Canada refuse to engage in discussions of how to maximize benefit while minimizing risk remains a mystery. Several surveys in North America and the U.K. have found that perceptions of trust in government regulation (and industry), regarding either pesticides or the products of agricultural biotechnology, are the strongest predictors for consumer support.[66] People either trust that pesticides and agricultural biotech products are adequately regulated or they do not, and those with low trust have the highest concern about possible risks. Those with high trust perceive greater benefits from both products. In a recent article van Ravenswaay concluded that trust in government and industry may be a more important influence on risk perception than the inherent safety or the danger of a particular agrichemical.[67]

At the U.K. Ministry of Agriculture, Fisheries and Food's Institute of Food Research in Reading, Frewer *et al.* have conducted numerous experiments to elucidate the best way to discuss agricultural biotechnology publicly.[68] Among their findings are:

- the most important and frequently cited source of information about food-related information was the media, far ahead of any other source;
- while scientists and medical sources were rated as trusted but not distrusted (media were often trusted and distrusted), they were infrequently named as sources of food-related information;
- the single most important determinant of gain or loss of trust in a source is whether the information is subsequently proven right or wrong, and that the source is subsequently demonstrated to be unbiased;
- information about natural toxins, genetic engineering, and pesticide residues was more distrusted than information about high fat diets, microwave ovens, etc.;
- medical sources are likely to be viewed as expert in medically related areas but having little knowledge in technological risk assessment, and therefore are poor sources of information about technological hazards;
- trust is clearly multidimensional and cannot be predicted by single items or psychological constructs;

- trust appears linked with perceptions of accuracy, knowledge, and concern with public welfare;
- if government sources and risk regulators are seen to be proactive in their interactions with the media and other trusted sources, this may positively influence the way in which risk information is reported, as well as increasing trust in government regulation;
- admitting to uncertainty, or facilitating public understanding of science as a "process," could increase communicators' trustworthiness;
- people seem to be adverse to ambiguous risks, and trust is all the more likely to be important where there is a perception that accurate estimates of risk are not available, as with genetically engineered foods.

Given that uncertainty is a normal component of science, we argue that, at a minimum, industry, government, academics, and others should endorse such scientifically grounded communication guidelines, to capture the benefits of agricultural biotechnology and to work actively to mitigate the risks.

ADDENDUM

by Angela Griffiths and Katherine Barrett

During the process of researching and writing this chapter, significant philosophical differences among the four contributing authors became apparent. Rather than leave these points of contention unacknowledged, we felt an explicit account of the controversy might be of interest to readers.

Simply stated, while we, the authors of this addendum, concur with analysis presented in the first sections of the chapter, we do not support the conclusions drawn in the final section, "Maximizing Benefits and Minimizing Risks." What follows is an alternative point of view. Interestingly, the controversy presented here well-illustrates a source of current debate in the field of risk studies – namely, that widely divergent prescriptions can be drawn from the same facts. Clearly, *what we ought to do* is a question of profound complexity, perhaps indicative of our technological age.

As the opening paragraphs of this chapter point out, the discussion of agricultural biotechnology has been framed narrowly in terms of risk versus benefits. While this chapter aims to present a broader framework through maximizing benefits and minimizing risks, we propose that *any* decision framework that advocates trading risks and benefits as a necessary starting point does not adequately address the social and ethical issues inherent in technologies such as agricultural biotechnology. On the contrary, setting minimum risks as a goal perpetuates several powerful and, we would suggest, ill-founded assumptions about biotechnology:

1 Biotechnology is the only solution to present and future agricultural problems;
2 Biotechnology is inevitable; we can only hope, and thus aim, to minimize the risks;
3 Risks and benefits can be accurately calculated and fairly traded.

While all three assumptions are closely related, the third is most relevant to the subject of this chapter.

That the risks and benefits claimed for agricultural biotechnology can be effectively and meaningfully stripped of local context, generalized to all foreseeable (and unforeseeable) situations, and subsequently weighed and balanced is belied by several important characteristics of these technologies:[69]

- *Scientific uncertainty.* As the first part of this chapter illustrates, the scientific literature regarding the risks and benefits of releasing genetically modified plants (GMPs) is rife with uncertainty.[70] For example, a chronic lack of, and inconsistency in, scientific data reflects uncertainty at a technical level. Lack of consensus about how data should be gathered and assessed reflects uncertainty at the level of scientific methods. Finally, and more fundamentally, uncertainty exists regarding the very nature of scientific knowledge which appears, as yet, inadequate to address the full extent of technological hazards.
- *Complexity.* One reason for persistent scientific uncertainty is that the release of GMPs into the environment involves, and affects, many interrelated systems: the modified genetic system of the plants, the ecosystems where the plants are released, and the social systems where the plants are farmed, sold, and regulated, for example. The interactions among these systems are highly complex and notoriously unpredictable.[71]
- *Scale and distribution of hazards.* Ecosystem damage resulting from the release of genetically modified organisms may be large scale, long term and irreversible – plants and micro-organisms are not easily recalled. Such damage may therefore affect people who have not explicitly chosen to adopt the technologies, such as future generations. How can risks and benefits that cannot be controlled in time

or space be measured, balanced, or compensated for? What is the role of government in protecting consumers or the public against risks? We believe that introducing risky new technologies subject to *caveat emptor* (buyer beware) is irresponsible. The Seeds Act (under which plant biotechnologies are regulated) was originally introduced to protect farmers from unscrupulous seed sellers making false claims. Now is not the time to abandon that protection.

Brian Wynne's idea of indeterminacy provides an insightful concept through which the above points may be acknowledged.[72] Indeterminate situations are not simply very uncertain; they are essentially open-ended and ultimately dependent upon the *social commitments* (e.g., values, biases, experiences) of all parties who help to define and shape the risk debate. This point seems particularly cogent with respect to GMP release. Clearly, the various social commitments of scientists, AAFC, industry, and the public have played, and will continue to play, critical roles in the way risks and benefits are defined, and thereby measured and allotted.

To summarize, the issues raised here suggest a breakdown, or perhaps a transcendence, of risk/benefit as a technically and morally appropriate framework for structuring discussions and forming decisions about agricultural biotechnology. However, we must interject an important qualification: this breakdown does not imply that we ought therefore to simply go ahead with technologies that cannot be assessed through traditional means. Rather, this breakdown points to the need for a new framework for acknowledging and communicating potential hazards of technologies. We propose that a more inclusive framework would 1) question the current boundaries of expertise and authority, and thereby open the discussion to all concerned parties and their own expert knowledge; 2) communicate what is not known (uncertainty) and cannot be known (interdeterminacy), as well as what is currently known; and, as a result, 3) focus not on questions of *how* but on *if* a technology ought to be employed.

8 Mother's Milk: Communicating the Risks of PCBs in Canada and the Far North

PASCAL MILLY, WITH THE ASSISTANCE OF WILLIAM LEISS

Polychlorinated biphenyls (PCBs) is the common name for a family of chlorinated hydrocarbon compounds used in a wide range of industrial and consumer products for about forty years. The commercial manufacture of PCBs began in the United States in 1929 in response to concern over the risk of fires created by oil-filled transformers and capacitors. The increasing occurrences of fires caused by power surges igniting mineral oil prompted the electrical industry to search for an alternative dielectric (isolating) fluid. Beginning in the 1930s a generic fluid called "askarel" – containing from 40 to 70 per cent PCBs – was introduced as a replacement product for mineral oil in equipment located in public or enclosed spaces. PCBs are viscous liquids that are relatively fire-resistant, noncorrosive, and possess excellent electrical and thermal properties. They are also very stable and do not decompose easily.[1]

By 1940 PCBs were widely utilized as insulating fluids in electrical and accessory equipment. Their main use was as dielectric fluid in "closed-system" applications (in transformers, capacitors, and heat exchange systems)[2] but their extreme stability and resistance to breakdown by heat and most chemical and physical agents made them desirable components in a wide range of other applications. PCBs served as volatilization suppressants in pesticide formulations, as dust suppressants on roads, as flame retardants in lubricating oils, and as plasticizers in synthetic resins, rubbers, and paints. They were also used as components in many consumer products and processes, such as in carbonless copy paper, printing ink and de-inking fluid for newsprint, or as surface coating for washable wall coverings and upholstery fabrics.[3] In these and many other "open-ended" applications, PCBs were in direct contact with the environment. The proliferation of open uses throughout the 1940s, 1950s, and 1960s, added to their widespread utilization as dielectric fluid in electrical equipment, contributed significantly to their environmental dispersion.[4]

For the first thirty-five years few questions were raised about any negative impacts resulting from their extensive usage. But in 1966 Sören Jensen, a Swedish scientist looking for traces of DDT in wildlife samples, discovered traces of PCBs in the fatty tissues of fish and wild birds.[5] This unexpected finding alerted the scientific community to the possible existence of a new and unrecognized environmental contaminant. Subsequent studies soon confirmed the presence of PCBs in the ecosystems of various parts of the world, which increased scientific and political concern. A number of scientific reviews were mandated by various government agencies, and several conferences were held to assess the extent of the problem.[6] Monitoring for evidence of PCB residues in the United States' food supply during 1970 and 1971 resulted in a series of food and feed seizures. At this same time, articles dealing with PCB contamination began to appear in the popular press.[7]

In 1968 an undetected leak from a heat exchanger used in a food processing plant in southern Japan led to the contamination of cooking oil with PCBs and the poisoning of approximately sixteen hundred people. A broad spectrum of toxic effects including severe chloracne and related dermal symptoms was observed among the victims. Developmental problems in infants born from mothers having consumed the contaminated rice oil were observed (although it was later established that some of the acute and chronic effects reported in this mass poisoning had been caused by the ingestion of chemicals other than PCBs).[8] The severity of the health effects observed in the wake of this incident (known as Yusho), coupled with the widespread finding of trace quantities of PCBs in the environment, provided additional impetus for moving PCBs onto national and international risk management agendas.[9]

It is often noted with irony that the very properties which made PCBs such superior industrial chemicals, namely, their stability and resistance to chemical and biological breakdown, also made them environmentally hazardous. When discarded in urban or industrial areas or burned at temperatures too low to destroy them, PCBs can be emitted and spread by airborne transport and ocean currents to the most remote locations.[10] Their low water solubility causes them to become attached to sediments at the bottom of rivers, lakes, and oceans where they can be absorbed by fish and other aquatic organisms. Though only slightly soluble in water, PCBs dissolve readily in oils and the fatty tissues of living creatures where they tend to accumulate. As PCBs travel the food chain, they become more concentrated, because they tend to be stored rather than metabolized or excreted; minute quantities of the compounds can build over time to levels high enough to cause biological injuries. Deleterious effects have been observed in marine organisms at all trophic levels, ranging from algae to bacteria and invertebrates to fish and fish-eating birds.[11] Recent estimates point to the environmental load of PCBs being gradually redistributed towards the marine environment, suggesting an increasing hazard for sea mammals in the future.[12]

1 THE PUBLIC CONTROVERSY

Scientific and political concerns about PCBs arising in the late 1960s propelled regulatory actions prohibiting the further manufacture and sale of these compounds. In Canada as in most countries, strict maintenance and handling procedures were also introduced to ensure the safe operation of authorized PCB-filled electrical equipment until the end of its service life. In the United States, PCB-contaminated material cannot be kept in storage for more than one year, and discarded PCBs have either been routed to approved chemical waste landfills or incinerated.[13] The Canadian situation is much different. Here public opposition to even temporary incineration facilities has meant the piling-up of PCB wastes in over three thousand storage sites across the land.[14]

Problems encountered in disposing of PCB wastes in Canada are the outcome of a series of incidents that have shaped public attitudes towards these chemicals and led to much public scepticism about the ability of governments and industry to dispose of them effectively. This section retraces the main events that made PCBs a household term for the Canadian public and goes on to argue that the failure to manage risk communication processes adequately is the chief source of the current difficulties in disposing of these wastes.

The 1985 Kenora Spill

On Saturday, 13 April 1985, a flatbed truck carrying a set of undrained electrical transformers was travelling the Trans-Canada Highway from the Montreal area to an Alberta storage site. Near Kenora, a northwestern Ontario community, one of the transformers sprang a leak and splashed about four hundred litres of PCB-contaminated oil along what was initially thought to be seventy km of asphalt. The media coverage of the spill immediately emphasized the "human angle" (which of course makes for a more compelling story) by stressing the plight of the Eyjolfson family who, while en route to a family reunion in Winnipeg, found themselves caught behind the tractor-trailer for a distance of twenty-five km before being able to pass. When Lloyd Eyjolfson picked up a newspaper at his in-laws' breakfast table the next morning, he learned that he, his pregnant wife, and his two toddler sons had been exposed to "mass quantities" of PCBs.

The official reaction to the spill was confusing and went on for about two weeks under intense media scrutiny. By the time provincial officials decided to close down the highway to apply an asphalt sealer over the polluted portions of the road, thousands of motorists had already driven on the PCB splotches. Then it was announced that the spill was at least 150 km longer than originally thought. Another event that seemed to undermine definitively the reassuring messages of public officials was the order given by the federal government to five commercial airlines to decontaminate planes that had carried tainted soil samples for testing by a Toronto laboratory. The incident received extensive national media coverage[15] which, perhaps because of its ready-made human dimension, concentrated on PCBs' most dramatic alleged health effects, namely cancer and birth defects. For example, on 29 April 1985 the weekly magazine *Maclean's* published a special issue on the spill with a cover picture of the skull-and-crossbones emblem over an oil barrel with the following headline: "PCBs: what they are, where they come from ... and how they can kill."

The 1988 St-Basile-le-Grand Fire

About three years later, on Tuesday, 23 August 1988, a privately owned chemical storage warehouse filled with about fifteen hundred barrels of PCB-containing oil burst into flames near St-Basile-le-Grand, forty kilometres southeast of Montreal. Because the uncontrolled burning of PCBs can cause their conversion into the more toxic PCDDs and PCDFs, local officials decided to evacuate the population living within a forty-km radius of the fire. About three thousand residents located in the path of possibly hazardous smoke and fallout had to leave their homes in the middle of the night.

Although the fire was rapidly brought under control, its potential health and environmental effects became the focus of considerable speculation and uncertainty. The next day, nursing mothers were warned to stop breast-feeding, and the Quebec government placed an embargo on produce grown on about six hundred hectares of neighbouring farmland. Warnings of potential hazardous effects were issued to residents as far away as east-end Montreal. During the following weekend about three thousand people were examined at the regional hospital and another five hundred people were ordered out of their homes because changing winds were bringing dust from the site of the fire to a trailer park on the east side of St-Basile.

By September, results from testing were deemed satisfactory, and nursing mothers were told they could resume breast-feeding. However, because some results were conflicting with others, the environment ministry decided to bring in a team of international experts to assess the situation before residents were allowed to return home. On 10 September, at a press conference attended by five cabinet ministers, the panel of international scientists submitted a unanimous report to the effect that the concentrations of PCBs, dioxins, and furans inside the houses of St-Basile residents were no higher than those usually found in uncontaminated buildings. Thus after eighteen days of wrenching uncertainty the 3,500 evacuees were finally told it was safe to return home.

Although only 8 per cent of the PCB-contaminated material actually burned, the St-Basile fire was probably the largest-ever uncontained PCB fire worldwide and effectively drew attention to the potential risks associated with the long-term storage of PCBs. The incident quickly became politically volatile in Quebec and outside the province. For several days PCB-related accusations and charges dominated Question Period in the House of Commons as all parties and both levels of government sought to control the issue. On 16 September the federal government issued an Interim Order stipulating proper storage methods for PCB wastes and made the implementation of those security measures mandatory in all provinces.

Three years after the fire there was no evidence that the fallout had any long-lasting effects on the health of area residents or on the firefighters who had fought the blaze. However, the dearth of information released by public officials during the mass evacuation, and the climate of secrecy that surrounded the expert interpretation of tests results, created an information vacuum that fueled rampant speculation. Some of the more sensational versions of events in the media coverage certainly led to the diffusion of inaccurate information and rumours. Many reports continued to play up PCBs' most dramatic health effects long after the events themselves had come and gone.[16] More generally, the St-Basile fire became a seminal event in Canada in terms of health and environmental risk issues, in part because it

coincided with the emergence in public-opinion polling of environmental concerns as a top priority for citizens.

The 1989 Baie Comeau Controversy

In July 1989 Quebec environment officials signed a contract with a
Montreal-based company to ship 206 large metal containers to a PCB
incinerator in Pontypool, Wales. This agreement, which was similar to
others reached between Canadian owners of PCBs and several active
disposal facilities in Europe, was to dispose of the remaining 3,500
tonnes of waste not consumed by the St-Basile fire. But whereas earlier
shipments had arrived without incident, Quebec's agreement coincided with a mounting campaign by the British wing of Greenpeace
against the international trade in hazardous wastes.

After British Greenpeace activists and Liverpool dockworkers forced
port authorities to order the freighter carrying PCBs back to Canada,
the provincial government made a hurried and controversial arrangement to store the wastes near the town of Baie Comeau, on Quebec's
lower north shore. When the first PCB shipment returning from
England arrived in the paper-mill town of 26,000 people, more than
two thousand protesters were awaiting the freighter at the dock with
an injunction against the unloading of the PCBs. But the injunction
was ignored, and the shipment was unloaded in the middle of the
night while police kept protesters at bay. In response, Baie Comeau
residents presented their town's council with a petition containing ten
thousand names, seeking a second injunction to have the storage site
declared illegal because it contravened the region's waste management plan. In the meantime the freighter was gone, and the PCBs
remained stuck on the town's wharf under the guard of provincial
police, angry residents, and television cameras.

After two weeks of political manoeuvring and court battles, a
Quebec Superior Court judge finally ended the stand-off by lifting the
injunction banning the removal of the unwelcome PCB cargo from
the dock, thus permitting its transfer to the storage site. Within minutes of the judge's decision, the provincial police ended citizens'
attempt to block the road with a show of force. Television newscasts
across the country showed images of the riot squad wielding trun-
cheons rushing into a crowd of protesters to clear the way for trucks
to move the PCB-laden wastes to their new storage site. The aborted
shipment of PCBs to Wales, and the highly visible episode in dealing
with them upon their return, tarnished Canada's reputation as an
environmentally responsible nation both at home and abroad and led
to widespread criticism of the export of toxic wastes as a socially and

morally unacceptable practice.[17] In August 1990 the federal government introduced regulations outlawing the overseas export of PCBs, thereby expressing a national commitment to the domestic management of all PCB wastes within Canada.

The above account would be misleading if it gave the impression that concern over PCBs has been limited to the three episodes described above. In fact, even a cursory examination of the press coverage on this issue shows that since 1985 local PCB controversies have erupted in every part of the country, involving just about every possible segment and organized group in Canadian society. Because of the extensive and alarming media coverage it generated, the 1985 Kenora spill was the decisive event in permanently associating PCBs with serious degenerative diseases in the mind of the Canadian public. Reports of the events surrounding the St-Basile fire and the Baie Comeau blockade certainly did nothing to dispel this perception. Still today, hardly any mention of PCBs occurs in the media without reference being made to their link with cancer. Despite the absence of any definite proof that PCBs may cause cancer in humans or are responsible for *any* human death, the repeated assertion of a link between PCBs and serious health effects has remained an ongoing and very suggestive feature of PCB media coverage.[18]

2 PCB RISK ASSESSMENT AND MANAGEMENT

Spanning more than a quarter of a century, the scientific investigation of the adverse health effects of PCBs has yet to reach any definitive conclusion as to the full extent of health implications resulting from PCB exposure, largely due to four major analytical complexities. The first analytical hurdle was to determine the compound's chemical composition: commercial PCBs are complex mixtures of up to 209 different but related PCB congeners (chemical variants) which, depending on the degree of chlorination and the position of the chlorine atom on the biphenyl nucleus, have different physical and chemical properties. In the environment different congeners undergo different environmental alterations and, once absorbed by living organisms, are metabolized differently. In the end the biologic and toxic effects of PCBs are highly dependent on the chemical composition of individual congeners.[19] While substantial improvements in analytical techniques have made possible the measurement of PCBs in a congener-specific fashion, most PCB levels in environmental extracts have been reported as an approximation of "total" PCB content. Inconsistencies in sampling and quantitation procedures and subsequent modifications in analytical methodologies have often produced equivocal PCB residue data and inhibited the comparison and compilation of analytical results from different laboratories.[20]

Second, the analysis of PCBs' adverse effects on living organisms has proceeded largely on the basis of experimental studies. The great variability observed across animal species in their susceptibility to PCB intoxication has made the interpretation of laboratory results and their extrapolation to humans particularly difficult.[21] Third, most testing procedures have focused on the most sensitive strain of the most sensitive animal species, using the most toxic PCB congeners.[22] While this approach can be useful to maximize the chances of detecting adverse effects, some scientists are concerned that experimental evidence of PCB toxicity based on worst-case scenarios has led to overestimates of the likely human health risks associated with PCBs.[23] Finally, it has been difficult to reconcile the extreme sensitivity of some animal species to PCBs with the lack of clear and consistent evidence of adverse health effects observed in human populations exposed to high concentrations of PCBs for extended periods of time.[24]

Because it is vast, complex, and rich in qualifying statements, the scientific literature on the health effects of PCBs is difficult to summarize. PCB accumulations in some animal species have been shown to produce a spectrum of pathologies, including birth defects, and to affect reproductive processes, hormonal balance, and enzyme and immune systems.[25] Cancer of the liver has been observed in rats fed diets containing large amounts of PCBs.[26] However, the anti-carcinogenic activity of PCBs on rodents pretreated with hepatocarcinogens has also been demonstrated. This indicates that under some conditions PCBs may protect against injury initiated by other compounds.[27]

Known toxic effects in humans result primarily from occupational and accidental exposure. Chloracne, hyper-pigmentation of the nails and mucuous membranes, and altered liver function are among the symptoms most often observed. Other possible signs of toxic responses include respiratory disorders, immunosuppressive changes, and impaired child development,[28] but the significance of these findings is unclear.[29] Less specific symptoms such as headaches, sleep and memory disturbances, fatigue, and impotence have also been reported. No conclusive relationship between human exposure to PCBs and cancer has been established in the studies that have addressed directly this matter.[30] Prolonged occupational exposure to high PCB concentrations may have a variety of effects on the skin and the liver.[31]

While it is unlikely that exposure to PCBs at typical environmental levels affects human health,[32] most people living in industrialized nations have measurable concentrations of these chemicals in their bodies.[33] The major route of PCB exposure is through dietary intake of milk, meats, poultry, and especially fish.[34] Subsistence fishermen who eat large quantities of seafood, and northern native people who consume large quantities of marine mammal fats as part of their traditional diet – also known as country food – have PCB body burdens several times higher than the general population.[35] No adverse health effects have been observed in adult aboriginal northerners with elevated PCB levels,[36] but the possible developmental effects on fetuses and breast-fed infants continues to be investigated.[37] Researchers have underscored that the overall benefits associated with breast-feeding and the harvesting and consumption of traditional foods clearly outweigh the uncertain risks of dietary exposure to PCBs. In most instances public health professionals have recommended that northern residents continue to consume country food and breast-feed their babies.[38]

When compared to other hazardous substances, the toxicity of PCBs ranks fairly low, but concerns regarding possible adverse effects due to long-term exposure at low concentrations have been significant enough to warrant strict regulatory controls.[39] From the 1930s to the early 1970s the industrial and commercial uses of PCBs resulted in a world-wide production of about one million tonnes. Of this amount approximately 635,000 tonnes were produced in the United States by Monsanto Chemical, the world's largest manufacturer of PCBs. Canada, which never produced PCBs, imported approximately 40,000 tonnes in total. Between 1930 and 1970 most wastes generated by the scrapping of PCB-contaminated equipment and products were disposed of without special precautions, and so large amounts of PCBs were released in the environment. In 1985 Environment Canada's inventory showed a total of 24,300 tonnes of PCBs either in use or in storage across the country. The remainder – equivalent to approximately sixteen thousand tonnes – can no longer be accounted for and is assumed to be disposed in landfills or dispersed in the environment.[40]

Risk management measures introduced from the 1970s onward have succeeded in drastically reducing PCB entry into the environment. Because of their persistence and stability, no corresponding decline in environmental PCB concentrations has been observed. Still, using concentrations in fish and birds as an indicator, studies carried out in the Great Lakes and other major surface waters show a slight diminution in PCB environmental levels.[41] While PCB natural degradation does take place very slowly,[42] long-range atmospheric movements (i.e., air/snow deposition and ocean currents) are redistributing some of the environmental PCB loads from the most contaminated areas (e.g., Lake

Ontario) to less contaminated regions (the Arctic).[43] On a positive note, breast-milk PCB concentrations collected throughout Canada appear to compare favourably with those reported in other western countries, and since 1982 these concentrations are on the decline.[44]

PCB Regulation

Concerns about PCBs' environmental pervasiveness and potential adverse health effects have spurred an array of national and international risk management initiatives. At first the thrust of these efforts focused on outlawing PCB production and curtailing their approved uses. In 1971, in response to informal pressure by the U.S. government, Monsanto "voluntarily" began to limit its sale of PCBs intended for open-ended use and for applications directly related to food or animal feed.[45] In 1973 the Organization for Economic Co-operation and Development (OECD) recommended that PCB usage be limited to essential closed-systems applications and urged member nations to provide a safe means for PCB disposal. Ongoing preoccupation with PCBs in the United States[46] led to the promulgation of the 1976 Toxic Substance Control Act (TSCA) and the issuance of EPA regulations prohibiting the manufacture, importation, and most non-electrical uses of PCBs.[47]

Encouraged by the OECD recommendations and its own reviews of the situation,[48] Canada began to introduce regulatory controls for PCBs in 1977. The Canadian strategy to deal with the problem has since evolved into a complex and intricate regulatory framework encompassing several layers of legislation, regulations, and guidelines, a "PCB Action Plan," and a "Federal PCB Destruction Program."

PCBs were the first class of substances to be regulated under Canada's Environmental Contaminants Act (ECA). Beginning in 1977 three sets of PCB regulations were promulgated under the ECA; essentially, PCB Regulations No. 1, 2, and 3 restricted the permissible uses of PCBs to closed (largely electrical) equipment already in service, set limits as to the maximum PCB concentration that could be contained in equipment to be imported or offered for sale, and established specific prohibitions regarding PCB releases in the environment.[49] Since 1980 no new supplies of PCBs have legally been put into service in Canada, but the normal life expectancy of transformers and capacitors (thirty to forty years or longer) means that some PCBs are still in use in electrical equipment. These are only gradually phased out as the equipment reaches the end of its service life.[50]

The Kenora incident prompted the passing of new regulations specifying requirements for the interprovincial and international transport of hazardous goods and wastes. The regulations, promulgated under the Transportation of Dangerous Goods Act (TDGA), made specific reference to PCBs; procedures to improve the efficiency of spill response and cleanup activities in case of accidents were included. After the fire at St-Basile-le-Grand Environment Canada issued three more sets of regulations, designed to ensure proper storage of PCB material (1989), to govern the safe operation of mobile PCB incinerators (1990), and to prohibit the oversea export of PCB wastes (1990).[51]

While federal regulations serve as a minimum standard across Canada, provincial and territorial governments have the option to introduce further obligations for controlling these substances within their own borders. In several areas of PCB management (e.g., transportation and releases to aquatic environments), both federal and provincial legislations apply.[52] The authorization to operate PCB waste treatment facilities is a provincial responsibility.[53] Only one stationary incinerator for PCB destruction, located near Swan Hills, Alberta, has been approved in Canada, and until 1994 it was restricted to handling Alberta wastes only. Atop this legally enforceable regulatory framework, several sets of voluntary administrative guidelines have been adopted by federal and provincial agencies. Voluntary standards, however, are not uniformly endorsed and can differ in value and/or specificity across provinces.[54]

After the 1988 fire at St-Basile-le-Grand, the ministers agreed to emphasize PCB destruction over long-term storage and to phase out all PCBs in Canada by 1993.[55] Introduced in 1988 shortly after the St-Basile fire, the federal government's PCB Destruction Program was designed to remediate the problems encountered by several provinces in finding suitable locations for destruction facilities. In 1989 federal lands and federally sponsored mobile PCB incinerators were made available on a cost-recovery basis to any community in Canada with sufficient volumes of privately or publicly owned PCB wastes. The program's initial objective was to rid Canadian society of PCBs by 1993.[56] As of early 1997, however, most attempts at eliminating the Canadian PCB waste inventory via mobile incinerators – the safest, most effective, and socially acceptable method of PCB disposal, according to government experts – have been stalled by the systematic opposition by local communities to the siting of PCB destruction facilities in their vicinity. Since 1988 federal attempts at siting transportable/mobile incinerators have succeeded in overcoming public opposition at only three locations: Goose Bay (Labrador) in 1990, Smithville (Ontario) in 1991, and, for a series of test burns, Baie Comeau (Quebec) in 1992.

Since the early 1980s PCB-containing equipment continues to be removed from service, and therefore PCB wastes are now accumulating in thousands of sites across the country. Federal regulations enacted in the wake of the 1988 fire in St-Basile-le-Grand have been successful in preventing major incidents or releases of PCBs from storage sites. Still, an accidental fire remains a possibility, and since the uncontrolled burning of PCBs can be a source of toxic by-products, regulatory agencies do not consider permanent storage of PCBs to be a viable waste management solution. In addition, the cost of secure storage constitutes an ongoing burden for both taxpayers and PCB owners and can encourage illegal dumping. Complete destruction of PCBs is thus the ultimate goal of PCB risk management, and it is the goal to which federal and provincial governments have repeatedly and emphatically committed themselves.

3 THE RISK COMMUNICATION VACUUM

Like dioxins, PCBs have been represented as major environmental threats in most of the accounts reaching the general public. The following statement, which can be found repeated without much variation in a great number of press articles, is typical of the characterization of PCB risks: "PCBs were banned in 1977, after they were linked to cancer in mice and to liver, skin, and nerve disorders in humans." Although factually true, this information is at least incomplete and at worst could give rise to unwarranted fears about PCBs – especially since related information about the dose necessary to cause those effects in humans, and the low probability of any person in Canada being subjected to such a dose, almost never seemed to find its way into the story. The net result of associating in the same sentence *without any further qualification* the carcinogenic potential of PCBs in rodents with reported human health effects is to blur critical differences between laboratory animals and humans in regard to their conditions of exposure and susceptibility to PCBs. In this regard the PCB case mirrors that of dioxins.

The failure in most media reports to make a clear distinction between the different settings in which the scientific assessments on the effects of PCBs were being undertaken – in ecosystems, laboratory animals, and humans – kept alive the possible confusions about the toxic potential of these compounds. A full review of the extensive collection of media stories on PCBs reveals that few attempts were made to offer a balanced view of the dangers represented by PCBs. One of these rare instances was a CBC Television documentary with the revealing title "Public Enemy No. 1." The segment, which looked back at the Kenora, St-Basile and Baie Comeau incidents, featured a lead-in by toxicologist Stephen Safe: "They [PCBs] are not deadly, dangerous, toxic to humans because if that were the case, then we'd have lots of bodies around that would have died from PCB poisoning, and we just don't have that." The program concluded with the toxicologist lamenting that where PCBs are concerned, "public opinion is very misinformed."[57] We shall return to this latter comment.

The extensive media coverage of PCB-related stories even gave rise to the unusual situation whereby on two separate occasions Canada's national newspaper commented editorially on what it described as its own unbalanced coverage of risk issues. In 1991 a *Globe and Mail* editorial noted that during the six years following the Kenora spill, the paper published a total of 386 stories on PCBs, "whose only proven health effect is to cause chloracne, eye discharge and vomiting in people who *ingest* them." For the same period, the paper said it had run 222 stories on the health risks of smoking, "a habit that killed 38,357 Canadians in 1989." "It is our job," the editorial concluded, "to maintain a sense of proportion when reporting environmental threats. So far, we are failing." Three years later the very same paper informed its readers that, for the past sixteen years, it had published on average about one story every two weeks on PCBs, "the bulk of them concerning PCB scares of one kind or another."[58]

This case of self-criticism by the print media is curious, to say the least, but it does dovetail nicely with the widespread perception among some risk experts that the media is guilty of regular "sensationalism" in its reporting on risk-type stories. "Blaming the media" for distorting risk events and their meaning for citizens takes second place only to blaming those same citizens directly for their ill-informed views. Recently the perception of sensationalism was subjected to a careful scrutiny in a scholarly study on media coverage of hazard events; the main finding was that, on the whole, media reporting underplayed the latent emotionalism associated with hazardous events.[59]

Stephen Safe's comment about a misinformed public begs the question of just how misinformation might arise and who ought to be held responsible for trying to correct the situation. In the present case there is no candidate for this role in Canada other than the federal government, in particular the departments of Health and Environment. The phase-out of commercial PCBs meant that there was no longer a manufacturing industry with an interest in defending these substances; the only issue before the public was the dual one of safe containment of existing stocks so as to prevent any further environmental releases, and safe and cost-effective disposal of those stocks according to acceptable criteria for PCB destruction. Since the regulatory overseeing of these processes falls entirely on the shoulders of governments, so too must the obtaining of public acceptance fall there. If public attitudes make that disposal process more difficult than it should be ideally, or even prevent it from happening, should we blame the public?

We think that in this case at least neither blaming the media nor blaming the public is appropriate. If PCBs share with dioxins the dubious distinction of being stigmatized substances, the explanation for this lies in an identical set of circumstances: the emergence of an information vacuum about these risks, so that – in the case of PCBs – nothing was provided in publicly understandable terms to supplement the diet of media stories about PCB-related incidents. Of course, virtually every time such an incident made the news, all of the truncated and therefore misleading one-liners about the emerging scientific findings on health effects in various contexts were trotted out. So it is odd that at least one major media outlet should question the number of those stories published in its own pages, or that others should lament the sorry state of the public mind which had been nourished on them. The essence of the matter, which was not touched on by the editorial writer for the *Globe*, is: What else was there for the hungry reader to feed on?

For more than two decades neither Environment Canada nor Health Canada, the two regulatory bodies responsible for the risk assessment of PCBs, made a concerted attempt to challenge the standard characterization of PCBs in media stories as "cancer-causing" or to communicate the fact that, at current levels of exposure, most people are very unlikely to be affected adversely by these compounds. This lack of effort on the part of regulatory agencies to inform citizens effectively is surprising since, as of 1985, it was clear that interest in PCBs and regulatory efforts to dispose of them was not about to dwindle. However, there is no evidence that the government made any concerted attempt to counteract the alarming messages about PCBs widely dispersed in the information environment.

The enormous amount of press coverage on PCBs in Canada, extending over a period of twenty years now, presents a unique challenge for those who might be said to bear the responsibility for the creation and maintenance of the PCB risk information vacuum. We readily concede that any determined attempt to remedy this situation would have been time-consuming, difficult, and perhaps even a bit expensive. However, to rule out such an effort on the grounds of the demands from other pressing business, or inadequate resources, or whatever, would overlook the simple fact that the limited public understanding of PCB risk has entailed substantial costs of its own in Canada. The monetary costs arise because the most cost-effective disposal technologies cannot be easily used, and more expensive ones must be employed. The psychological costs are no less significant, and may be greater still, as we seek to show in the concluding section. In any case the effort was never made, and the risk management agencies let the media act, in effect, as the *only* communication channel for PCB risk information.

As already mentioned, the inability of regulatory agencies to create circumstances for the exchange of PCB-related information in ways that could promote their effective management is most pronounced in the area of PCB waste disposal. From the beginning the federal government failed to communicate adequately its rationale for developing the PCB destruction strategy. When the Federal PCB Destruction Program was launched in 1988, part of the federal Cabinet decision to commit funds to the program was conditional upon Environment Canada seeking the advice of the Canadian Environmental Advisory Council (CEAC) on the most appropriate process for siting mobile PCB facilities. The CEAC report, *PCBs: A Burning Issue*, submitted one year later to Environment Canada, contained a number of recommendations but most emphatically stressed that public consultation be fully integrated into the process of finding a permanent solution for the disposal of these wastes.[60]

Despite this recommendation, only one stakeholder workshop was organized at the national level for Environment Canada to consult with organizations and industries concerned with PCB disposal.[61] And since the workshop was held after the federal PCB destruction program had already been announced, the one-day meeting appears to have been little more than a ritual in consultation. Many participants at the 1989 workshop seized the opportunity to tell their government that the information in their possession did not lead them to support the government's strategy. Yet there is no indication whatsoever that the concerns formulated during this meeting resulted in any modification of the program's content or in any renewed attempt by the government to develop a constituency to support its implementation.

Only two temporary mobile units have been successfully sited and operated in Canada under the federal program. A chief reason is that, in spite of the CEAC recommendations, the site selection process has been essentially predicated upon purely technical criteria. An independent review of the government's efforts in that region clearly spells out what happened:

The effort to destroy Atlantic Canada's stored PCBs has focused largely on finding the "best" site from technical and scientific considerations as viewed by technically trained people. The search for a destruction site was carried out by assessing each Federal property in Atlantic Canada against an extensive set of criteria. Although one of the criteria was the willingness of the community to host the facility, this criteria played virtually no role in choosing a short list of two potential sites. The process did not afford those who live nearest the two potential sites any formal or structured opportunity for meaningful community input before their locations were selected. The process failed to provide for the local community to shape a destruction proposal in a way that responded to the particular concerns or needs of the community. The result is that the people who live nearest the two candidate sites are vehemently opposed to the siting of a temporary destruction facility in their areas.[62]

Apart from forewarning the government that, to be successful, its siting program would have to be focused on the issue of community acceptance, the CEAC recommended that before moving ahead on siting, differences in federal and provincial jurisdictions should be harmonized. As shown, the regulatory response to PCBs has been essentially reactive and piecemeal, progressively submitting their storage, handling, and disposal to an intricate and unwieldy set of uncoordinated legislations, regulations, and guidelines. Government made no sustained efforts to encourage a more concise and consistent regulatory framework. Ironically, all this makes it difficult to convince the public that a group of chemicals which must be subject to such an elaborate set of regulations is not extremely hazardous.

Finally, the CEAC warned Environment Canada that acting as both a promoter and regulator of incineration would likely result in a conflict of interest and compromise the viability of its project. Indeed, the federal department seemed uncomfortable with both of these roles and, as expected, the federal PCB destruction program was abundantly criticized for being motivated by political expediency and convenience rather than by the minimization of environmental and health impacts.[63] As a proponent of incineration, the government was also unsuccessful in communicating its opinion that, even though there are no perfect solutions to the PCB waste disposal problem, several thorough assessments of this technology had shown that, on balance, incineration provides a safe and effective means of destroying PCBs. Little information was provided for citizens to weigh the relative benefits of the incineration option compared with alternatives. The government's blithe disregard for the alternative framings of the problem, which could have been easily deduced from a cursory reading of the media stories, was fatal to the prospects for broad public acceptance.

The attempt to destroy Atlantic Canada's stored PCBs was the last effort by the federal government to site a mobile PCB incinerator in this country. As of 31 March 1995 the Federal PCB Destruction Program was cancelled. The government has now entered an agreement with the Swan Hills facility in Alberta for the treatment of all federally owned PCB wastes. While this agreement concerned the disposal of the portion of the Canadian PCB inventory in the hands of the federal government, much uncertainty remained regarding the fate of those PCBs owned by provincial governments, electrical utilities, private industries, and semi-public organizations (e.g., municipalities, schools, hospitals).[64]

When in the fall of 1995, after fifteen years of closure, the United States decided to open its border to allow PCB imports from Canada destined for destruction, the Canadian minister of the Environment immediately responded by an Interim Order under the authority of the Canadian Environmental Protection Act prohibiting the export of PCB wastes to that country.[65] One year later the Canadian government decided to rescind the order.[66] The news release announcing the federal government's latest stand on PCBs indicated that "[w]ith the border open for export for destruction, Canadian PCB waste owners should be able to eliminate all of the PCB wastes in storage in Canada by the year 2000."

4 PCBs IN HUMAN MILK AND COUNTRY FOOD IN THE FAR NORTH

The contention that sound risk communication practices are critical to effective risk management can be further illustrated in the context of recent efforts aimed at mitigating the effects of PCB contamination on aboriginal people living in the Canadian Arctic (north of 55° latitude). In this instance the differences in world views between scientific experts and lay population which, many analysts claim, are key impediments to successful risk management, are particularly striking. Indeed, the gap between experts' and laypersons' perspectives on health and environmental risk is perhaps nowhere so pronounced as in the differences between the professional knowledge of southern risk assessors and managers and the cultural universe of aboriginal northerners.

Background

Although levels of environmental contaminants are generally low across the Canadian Arctic, isolated Inuit populations living off marine resources exhibit relatively high body burdens of various contaminants, including PCBs. Whereas there is no indication that current PCB body burdens have had adverse health effects on adult populations, the ability of these compounds to cross the placental barrier and to bio-concentrate in milk fat have raised concern over possible developmental effects on fetuses and breast-fed infants. So far evidence concerning the possible effects of PCBs on human reproduction and development has been inconclusive.[67] Yet revelations about elevated PCB levels at Broughton Island in 1988 and in Nunavik in 1989 created alarm among Inuit, undermined their confidence in the integrity of traditionally harvested foods, and raised concern among Inuit officials that frightened mothers might stop nursing their babies.

The disruptive impacts created by information linking elevated PCB body burdens among the Inuit with their traditional diet of fish, seal, walrus, and whale stems from the unique qualities that aboriginal northerners attribute to wild foods. Understandably, the availability of food has always been an overriding preoccupation for small Inuit communities living in the frigid Arctic climate.[68] But while good food is clearly indispensable for good health, the heat and strength-giving properties that come from the animals the Inuit hunt and fish are viewed as much superior to what is provided by imported food. For aboriginal northerners the inherent relationship between food and health extends far beyond the nutritional value of the food they consume. Whereas for most people living in southern Canada the production and distribution of food is divorced from its consumption, the capture, processing, and consumption of country food are deeply rooted in the culture of aboriginal communities and are key elements of their social organization.[69] Thus aboriginal northerners value their traditional diet not simply as a source of sustenance but also as the prime component of good health, which includes a sense of personal identity and social well-being.

While the levels of risk caused by the intake of PCBs in country food are uncertain, the health benefits associated with breast-feeding in particular and the Inuit's traditional diet in general are known to be substantial. For instance, a diet rich in fish and sea mammals during pregnancy helps fetuses develop more fully and may account for the fact that Inuit babies are rarely born prematurely.[70] Certain fatty acids derived from the consumption of marine products, thought to be responsible for these beneficial effects, also provide protection against cardiovascular diseases and may counteract mercury and PCB-induced toxicity.[71] Retinol, a vitamin present at high levels in the fat of marine animals, has many benefits including defence against upper respiratory infection and promotion of visual and auditory acuity. Selenium, a trace metal also found in these animals, has recognized anticarcinogenic properties. Additionally, Inuit meats and blubber are known to provide large amounts of high quality proteins and to be a source of many indispensable minerals such as iron and zinc.[72]

Moreover, whereas the harvesting of country food is a net contribution to household income, for many northerners the cost of imported food and milk substitute is prohibitive. The limited availability, freshness, and quality of southern food in northern communities, as well as the risks of cardiovascular disease, cancer, and diabetes associated with a southern diet, further make the substitution of country food with imported food impractical and undesirable.[73] Similarly, breast-feeding and breast milk are widely recognized to convey enormous benefits to developing infants and to be particularly effective against children's infectious diseases. In sum, despite country food and breast milk being major sources of PCB intake, the nutritional benefits they provide compensate for the potential toxic effects of the contaminants they contain. Hence, in most cases, health professionals encourage northerners to continue breast-feeding and to consume country food.[74]

A number of other pressing challenges face northern aboriginal communities with respect to their health status. For instance, a review of several studies carried out by Grondin et al.[75] reveals that mortality rates caused by trauma are five times higher among the Inuit from northern Quebec (also referred to as Nunavimmiut) than among the province's general population. Rates for sexually transmitted diseases in this population are of epidemic proportion, amounting to thirty to fifty times those in the south. Other specific problems affecting the health of the Nunavimmiut include chronic middle ear infections, a widespread condition which results in one-quarter of school age children suffering some kind of hearing loss, and dental cavities which affect 80 per cent of children by the age of five and render more than one in five adult Inuit functionally incapable of chewing food.[76]

The propensity of the Inuit to court other well-known risk factors (tobacco, alcohol, illegal drugs) is also of concern. For instance, the average smoking rate among inhabitants of Nunavik is 70 per cent (as compared to 35 per cent in Quebec) and reaches 80 per cent among women aged fifteen to twenty-four. Finally, suicide attempts are seven times higher in Nunavik than elsewhere in the province. All in all, despite the fact that recent improvements in basic socio-sanitary conditions and health services have resulted in tremendous gains in life expectancy (from thirty-one years in the early 1950s to sixty-six years in the early 1970s – probably mostly due to reduced infant mortality), the Inuit population appears to have serious reservations about its health status. Whereas 74.5 per cent of Quebec Crees and 68.5 per cent of southern Quebeckers say they are in good or very good health, only 47 per cent of Inuit share the same opinion.[77]

These and other findings have led researchers to conclude that it is unlikely that exposure to environmental contaminants like PCBs contributes significantly to mortality and morbidity in Nunavik.[78] Yet, while the physical impact of contaminants on the health of northerners may be minimal, health professionals and Inuit officials are concerned that the information about contaminants which circulates in the Arctic may induce aboriginal populations to alter their lifestyle and traditional eating habits in ways that could be detrimental to their health and well-being.

PCBs in Broughton Island

In 1985 trace findings of PCBs in various species of land and sea mammals across the Canadian Arctic prompted scientists from Health Canada and McGill University to undertake a study of the extent and implications of PCB exposure among northern residents dependent upon a subsistence diet.[79] Because of its high per capita intake of country food, the community of Broughton Island (population 500) in the Baffin Island region was selected. Consent was obtained from the mayor and council of Broughton Island to conduct a pilot study, and it was agreed that they would be the first to be informed of the study's conclusions. The study involved an investigation of the amount of PCBs consumed in the diet and an analysis of PCB levels in blood and breast milk.[80]

The pilot study revealed that one in five islanders tested was ingesting a higher level of PCBs than Health Canada's "tolerable" daily intake of one microgram per kilogram of body weight. PCBs in blood exceeded Canadian guidelines in 63 per cent of the children tested and in 39 per cent of the women of child-bearing age. One of the four samples of breast milk obtained also contained PCBs at levels exceeding the guidelines. Shortcomings in laboratory techniques, however, prevented the drawing of firm conclusions from these results, and no dietary advice was issued.[81] Not surprisingly, local residents were distressed by these findings. Broughton Island's council and mayor agreed to further studies on these issues, and between 1987 and 1988 seven dietary assessments were carried out in the community. The purpose was to obtain an improved determination of contaminant intake and to examine the nutritional benefits of Inuit foods in order to make a benefit-risk assessment of the islanders' diet. The studies showed that traditionally harvested foods contained many essential nutrients. The scientists concluded that substituting country food with imported food could place the Inuit of Broughton Island at risk of nutritional deficiencies, "especially during the nutritionally vulnerable periods of pregnancy, lactation and infancy."[82]

During the fall of 1988, however, while the scientists were analysing the results of their field research, rumours that alarmingly high levels of PCBs had been discovered began to circulate and were soon amplified by a barrage of sensational media reports. When the scientists finally released their findings in the spring of 1989, recommending that Broughton Island's residents carry on with their traditional eating habits, the islanders' anxiety turned to confusion. For three months, media reports had been forewarning them that the amounts of contaminants the scientists had found in their bodies were such that they had to brace themselves for "huge diet and cultural change."[83] In the fall of 1989 the mayor of the hamlet complained that after the results had been officially released his community had been left in limbo as to their actual significance, and he expressed dismay at the lack of adequate explanation and follow-up to the research findings.[84] Two years later the chief medical officer for the Baffin Region indicated that the islanders were now assuming that PCBs were responsible for many of their health concerns including cancers, suicides, and premature births.[85] Residents of Broughton Island are still awaiting assessments of the risks posed by other contaminants (e.g., toxaphenes) which, along with PCBs, had been found in their blood during the 1987–88 studies.[86]

PCBs in Nunavik

In 1988 the Community Health Department of Laval University Hospital discovered PCB concentrations in the milk of Inuit women from northern Quebec that were among the highest ever found in a general population.[87] Average levels found in Inuit milk fat samples were about five times those of southern Canadian Caucasian women, with some samples containing about ten times the amount of PCBs deemed tolerable by Health Canada. Although these findings were preoccupying, they had to be interpreted in the broader context of Nunavik's nursing policy aimed at curbing the high incidence of infectious diseases among Inuit children by promoting the healthful effects of breast feeding. Enforcing Canadian guidelines would have meant discouraging breast-feeding for 70 to 80 per cent of Nunavik mothers.[88]

In close cooperation with Laval the Kativik Regional Council of Health and Social Services (KRCHSS) – the Inuit organization responsible for public health in Nunavik – decided not to issue any health advisory but instead to expand the database to better assess the health risk involved. A research program was initiated to monitor the breast milk of Inuit women in fourteen villages of Ungava and Hudson Bay regions (population 6,500) and to specifically assess the risks of breast-milk contamination to the children of Nunavik. The results showed total PCB levels in the milk fat of Inuit women to be seven times higher than those measured in a control group from southern Quebec, with concentrations ten times as high for some persistent PCB congeners.[89] A cohort study of Inuit newborn followed up to age two revealed that "breast-fed children had generally less ear infections at two months, as many at six months and more at twelve months than bottle-fed children."[90] Research on the health effects of PCBs and other orga-nochlorine compounds continues in northern Quebec; so far, how-ever, scientists have stressed that for the great majority of women in Nunavik, breast-feeding should continue to be encouraged as the healthiest choice.[91]

To calm fears created by media reports on the initial discovery of high PCB concentrations in Inuit milk and to avoid an overreaction on the part of the Nunavimmiut, the Inuit-controlled KRCHSS established the PCB Resource Committee to act as a link between the scientific researchers and the population. Based in Nunavik, the seven-member committee was made up of a field coordinator from Laval and local health workers and representatives. Members of the committee appeared on open-line radio and television programs to keep the people of Nunavik informed of ongoing studies, developed communi-cation materials promoting breast-feeding and country food, and pre-pared the release of new research findings to the population as these became available. The health personnel of the two regional hospitals who were part of the PCB committee played an active role in the col-lection of study data. As well, they contributed to communicating the known value of breast-feeding and country food while caring for patients and in informal discussions with community members.[92]

Although a formal evaluation of the communication activities con-ducted by the PCB committee has yet to be performed, there is a sense among its members that their stable presence and strong community involvement made it possible to gain the confidence of the Quebec Inuit and to communicate their message effectively to the population of Nunavik.[93] Still, there are indications that the information concern-ing PCB contamination which is circulating in northern Quebec has affected the perceptions that northerners have of their traditional diet and led to some undesirable lifestyle changes. Results of a 1992 survey show one in five Quebec Inuit to believe that, because of their lower PCB content, imported foods are healthier than country food. Like-wise, more than one individual in seven indicated having altered his or her lifestyle (e.g., decreased or discontinued marine mammal consumption) after learning that traditionally harvested foods and human milk were contaminated with PCBs.[94]

Managing and Communicating PCB Risk in the Far North

Because of the centrality of country food in the health, economy, and life of aboriginal communities, Arctic residents have found revelations concerning food-chain contamination particularly unsettling. So far the impact of these revelations on the actual harvesting and consumption of traditional foods appears to be relatively subtle and to vary among individuals and from one community to the next.[95] Yet there is no doubt that information concerning the presence of trace contaminants in traditional food sources has led to pervasive unease and anxiety among indigenous northerners.

Inasmuch as the notion of industrial contaminants and of their detection by scientific means falls outside the sphere of traditional experiences, indigenous populations have been inclined to interpret contaminant information in the light of their past experiences with outsiders. Because the contact with southern visitors and the transition from living on the land to settlement life that followed brought about profound disruptions and radical changes in the living conditions of northern aboriginals, they have grown wary about external interventions.[96] As a result, contaminant information and advice provided by scientists and other outside experts tends to be received with various degrees of scepticism, suspicion, and mistrust.[97] As the Broughton Island episode illustrates, indigenous northerners may have good reason to fear that efforts by southern scientists and authorities to assess and manage the risks of contaminants in the Far North will result in further disruptions and little benefits for local inhabitants.

During the 1970s public health agencies generally responded to the problem of northern contamination by recommending that aboriginal residents limit or avoid consuming contaminated species. The growing recognition of the multiple benefits that country food brings to northerners, coupled with a scarcity of straightforward information on the health consequences of current levels of contaminant intake, has convinced public health authorities to reverse their earlier stance and to support rather than discourage the consumption of traditional foods.[98] At present, however, the multiplication of information sources generating competing and often contradictory messages on contaminant issues makes it difficult for northern inhabitants to know just who to believe or what information is most relevant to their situation.

For a very long time the most credible sources in the communities on matters of country food have been elders and experienced hunters. In recent years the prominence and multiplication of vivid media reports attributing dire consequences to the presence of contaminants in the Arctic have cast doubts on the integrity of traditional food sources. Concurrently, the intensification and visibility of scientific activities designed to evaluate the extent and implications of northern contamination have further increased speculation regarding country food consumption. Between 1991 and 1995, for example, more than one hundred discrete research projects were conducted under the auspices of Canada's Arctic Environmental Strategy.[99] The comings and goings of scientists conducting sample collections in fauna, food/dietary studies, and human-health related research and surveys have stimulated concerns and rumours among the small communities of the sparsely populated Canadian Arctic.[100] Today, information about PCBs and other contaminants found in the traditionally harvested diet comes from radio and television broadcasts and from encounters with health personnel and researchers. In addition, contaminant information is disseminated through word of mouth, a process sometimes referred to as "contaminant gossip."[101]

Besides the legacy of past experiences and the recent increase in the amount of contaminant information circulating in the Arctic, attempts by southern experts to mitigate the effects of environmental contamination on northern natives have been complicated by difficulties in communicating across linguistic and cultural boundaries. Inuktitut, the preferred language of most Inuit living in the Eastern and Central Arctic, has no equivalent for many of the scientific concepts and terms used as a matter of course in discussing chemical contaminants. For instance, some of the translations of the word "contaminant" itself are so approximate that they do not allow northerners to distinguish between contaminants and other food spoilage caused by parasites, bacteria, or animal diseases.[102] While the adverse effects of contaminants is a matter of dose, calling contaminants diseases suggests that their harmfulness is independent of the concentrations in which they are found – and that they may be communicable. Frequent misunderstandings caused by the absence of adequate terminology for conveying the meaning of terms such as "PCBs" or "parts per million" are further compounded by sharp differences in the conceptual universe of the Inuit and that of Canadian scientists, and their respective outlooks on areas such as food, health, and relationships with animals and the land, which are essentially culture-specific.[103]

The perspectives of northern aboriginals and those of southern scientists on what constitutes useful knowledge on matters related to country food are thus strikingly different. Living and hunting in the Far North for thousands of years, the Inuit have accumulated an enormous amount of close observational knowledge about Arctic animals, and their behaviour, distribution, and ecology. Based on this understanding and on a number of visual and physical cues (smell, appearance, colouring, texture) they have developed a detailed system for diagnosing the quality and safety of wild foods. Yet the traditional knowledge which for centuries made it possible to determine reliably the fitness of country food is ineffective in the presence of invisible trace contaminants.[104]

At the same time, the scientific language used by southern experts to determine food safety is very much at odds with indigenous knowledge and experience.[105] The expert diagnosis expressed in parts per trillion of blood and grams per kilo of body weight and delivered in the form of probabilities of harm fluctuating according to the age, sex, and other characteristics of the individual exposed are inherently difficult for indigenous northerners to understand. The risks that concern northern natives are those they must confront in reality, not those that emerge from the micro-world approach of scientific risk assessors, as this elder's reaction to a presentation on environmental contamination suggests:

You people go to school. You should know as a result. But when you come up here, we find that you don't. But you went to school. But what of us? We know things. But no one asks us! We know how the rivers work. We know where the dumps are. But scientists come up here and they look at what they want to look at. But they look at [he gestures with his fingers] just a little bit of the fish. What about the other fish. No one talks about all of the environment.[106]

From a northern aboriginal perspective, the linear-analytical approach of southern scientists – narrowly focused on the cause and effects of each contaminant independent of the multi-dimensional factors affecting the quality of wild foods and the situation of those who consume them – is profoundly unsatisfying.[107] This in turn compromises the credibility of the risk management options put forward by southern experts.

Moreover, some concern has arisen that, in spite of its marginal usefulness to local populations, scientific effort to assess and mitigate the impact of contaminants on northern aboriginals may devalue their sense of self and undermine their confidence in the reliability of traditional knowledge to diagnose the fitness of country food. This could affect the status of elders, induce a decline in hunting skills, and disrupt family roles and traditional activities. Pointing to behaviours that have high positive value in northern aboriginal communities as possible sources of danger could thus have a more adverse impact on the well-being of northern natives than that which may result from their mere exposure to the contaminants themselves.[108]

From a risk management perspective, there is increasing agreement that public authorities cannot effectively assist northern populations in mitigating the risks of contamination without managing their scientific capabilities in ways that are directly relevant to the present situation of northerners and that explicitly reflect and validate their specific concerns and interests. So far, the diagnosis of the contaminant problem by outside experts has made it very difficult for aboriginal northerners to receive scientific advice on contaminants that relates to their specific circumstances. For instance, experts' characterization of PCB health risks to the Inuit of Broughton Island and Nunavik by reference to southern exposure standards created unwarranted alarm because it failed to consider the particular risk/benefit trade-offs of country food consumption by Arctic residents.

Greater participation and control by Arctic inhabitants over problem definition, data analysis, and development of risk control options can improve risk management response to northern contaminants and better benefit the people living in the Far North. Variations in eating habits from one community to another and from one age group to the next suggest, for instance, that because of their first-hand knowledge of local eating patterns, community members may possess critical information regarding contaminant exposure. Similarly, since northern communities react to the contaminant problem in a manner that is contingent upon their specific history and the degree to which the contaminant issue competes with more immediate concerns, risk management strategies need to be tailored to each community's degree of interest (or sensitivity) in the subject. A community-based approach to the contaminant issue that builds upon local knowledge is most likely to enhance the relevance of risk management actions.[109]

From a risk communication perspective, much uncertainty remains about what should be communicated and how. On one hand, there are still substantial scientific uncertainties over the long-term effects of chronic exposure to low level contaminants. For instance, although scientific experts agree that current levels of contamination do not warrant changes in nursing and country food consumption, no scientific consensus exists as to what concentration of PCBs in human milk constitutes a threshold that would contraindicate breast-feeding.[110] What is typical of so many risk situations holds here as well: after the one hundred studies and beyond, the information most frequently requested by aboriginal northerners – namely, clear and consistent answers regarding the sources of contamination and whether their foods are safe to eat or not[111] – cannot be supplied. Some field practitioners have emphasized that the efficacy of future contaminant information will depend squarely upon a better prior understanding of the actual perceptions and information expectations of northern communities.[112]

There is now a recognition among governments and other key players that political circumstances are changing in the North. Spearheaded by land-claims agreements, devolution of decision-making power to northern residents is taking place in all areas of northern development, whether economic, political, or social.[113] The trend is for local aboriginal organizations progressively to take the lead role in information management over the relative risks/benefits of country food consumption and breast-feeding. The successive names of the Nunavik liaison committee established to respond to the discovery of high levels PCBs in breast milk – the PCB Resource Committee (1989), the Food Contaminant and Health Committee (1994), the Nunavik Committee on Nutrition and Health (1996) – are indicative of this broader trend towards local problem definition and decision-making.

Yet while greater control by northern communities over the management and communication of research is clearly desirable, it is also important that the unique contribution southern science can make to detect and assess invisible contaminants be unambiguously acknowledged and enhanced. For example, some scientists have expressed concerns that in light of the existing licensing and permitting requirements already regulating the conduct of research in the North, new jurisdictional arrangements that would further raise bureaucratic barriers could drive scientists away from the Canadian Arctic.[114] Deterring the conduct of science in the North would ultimately diminish the quality of risk information available to aboriginal residents. Again, effective communication between interested parties is essential at this stage to ensure that new administrative arrangements promote the successful articulation of scientific and traditional knowledge and maximize the respective contributions various parties can make to assess and mitigate the impact of northern contaminants.

We end this long story on an unpleasant note. According to the authors of a major study published in 1995, *Communicating about Contaminants in Country Food*, findings from the PCB studies in the Far North in 1988 and again in 1989 were given to the media before the communities involved in those studies had been briefed on them. Community members, therefore, first learned about them in alarming media reports. The studies include the ones about elevated PCB concentrations in Broughton Island and Nunavik, and those reports contained accurate summaries of the study findings.[115]

Among those who have borne the costs of the risk communication failures we have discussed in the foregoing case studies, the Inuit in Canada's Far North may have experienced the severest impacts of all. They first read about, then heard from the researchers, comparisons of their PCB body burdens – the result of the long-range transport of pollutants from industrialized zones far away – with those of southerners; they learned how at least some of their diets exceeded Health Canada's number for acceptable daily intake (ADI). After the damage was done, a Health Canada official scrambled to explain that the ADI was based on risk estimate and that exceeding the number was not necessarily worrisome: "Once you exceed that number, it means you are eroding the safety factor [which could be as high as one thousand] … but it is not necessarily an indication for action."[116] Far too little, far too late in the game to do any good. Like the pollutants themselves, the risk communication failures originating in the industrialized South had undergone a process of long-range transport, as well as the social analogue of biomagnification (risk amplification), coming to rest among some of the most vulnerable people in Canada.

9 Ten Lessons

Prologue

As the people wandered in the desert, fretting about risks, and the voices clamouring for relief grew, the elders retained three consultants to examine some entrails and tell them what to do.

The First Night

The Diagnosis: "Your people suffer from severe ignorance."
The Referral: "You must see a risk expert at once."
The Medicine: "My cathartic of comparative risk statistics should do the trick."
The Specialist's Bedside Chatter: "Lady, if you really must worry about something, worry about peanut butter, not nuclear power."
The Patient's Response: "Don't patronize me, you arrogant bastard!"
The Prognosis: The patients won't take the medication. So despite offering his services for free, the first consultant was thrown out of the tent.

The Second Night

The Diagnosis: "Your elders suffer from an inability to communicate with their people."

The Referral: "You must see a marketing communications expert at once."

The Medicine: "These new empathy drugs should do the trick, but if complications develop, an intravenous solution of third-party credibility may be needed."

The Specialist's Bedside Chatter: "Lady, trust me, I share deeply your concerns about all possible harmful effects on your children and your children's children, even unto the seventh generation."

The Patient's Response: "That's a good line, but I still don't trust you, and I still don't want your camel waste in my back yard."

The Prognosis: The medication doesn't help, but since everyone feels better taking pills, the second consultant was invited to stay in the tent.

The Third Night

The Diagnosis: "Everyone carries the bacterium, and an outbreak of the disease of worrying about risks can erupt at any time."

The Referral: "Try counselling instead of drugs."

The Counsel: "I can't cure you, but I may be able to relieve the symptoms a bit."

The Specialist's Bedside Chatter: "Talking about it might help."

The Patient's Response: "Are you sure there aren't any pills you can prescribe?"

The Prognosis: The outbreaks of the disease should be monitored closely; the infectious agent may mutate into a benign form over time.

Epilogue

The elders wondered why they should pay good money for this kind of advice anyway, and sent their lobbyists off to Parliament with instructions to pass a law outlawing the bacterium.

In chapter 2 we depicted the emergence of good risk communication practice as a three-phase process. Phase one was influenced by the risk expert's belief that educating the public about risk assessment methods and statistical outcomes would allow publicly acceptable risk management to be based squarely on comparative risk numbers. The bottom line was: the higher the confirmed body count, the more attention the risk deserves. In phase one many risk experts were indifferent at best, and contemptuous at worst, towards contrary relative risk judgments emanating from the public domain.

Phase two sought to repair some of the resultant damage by addressing directly the concerns voiced by ordinary citizens, regardless of whether or not the nature of those concerns matched the results of calculated risk estimates. Risk managers were advised to locate the psychological sources of public concerns and to express empathy with the underlying fears on which they were based. The strategy was adapted from what had been learned in the field of marketing communications about effective message delivery; the advice was implemented through the training of executives in techniques for information delivery that were intended to make those executives trusted and credible communicators of risk-based messages.

What was fundamentally incomplete about the first two phases, considered in isolation, was that both unwittingly depended on a "magic bullet" effect to resolve risk controversies. In phase one the exquisitely calculated risk estimates themselves were expected to be capable of having a salutory impact on public thinking: If catastrophic reactor failure in a nuclear power station could be shown to be a ridiculously low-probability event, whereas poor nutrition or smoking were known with great confidence to be significant risk factors for human health, why would anyone in his or her right mind worry about the former rather than the latter two? The expectation was frustrated, for the most part, but a general commitment to risk assessment was won, and as a result a well-tested set of numbers for a wide variety of significant risk factors is accumulating, from which both society and individuals can derive good guidance in decision making.

In phase two the marketing-based communications exercise itself was the hoped-for magic bullet: if the techniques were powerful enough, even though they were designed originally to sell toothpaste and politicians, perhaps they could make unpalatable risk messages acceptable as well. Alas, there is no evidence to suggest that the outcomes of any of the larger risk issues (such as the ones reviewed in our case studies) have been influenced by the applications of such techniques alone. On the other hand, this new orientation encouraged public affairs and communications professionals working for industry and governments to make an honest effort to listen carefully to the concerns raised by the public, to provide responses to them in understandable terms, and to make prompt disclosure of relevant information. Many such professionals are now solidly committed to this way of carrying out their business, and this is all to the good.

However, there is a growing realization that there will be no "quick fix" to the inherent difficulties in communicating about risks. This is why phase three stresses the need for a long-term institutional commitment to the gradual development and application of good risk communication practices. The lessons we seek to draw from our case studies in the following pages represent our contribution to the task of identifying those practices.[1]

THE LESSONS

Our case studies show that risk communication is serious business and that failures in risk communication practices can be costly. In Great Britain that portion of the population who may worry about risks more than others now must wait another twenty years to see how many cases of nvcJD will emerge and whether those cases will, finally and definitively, be linked by science to transmissable bovine spongiform encephalopathy. British press reports show a clear sense of betrayal of the public by the politicians and civil servants who insisted for so long that there was "no conceivable risk" of contracting cJD by eating beef. The financial consequences to E.U. nations for additional farm price supports for beef (due to falling demand) and the costs of the mass cattle cull in the British herd may be as high as five billion dollars. Much of this bill can be assigned to risk communication failure. This is because, when (after another twenty years or so) the number of human nvcJD fatalities attributable to transmissable BSE is finally known, it may turn out to be a relatively low number (it even *could* be zero) – but now, in 1997, the confidence of beef importing nations in the British risk management system has been utterly destroyed. In large part this is because of the patently unwise "no risk" assurances issued between 1990 and 1995; confidence can only be rebuilt through drastic measures.

Risk communication failures involving PCBs have been very costly for the Canadian Inuit, as we have shown. To this must be added some incremental monetary cost – possibly significant, but impossible to measure – for the eventual total destruction of existing PCBs stocks, because it has taken far longer than it should have to win public acceptability for technically feasible disposal technologies, capable of rendering 99.99+ per cent of those compounds into environmentally benign substances.

Whatever the final outcome of the class-action lawsuits against Dow Corning, the company's risk communication failures have so far cost it tens of millions of dollars in staff, public relations, and legal costs, and the final bill will be much higher. Monsanto Canada has also paid a financial penalty for risk communication failures (its own and others') in the case of rBST – but, although it may seem odd to say so, the public has paid a high price here too. That price is the damage done to the science-based risk assessment process by the silence of some parties and the mischief of others, who so thoroughly intermixed peripheral issues with the health risk ones that no reasonable risk discussion was possible. Since it is hard to imagine how citizens can decide what to worry about (and what not to) without the assistance of science-based risk assessments, anything like Canada's rBST experience is disquieting.

It is hard to say whether or not the chemical and other industries have paid a significant "risk premium" for dioxins yet – that is, the premium for the stigma which dioxins carry – in the sense that expenditures have been made for risk control measures which are not justified in terms of a common yardstick for acceptable risk. But almost certainly they will pay this premium in the coming years, at least in countries such as Canada, where the promise of "virtual elimination" is likely to be interpreted as legitimizing the hunt for the last molecule in industrial processes. But what less vigilant stance would be appropriate when public policy has hung the label "mega-ugly" on these substances?

Lesson 1: A risk information vacuum is a primary factor in the social amplification of risk. Risk communication failures can initiate a cascade of events that exacerbate risk controversies and render risk issues difficult to manage. At the core of all risk issues there are problematic aspects – lack of timely information, uncertainties in the risk estimates, lack of trust, lack of credibility, complexity of the scientific descriptions, and so forth – which breed apprehensiveness, suspicion, and concern over personal safety among the public. In a risk information vacuum, this latent apprehensiveness, suspicion, and concern feeds upon itself and, in the absence of the dampening effect that good risk communication practices might supply, may be amplified to the point where credible and pertinent information makes no difference in the formation of popular opinion.

Where transmissable spongiform encephalopathy (TSE) is concerned, the public fears and suspicions in Britain grew in direct proportion to the unequivocal denials of politicians, who unwisely chose to exploit the unavoidable uncertainties in the ongoing scientific detective work to justify an appalling lack of concern about the seriousness of the emerging risk factors. The case study materials demonstrate that, in each year after 1990, enough relevant new science was being reported to form the basis of prudent and measured messages of a very different sort than what was actually sent: the possibility that there would emerge a (probably) relatively small human health risk from BSE, which would be aggressively monitored by a concerned government that would promptly report what it found to the public.

The matter of dioxins as a pre-eminent risk issue should have declined steadily after 1985, when governments had formed their resolve to work steadily towards reducing emissions from anthropogenic sources, and when major industries had signalled that they would cooperate with this agenda. The issue amplification that occurred instead can be attributed directly to the vast risk information vacuum that was permitted to develop: just compare the enormity of the accumulated international scientific research productions on the one hand with the dearth of credible, publicly accessible accounts of the meaning of that great effort on the other. Add to this the proclivity of some senior politicians in environmental portfolios for making offhand, inflammatory statements about dioxins, and a few other factors, and there is no need to search further to ascertain why dioxins will continue to be a featured item on the public's risk issue plate in the coming decade.

Suspicions about the industry's lack of candour about complications in the functioning of silicone breast implants provided fertile ground for the sprouting of other, greater fears. And PCBs: one can sit and read the calm words in Health Canada's May 1989 pamphlet entitled *PCBs and Human Health*: "There is no evidence of any harmful effects of small amounts of PCBs found in breast milk." But those were not the first words the Inuit heard about the elevated levels of PCBs researchers found in their body tissue. What they first heard were the alarming media reports, for which they were totally unprepared, despite the fact that PCBs had been a high priority for scientific research and regulatory action for almost twenty years before the controversy broke in Canada's Far North. They were unprepared in large part because in all that time no agency stepped forward to take responsibility for ensuring that conclusions from the new knowledge were being regularly and effectively transmitted to audiences in the public domain which might some day need to know about them. Instead, one could encounter in the media periodic musings by experts about the public's inexplicable misunderstandings in the matter of PCB risks.

As we write, some serious risk information vacuums are just now developing, particularly in the areas of agricultural biotechnology and endocrine disruptors. And the now-familiar process of risk amplification in those areas is already firmly rooted.

Lesson 2: Regulators are responsible for effective risk communication. What agency in society has the primary responsibility for risk communication? By a process of elimination the answer is clearly that governments do, and in particular those agencies of governments having regulatory authority over a broad range of health and environmental risks. These agencies either already have – or are capable of acquiring through enabling legislation – the legal authority to manage risks. This means simply that they can devise and enforce rules that can modify behaviour across the entire range of risk situations: in the workplace, on the roads and highways, in emissions of substances to all environmental media, in product design and marketing, and so forth.

In general the objectives of these agencies are risk control and risk reduction, not risk elimination, because as a general rule risk – a certain probability of harm – is an inescapable part of activity in the environment. Some risks can be entirely eliminated, of course, such as those associated with specific consumer products (such as silicone breast implants), which can be done away with by banning them, so long as substances associated with them have not been dispersed irretrievably in the environment. But there is nothing we can do to get *E. coli* O157:H7 out of the cattle population, or dioxins and PCBs out of the environment; scientists have not yet even identified with certainty the infectious agent responsible for spongiform encephalopathies.

Risk control and risk reduction are inherently halfway measures, designed to limit the estimated harm that may be done to individuals, using some measure of safety (one-in-a-million, or "no detectable level," or some comparable yardstick) that ultimately must stand the test of public acceptability. Halfway measures – limiting rather than eliminating exposures – are much harder to explain to the public than the more dramatic "bans," but most of our risk management options do lie in this domain. Perhaps much of failures to date in the risk communication of halfway measures can be attributed to the fact that it is undeniably difficult to do this well. The upshot is that most responsible agencies would rather not try at all, rather than take the chance of getting it wrong.

Both the scientific research that describes particular hazards and the expert judgments that make up a risk assessment are devilishly complicated matters. What is more, the scientific understanding evolves continuously as research proceeds, and entirely new twists (as in the case of dioxins) may emerge. The risk reduction scenarios, built upon immense efforts in scientific detection and risk assessment, encapsulate many very difficult intellectual constructions. How is it conceivable, then, that the results of such efforts could be communicated effectively – especially to non-expert audiences – by the production of a three- or four-page newsletter, say, once every few years?

Health Canada has had an established practice of not announcing the issuance of a regulatory decision as a matter of policy, so unless practice changes, when its decision on rBST is finally made, someone else will have to tell the public about it. By way of contrast, in the United States the FDA regularly makes brief statements in conjunction with regulatory actions, outlining the reasons for the action. On 22 March 1996, two days after the storm broke in Britain over BSE and its possible link to nvCJD, the U.S. Department of Agriculture prepared a document analysing the implications of the British events for U.S. meat safety and announcing an enhanced BSE surveillance program in slaughterhouses. In late January 1997 President Clinton announced through his nationwide weekly radio program a huge new effort to create a comprehensive early-warning system for threats to food safety. Although Agriculture and Agri-Food Canada will reply to media questions, to the date of writing it has not formulated any general public statement about BSE and the safety of the Canadian meat supply.

Lesson 3: Industry is responsible for effective risk communication. Except for occurrences related to natural hazards, industry may become involved in some way with every risk controversy, because a product or process, or a substance used in either of them, is attached to the risk, directly or peripherally. Given the number of products, processes, and substances circulating in an industrial society, risk controversies – especially long-running ones – are relatively rare. That said, it is hard to predict where an intractable risk controversy will take root and blossom. There are some purely accidental features in the biographies of most (but not all) such controversies that have erupted to date.

One could safely wager before the fact that, say, the disposal of high-level radioactive waste was likely to be a distasteful affair, even among the most orderly peoples. The same is true of pesticides, given the very nature of those substances. On the other hand, it is quite possible that, under different conditions, neither PCBs, BSE, silicone breast implants, nor rBST may have given rise to any special concerns. Or even dioxins: suppose that there had never been such a thing as Agent Orange, and that no one had sold dioxin-contaminated still bottoms for use in a dust-suppressor mix across the Missouri countryside; or suppose that industry had figured out how to prevent the formation of dioxins in trichlorophenol. Suppose that Greenpeace had not made dioxins a *cause célèbre* just as the memory of Agent Orange was fading. These are all accidental features of what we know as the dioxin controversy, and in the absence of one or more of them, dioxins might have had a very different profile during the past twenty-five years.

Industry is in an unusual position with respect to the hazards its products and processes entail. On the one hand, these days the public assigns rather low credibility to anything said about such risks from that source. On the other hand, industry generally knows those hazards well, often better than anyone else simply because the substances themselves were invented in its labs. This can appear to be a "Catch-22" situation. Is there a way out?

The first step, which industry understands well at this point, is the scientific characterization of the most serious hazards associated with a newly created or newly understood industrial substance or process. But from the perspective of the present, the very next step should be to characterize these hazards from the standpoint of both public policy implications and communications responsibilities. When one approaches them with these considerations in mind, the hazards in question may fall into a number of different categories, such as:

- Primarily workplace hazards, governed by labour legislation, hazard warning protocols, emergency training requirements, and legal liabilities related to occupationally caused disease (asbestos, formaldehyde);
- Population health hazards resulting from biological processes (infectious diseases, food-borne pathogens);
- General environmental hazards from the dispersion of industrially generated substances through environmental media, including environmental fate characteristics (persistence, etc.) and impacts on different species (pesticides, ozone-depleting chemicals);
- Both workplace and general environmental hazards (metals, organochlorine compounds);
- Incremental risks produced as a byproduct of beneficial industrial products (pharmaceuticals, chlorination, modern transportation).

This is an illustrative list rather than an exhaustive or correctly categorized one. But some such list can help to guide thinking about what types of issues are involved and where the primary risk communications responsibilities ought to lie.

It is now generally accepted that industry must take primary risk communication responsibility for product-related risks and workplace hazards, as well as for community awareness in the vicinity of facilities where hazardous materials and processes are employed.[2] And in general there is a reasonably good appreciation today of what to do, and how to do it, in these situations. (Whether what is actually done or not done in specific instances is adequate, from the standpoint of affected parties, is a matter of particular cases.) But for anything involving general exposures of humans and other species as a result of environmentally dispersed hazards, industry has to tread carefully, on account of its credibility problem – one that can be solved eventually by the compilation of a proven track record in credible communications.

In these cases industry also should insist that governments step into the breach and assume primary responsibility for preventing the formation of the risk information vacuum. But because governments face unrelenting lobbying on dozens of issues from industry and other parties, the results that may be expected from such an insistence depend entirely on the relative priority which industry itself assigns to good risk communication practice. Governments will not step into the breach if weak pressure is applied, implying that the lobbyist is merely paying lip service to the task, since – as we have said – doing effective risk communication for risk management's halfway measures is an onerous and expensive process that will garner few laurels for the practitioners. Where so few rewards are in the offing, government officials will respond only to the most determined and persistent entreaties from industry risk managers to get the job done.

Lesson 4: If you are responsible, act early and often. Obviously an agency needs a great deal of discretion in deciding how to allocate among diverse risk issues its investments of significant risk communication resources, especially in an era of declining overall resources. But some astute forecasting capacity is absolutely essential, for timeliness is everything in effective risk communication: overcoming entrenched perceptions that are broadly dispersed in the social environment is a thankless task with almost no chance of succeeding. Of course it is possible to be ambushed by events, especially if they are extensively reported in the media, but on the other hand, governments (and the professionals whom they can consult) have a great deal more information now, as opposed to the quite recent past, about the range of principal environmental and health risk factors.

Doing good risk communication early is of little benefit if it not also done often, as often and as long as is needed to prevent a risk issue from being put into play – in the way in which dioxins risk was – by other interested parties. *How* often is a function of the sheer scale of the scientific research effort, in producing results requiring clear explanation, and of the chance events that intersect those efforts. This is a demanding task requiring special skills and the resources needed to reach key audiences and opinion leaders.[3] There is simply no cheap solution, and in an era of declining overall budgets this entails the reallocation of resources towards public communications endeavours.

Dozens of significant risk factors have elicited deep public concern in the past or may do so in the future. Issue management forecasting must be able to pick out those having traits with the potential to foment intractable risk controversies. More complete risk reporting in the general media, better dissemination of leading-edge scientific research in journals such as *Nature* and *Science*, and new information sources (such as the Internet) make possible a forward-looking surveillance of emerging risk issues today. Our own list of issues likely to engender long-term, endemic public controversies over the next ten years is:

- food safety generally;
- endocrine disruptors (including dioxins);
- greenhouse gases and global climate change;
- biotechnology, especially agricultural applications;
- health impacts of atmospheric pollutants.

These are not necessarily the only high-profile risk issues for the coming years, but they are among those which will be controversial, that is, ones involving high stakes for social interests but which also have no clear and simple risk management solutions.

One might say they are obvious candidates. So much the better, since there will be less reason to quibble over the ranking of them. And it is a long enough list indeed, if risk communication responsibilities are to be taken seriously at long last.

Lesson 5: There is always more to a risk issue than what science says. In defending bovine growth hormone, industry adamantly insisted that milk from rBST-treated cows is "exactly the same as" milk from untreated animals and moreover, the fact that rBST is classified as a drug is an unimportant detail, for it is merely a matter of the bureaucratic slot in which the government regulatory system places it. We are prepared to accept these as fair and appropriate judgments from a scientific point of view, but we still think that it is unwise to make them, and even more unwise to disparage the intelligence or motives of persons who do refuse to accept them. Milk is no ordinary commodity, as the imagery used in the regular advertising campaigns promoting milk consumption shows well. Its hoary status in culture as well as in human nutrition means that one should not approach it as just a mixture of chemical compounds.

Monsanto officials when quoted in press stories stressed repeatedly that rBST use is safe for both cows and humans, that rBST had been reviewed exhaustively and then endorsed by many medical and regulatory bodies, and indeed that rBST probably had undergone more scrutiny than any other animal health product in history. We accept all of the above as fair and honest representations – but they simply miss the point so far as the framing of this issue in the social arena is concerned.

The implicit contention in the purely scientific discourse about rBST is that the public should not care about the farmer's manipulation of bovine hormonal systems so long as the end product for the consumer is "exactly the same" – in terms of its chemical composition – as before. This is wrong. For it is not unreasonable to think that this implicit contention may be upsetting to people within the intuitive complex of associations that milk has in society ("natural" goodness, wholesomeness, purity, links to children, nutritive value, and so on). By ignoring these broader considerations and implicitly denying their legitimacy, the rBST promoters may have amplified anxieties and mistrust.

A related case is the labelling of genetically engineered foods. For Bt-containing potatoes as in milk from BST-treated cows, industry has insisted that special consumer information is unnecessary because the end products are no different from what has always been on the store shelves. This stance means that oft-expressed public concerns are simply irrelevant. A more enlightened position would be that in Canada full information is a consumer's basic right and that the matter is not one of *whether* to label but *how.* Labelling every ingredient in complex food mixes, such as prepared sauces, that may contain miniscule amounts of engineered plants, it is said, could overwhelm the shopper, and the full account might even exceed the dimensions of the container surface. Our answer is that this is simply a matter of thinking intelligently and sympathetically about how to respond to public concerns; for example, well-publicized 1-800 numbers or separate information kits rather than exhaustive lists on product packages could satisfy most of the demand. The important point is that the industry should be perceived to be solicitous of consumer inquiries and eager to provide a generous supply of pertinent data.

Lesson 6: Always put the science in a policy context. Almost any type of risk issue can turn into a seemingly intractable risk controversy, and it is the nature of such controversies inevitably to give rise to demands on governments to "do something" about controlling or eliminating the risks in question. In other words, although the scientific description of the hazards and probabilistic risk assessments can be matters of widespread public interest, in the final analysis the competing choices among risk management options – banning or restricting a substance, say – make up the contents of letters and calls to politicians. Inevitably, also, the demands for policy closure in the form of regulatory action will in many cases precede that other relevant closure, the one represented by a firm scientific consensus on the underlying biochemical mechanisms out of which the hazards emerge.

This means that the contents of effective risk communication cannot be limited to the scientific description of hazards or the risk numbers. Rather, the science should be put into a policy (action) context, which in the early stages of an emerging risk controversy might take the form of forecasting a range of policy options – including the "do nothing" option – and of exploring their consequences in terms of implications for economic and social interests, international developments, and obligations for environmental protection.

In other words, responsible agencies ought to begin discussing the possible policy responses to emerging risk controversies as soon as they arise, and continue to do so throughout their life history. Part of that discussion is, of course, a sketch of the scientific results already known and the research still under way, but this is not the whole of the risk communication mandate, nor indeed even the most important segment of it. Rather, the primary obligation is to explain the implications of policy choices in risk management.

Lesson 7: "Educating the public" about science is no substitute for good risk communication practice. Sanctimonious urgings for new programs designed to increase the public's awareness about the inner mysteries of scientific research are encountered frequently.[4] What appears to sustain this mission is the curious belief that the citizenry's ignorance of scientific method can best explain the observed differences between the expert assessment of risk and the public perception of the same. The ancillary apparent belief is that knowing more about current scientific research would calm the public's nerves in matters of risk. And, presumably, a quick course in the specialist jargon used by the various scientific disciplines is the right curative for both ignorance and worry.

Carrying the refrain that "knowing more about science is good for you" is a bit like trying to convince children to eat the vegetables they dislike. This is a vain hope founded on a misdiagnosis of the ailment, if – as we suspect – the underlying strategy is to reduce public anxiety about risks. For with rare exceptions specialist knowledge in its original form circulates inside ever-narrower confines, even within the major sub-groupings for academic learning (natural sciences, social sciences, fine arts). So if the producers of specialized research are disabled with respect to much of what circulates around them, why should the non-expert public be expected to do what the professionals themselves cannot nor, indeed, even try to do?

Whatever its advantages might be, the mission to "educate the public about science" is not a substitute for assuming responsibility to carry out good risk communication practice. Where risks are concerned, what the public wants to hear is what those charged with risk management responsibility think ought to be done, and why; the explanation of the scientific reasoning on which risk control measures are based is strictly of secondary interest. This is not to suggest that the scientific reasoning is irrelevant or unneeded – quite the contrary. It does mean that it is up to the risk communication practitioner to take the time and trouble to construct a fair and understandable representation of both the relevant science and its meaning for the choice of policy options. And to do so, as we said, early and often, whenever emerging new scientific results appear to alter the risk assessment or the policy consequences, or whenever other interested parties who are deeply involved in the issues develop well-articulated competing representations.

Lesson 8: Banish "no risk" messages.   Ironically, although citizens and environmentalists are often taken to task by government and industry officials for advocating "zero risk" scenarios, pronouncements of the "there is no risk" variety are a favourite of government ministers and sometimes of industry voices as well. In fact, at least some business sectors – the chemical industry in particular – do this less and less, which is a sea-change from what used to be their standard public relations practice.[5] To the extent that government ministers still indulge themselves in the practice, what they are undoubtedly hoping to accomplish thereby is just to get an annoying problem off their desks. But it is always a mistake to yield to this temptation.

A zero risk policy is the functional equivalent of exorcism. In both cases, alas, the offending agent is invisible to the naked eye, so that one can never be entirely sure that one is rid of it, no matter how furious the cathartic program is. Even an apparently sensible agenda such as "virtual elimination" may turn out to be an ill-advised concession to the stigmatizing urge, because it can appear to signal insufficient courage to take all the measures necessary to protect public health. Besides, something like dioxins will be virtually eliminated one day, and not the next – because inevitably a new technology will rediscover it everywhere in the environment at a lower level of concentration. And as soon as this happens there will be calls for renewed efforts to drive it away again, based solely on the fact that it is known to be there still, for at that point the harm that it does is simply a function of its continued existence and nothing more.[6]

Lesson 9: Risk messages should address directly the "contest of opinion" in society.   There is a curious reluctance, especially on the part of government risk managers, to address directly the various alternative representations of risk issues as they form and re-form in dialogue among interested parties in society. A charitable interpretation is that this reflects a wish not to appear to be "manipulating" public opinion, but if this indeed is the motivation, it is misguided. For if one accepts the contention made above, namely that government regulators have the primary responsibility for effective risk communication, these officials cannot avoid confronting the issues as they are posed in society, not how they appear in science-based risk assessments.[7]

Our cases are rife with examples of this failure. No one addressed the developing fears of immune-type diseases attributed to silicone breast implants until it was too late and opinion was already formed. We have already commented on the bizarre silence by Canadian regulators about alleged risks associated with rBST. In the case of dioxins, no Canadian regulator has confronted publicly and adequately the criticisms of Health Canada's allowable daily intake guideline. No one gave the Inuit a timely explanation of the meaning of the safety factor built into the exposure calculations for PCBs. And so far no responsible risk communicator in Canada is mounting a fair discussion of the environmental risks associated with plant biotechnology.

These failures imply a stubborn bent on the part of those regulators to recognize only those aspects of risk issues that flow directly from the terms of their own risk assessment protocols. The reluctance to become engaged in the social dialogue on risks is understandable, to be sure, because it is often a very messy affair. Plant biotechnology is a good case in point: for some time now claims about unusual adverse effects from genetic engineering that are totally at variance with the basic concepts that regulators use to evaluate biotechnology have been circulating among Internet news groups, and these claims are not contested by the regulators in the arena of public opinion. Greenpeace has started to put agricultural biotechnology into play as a risk issue, with direct actions in Europe against grain shipments and the beginnings of a series of publications.[8]

However messy these arenas may be, those responsible for effective risk communication practice will have either to get a bit dirty in them or take the chance of paying some of the other substantial costs of risk communication failures.

Lesson 10: Communicating well has benefits for good risk management. To date, good risk communication has been largely an afterthought in the risk management process, when it is remembered at all, and in resource allocation terms a mere footnote to the huge budgets assigned to primary scientific research. Those thrown into the fray when the communications tasks simply cannot be ignored are usually scientists

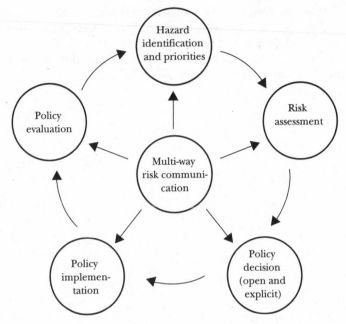

Figure 9.1
The risk management cycle with risk communication at the hub[9]

with little or no training for such tasks or public relations specialists who spend much of their time protecting others in the organization from excessive outside scrutiny. (Those who carry out these tasks well – and there are some – are mostly self-trained.) Underpinning this state of not-so-benign neglect is the implicit notion that risk communication is a distraction from the real business of risk assessment and control. The costs of risk communication failures are too high to allow this notion to persist. Good risk communication practice should be regarded as equal in importance to the other key elements – risk assessment and the evaluation of risk control options – in the overall risk management process. Accepting this contention also means that sufficient resources should be allocated to the risk communication effort, and opportunities must be found to provide adequate personnel training in the unique set of skills that these efforts demand.

In fact, far from being a distraction, good risk communication practice can be regarded as the causeway that links all the organizational elements in a well-functioning risk management process. We like Soby's diagrammatic representation of its place (fig. 9.1). In this conception multi-way risk communication is the causeway across which flow the exchanges linking the varied contributions of the two essential foci in risk management, namely science and risk assessment on the one hand, and policy processes on the other.

This causeway cannot function at all in the presence of a risk information vacuum.

PART THREE

New Perils for Risk Managers

10 Two Stinking Cows: The Mismanagement of BSE Risk in North America

WILLIAM LEISS

One stinking cow ...

Alberta Premier Ralph Klein (July 2003)[1]

THE STORY IN BRIEF

The discovery of two cases of BSE in the Canadian herd has had devastating impacts on Canadian farm families and the farm economy. Estimated direct and indirect economic costs from the first – single – case of BSE exceed $5 billion, as of November 2003, and those costs continue to rise with each passing month.[2] The personal and family costs among farm families are incalculable. How could this have happened, as a result of one or two sick cows? How could this have happened, since no one thinks that Canadians' health is seriously at risk if meat from a few cattle infected with BSE has entered our food supply?

The simple answer is, governments in Canada brought on this catastrophe by mismanaging the risk of BSE. Specifically, government officials failed to communicate to beef farmers and the larger agricultural industry the true risk, that is, the best estimate of the likelihood that BSE would show up in the Canadian herd. The risk was said by officials to be virtually nonexistent; yet they must have known that this was not the case, for reasons I will explain later. The truth is, there was always a fair likelihood that North America would see a few cases of BSE in its herds. There is still a fair likelihood that one or more additional cases will appear this year or next.

This whole episode is filled with terrible ironies. The normal excuse given by governments for failing to communicate risks effectively is that "the public may panic." Which is a case of blaming the victim, since more often those who panic are our politicians, who seize up at the thought of having to take the trouble of explaining to the public the nuances and subtleties of risk assessments. In the case of our troubles with beef, however, this excuse is unavailable. Canadians have responded to the terror of BSE by *increasing* their consumption of beef, which – since prices have not dropped – probably reflects a generous gesture of support to our ever-struggling farm sector. (A simpler reason may be that we love our beef, and the BSE story has kept our awareness of this preferred dietary option uppermost in mind.)

So, if the public didn't panic, what's the problem? And why do we have such catastrophic economic consequences? What this case shows is that when the need arises to communicate risks honestly and fearlessly, apparently trivial differences in wording and emphasis can be responsible for devastating outcomes. The answers to these two questions turn on two things: first, on the seemingly innocuous differences in the connotations of the words "negligible" and "low" (risk); and second, on not discriminating among the different types of risks faced by Canadian beef producers, who were expanding their export markets into a world where having a single indigenous case of BSE in the national herd could cause those markets to be shuttered in an instant – and stay shuttered for a full seven years. What befell Canadian beef producers in 2003 was a disaster waiting to happen. The origins of that disaster lie in a series of bad risk-policy judgments made by federal officials at the Canadian Food Inspection Agency, over almost a decade.

BSE – bovine spongiform encephalopathy or mad cow disease – is one of a larger class of animal diseases called transmissible spongiform encephalopathies (TSEs).[3] They may arise spontaneously (sporadic cases) or be acquired by transmission; they can also cross the species barrier. The best-known member of this class is scrapie, which affects sheep (BSE may have originated as a mutation of scrapie); others include CWD (chronic wasting disease) in deer and elk, and feline spongiform encephalopathy (seen in both domestic and wild cats). A number of the cases, such as those in mink, cats, and a wide variety of hoofed animals kept in zoos, are attributable to the feeding of animal protein infected with scrapie and BSE. CWD still presents challenges to science in terms of its origins and mode of transmission. The human form of sporadic TSE is Creuzfeldt-Jakob Disease (CJD), which is also transmissible through direct contact with infected nerve or pituitary gland tissue (corneal transplants, growth hormone implants). Another acquired form, caused by infection from BSE, is known as new-variant CJD.[4]

The most widely accepted explanation for the origins of these diseases is the "prion hypothesis" associated with the name of Stanley Prusiner. The hypothesis asserts that an abnormal form of a common protein in the brain of animals is infectious; that is, it can cause a normal prion protein (PrP) to convert to the abnormal conformation. In both sporadic and acquired forms, the disease spreads by positive feedback through this conversion process. The abnormal form has "slightly different amino acid sequences and, therefore, slightly different secondary and tertiary structures. The different structures will alter the stability of the three-dimensional shape of the molecule, and alter the probability with which it can undergo a spontaneous change in shape."[5] The progress of the disease causes amyloid plaques – small cavities or holes causing the diseased areas of the brain to appear sponge-like – to proliferate, destroying a wide range of brain functions affecting motor control, memory, mood (aggressiveness), and other faculties. It is incurable and inevitably results in premature death.

BSE has been one of the highest-profile issues in animal health and food safety around the world for over fifteen years now. The early history of the issue is traced in chapter 1. First, the British beef industry was decimated, giving rise to countless tragedies among farm families and running up costs against the public treasury in excess of £4 billion. Next, BSE spread to over twenty other countries, including most of the European continent and as far away as Japan, where the dual difficulties of farmers and public costs have been repeated. According to what I believe is the most plausible explanation for the global spread of BSE, this resulted from the exporting of infected feed, live cattle, and other bovine materials from Britain. The feed exports were the worst of these: the official *Report of the BSE Inquiry* (October 2000) in Britain confirmed that British officials permitted these exports to continue in full knowledge that some portion of the feed was certainly infected.

Almost certainly, BSE initially came to Canada – and, in all probability, to the United States as well – through imports from Britain of small numbers of infected live animals. What follows is a quotation from a draft risk-assessment document prepared by a Canadian federal department in mid-2000 (but never completed or released): "Therefore, live cattle and sheep imported from the U.K. during the early 1980s, and possibly before this, up until the time of import bans, could have served as a vector for the introduction of BSE to Canadian livestock either through direct animal contact or through consumption of animal feeds produced with rendered materials of imported animals."[6] Although an alternative hypothesis about the origins of the disease, supporting the contention that the two Canadian cases were spontaneous rather than acquired, is not entirely implausible, the "weight of evidence" accepted by scientific and government authorities around the world, including those in Canada, is that such cases arise by animal-to-animal recycling of infectious prions primarily through infected animal feed.[7]

The reader may ask, "Where is the mismanagement in all this? If what is described above is indeed how things unfolded, the occurrence of BSE cases in Canada is a tragedy, to be sure, but not one that could have been prevented." Indeed, the charge of "mismanagement of risk" implies that something could have – and should have – been done differently. I believe that the facts of the case justify this charge.

What was done wrong? The answer is that, led (or, more accurately, misled) by officials at the Canadian Food Inspection Agency (CFIA), governments in Canada seriously underestimated the risk that one or more indigenous cases of BSE would appear in the Canadian herd. For the entire period from 1997 to December 2003, the CFIA assessed the risk of BSE in Canada as "negligible." The dictionary definition of the word "negligible" is "so small or unimportant or of so little consequence as to warrant little or no attention: TRIFLING." And indeed, the CFIA paid little attention to the risk estimation of BSE: The agency had done an elaborate quantitative estimation of the risk of BSE in Canada for the period prior to 1997, but – inexplicably – stopped its work at that point. For the period after 1997, the agency simply asserted – *without any supporting argument whatsoever* – that, in view of policy choices made in 1997, the risk thereafter also was "negligible." No calculations at all were adduced in defence of this judgment. And yet, if you were a Canadian beef farmer in, say, the year 2000, what would you care about the risk as it was in 1990? What you needed, and should have had in hand from your government, was some solid estimate of the risk you were facing at that moment. No justification has ever been proffered by the CFIA for this bizarre behaviour.

Support for this strong criticism is easily found, because in 2000 many other government agencies, in the Canadian federal system, in the United States, and in Europe, were doing just what was called for – namely, working out a proper risk estimation for the period after 1997. The result was that the CFIA's pseudo-assessment was contradicted by a number of other reputable sources in this period. First, the never-completed and never-released Health Canada report from mid-2000 (referred to above), using a standard risk assessment protocol based on a very comprehensive exposure pathway analysis, estimated the risk not as negligible, but as "low." This report is incomplete for one simple reason: scattered throughout the document are questions addressed to the CFIA (by name), requesting further information that would allow the assessment to be brought to a conclusion. Since no later version has ever been prepared in the nearly four years since the original was done, one can only infer that the CFIA did not cooperate with Health Canada in seeing that the draft version was completed – and then publicly circulated. This is itself unacceptable, since a huge effort was invested by Health Canada and by the report's authors in compiling it. Furthermore, there is no indication that the CFIA took into account the complete package of evidence, the very careful reasoning, and the exhaustive analysis of exposure pathways contained in this report, in its own assessment of post-1997 risk.[8]

Exactly the same conclusion about Canada – namely, that the risk of BSE was low, not negligible – was reached by a report prepared (in July 2000) by the European Union: "the Canadian system was exposed to a very low or low challenge by cattle imports from U.K. It cannot be excluded that BSE-infectivity entered the country by this route and was recycled, reaching domestic cattle. A low-level domestic prevalence cannot therefore be fully excluded to exist since the early 90s. However, the level must be below the detection level of the rather good passive surveillance in place."[9]

The standard risk assessment protocol followed in the Health Canada study was also used by the Harvard Center for Risk Analysis, which was commissioned twice by the USFDA to conduct a detailed study of BSE risk in the United States. It came to the same conclusion: there is a risk of a small number of cases showing up in North America because of the exposure pathways (the second Harvard report, done in 2003, assumed that any BSE infectivity in the U.S. would have come from imports from Canada!).[10] The last sentence in the E.U. report quoted above indicates that the minimalist surveillance systems chosen by both the U.S. and Canada were unlikely to be able to find these cases. The bottom line is, we didn't want to find them and just kept our fingers crossed that they would never show up. Canada was unlucky.

What difference does all this make? A *huge* difference, in my opinion. During all this time, Canada subscribed to an international policy on BSE that is straightforward and brutal in its consequences: if you are a country exporting beef, and you have just one indigenous case of BSE in your herd, you're out of the beef export game *for seven years*. That's the policy we apply to other countries. So what on earth do we have to complain about when other countries shut their borders to our beef, after the Canadian cases showed up?

Did our authorities cover up the true nature of the risk – the possibility that a case of BSE would appear within our borders – because they were unwilling to describe clearly to Canadian beef farmers the disasters that would unfold for them should that possibility materialize? Remember, they called the risk "negligible," which means, in common-sense terms, "It won't happen here." What they should have said to farmers, in language that could not be misunderstood, was something like this:

- There's a fair likelihood that anywhere from one to a few indigenous cases of BSE will show up in the Canadian herd;
- Since Canada and other countries subscribe to a policy of "one cow and you're out," beef producers in Canada should be fully aware of the reality that others will shut their borders *immediately* to our beef if even one indigenous case of BSE is discovered here;
- You should also be aware that, in the event that even one indigenous case of BSE is found in our herd, international trade agreements to which Canada is a party provide that we will not be allowed to resume exports of beef and beef products until a full seven years have passed following the last case.

What would beef producers in Canada have done, in the years between 1997 and 2003, if they had received these three messages, loud and clear, from their industry and their governments? Would they have continued building up a huge beef herd, 75 per cent of which was destined for export after slaughter? In my opinion, this was an utterly unreasonable risk for producers to take – *provided that* they had been informed in clear language about this risk by the federal regulator, as they should have been, but were not. Beef producers in Canada were not told the truth about either the actual risk or the devastating long-term consequences that might follow.

The tragedy now unfolding on our farms arose in large part because the people who speak on behalf of our institutions, principally those in the federal and provincial governments, have never learned how to use the language of risk appropriately. Instead of telling Canadian beef producers that BSE wouldn't happen here, they ought to have said, "Yes, it could very well happen, and if it does, the economic consequences will be devastating." These officials knew that the first case (called the "index case") would bring an economic disaster to Canada's beef producers – this is clearly acknowledged in a CFIA technical publication published, ironically, shortly before May 2003.[11] I believe that, in the light of this knowledge, the appropriate risk management strategy – the one that should have been strongly recommended to beef producers between 1997 and 2003 – would have been to restrict the growth of the national herd until the risk had diminished (as it will with time).

Repeated and longstanding failures in the communication of risk are at the heart of what went wrong in the mismanagement of BSE risk in Canada. These failures occurred during the entire period after

1997, when Canada and the United States adopted a set of policy choices about BSE risk in response to the belated acknowledgment by the U.K. government, in 1996, of its own catastrophic failings in this regard. Unless we understand clearly what went wrong in our own country, and why, and draw the lessons that will enable us to avoid similar mistakes in the future, we are at risk of going through such painful processes again and again.

A word about the organization of the text that follows. Many technical matters are associated with an issue such as BSE – risk estimation, disease surveillance policy, risk management choices, and so on – which must be presented if the issue is to be grasped in its full complexity. The issue of BSE risk in Canada developed in two phases, following the discovery of the index case (May 2003) and then the second case (December 2003); the discussion takes advantage of this by breaking down the presentation of technical matters into two segments as well.

THE FIRST COW

When the public announcement came, on 20 May 2003, confirming the first indigenous case of BSE in the Canadian herd, the shutters fell instantly at our borders. For a country then exporting around 75 per cent of the beef it produced, the impacts on our farm sector were instantaneous and brutal. Unsurprisingly, perhaps, those who have convinced themselves that the public depends on them for enlightenment in such matters – federal and provincial politicians – scanned the horizons for another country that could be blamed for our problems. Their gaze quickly fixed on the Japanese – a curious choice, since most of our exports once crossed the border to the south; moreover, the Japanese had been procuring most of their beef imports not from us, but from the United States, for quite some time. The solution to this puzzle was that the Japanese, thoroughly spooked by their own cases of BSE, were telling the United States that, if that country continued to import Canadian beef without strictly segregating it from U.S. beef, the Japanese would embargo imports of U.S. beef as well.

Thus Canadian politicians, led by then federal agriculture minister Lyle Vanclief and Alberta's premier Ralph Klein, engaged in a campaign of escalating rhetorical frenzy about Japan's policy of refusing to lift the ban it had imposed on Canadian beef imports. The federal minister mused about retaliatory trade sanctions against Japan and implied that his Japanese counterpart, who met with him face-to-face in Ottawa, offered no reasons for Japan's decision: "He wasn't clear on his concerns, quite frankly," Vanclief told our media.[12] (Really? See below.) But, as might have been expected, Mr Klein took the rhetoric prize with his challenge to Japan issued on July 14: "I would offer a billion – well maybe five billion [dollars] to have a Japanese person come over here and eat nothing but Canadian beef for a year. If he gets mad-cow disease, we'd be glad to give him $5 billion – well, make that $10 billion. It ain't going to happen." For the irrepressible Alberta premier, who once, during the Kyoto debates, speculated that the warmer climates prevailing in Alberta eons ago might have been caused by "dinosaur farts," this was all about the dirty politics of international trade.

Was it indeed? A consensus emerged quickly in Canada in the summer of 2003. The politicians' rhetoric was echoed by legions of outraged editorial writers in Canada's national and regional newspapers, for whom this case was all about how the Japanese were insulting our wonderful food regulatory system. The *Globe and Mail* ended its July 15 editorial with this statement: "It is difficult not to conclude that Japan is playing protectionist politics with food, as it has so often in the past. Canada is in no position to retaliate. For now the only alternative is to continue pressing the case with science and facts." Ah, yes, "science and facts," the new magical incantation in our politicians' everyday vocabulary.

I shall return to the religion of science, as it is practised (and abused) by Canadian and u.s. officials in the international trade and regulatory arena. But first, a few elementary facts (called for by the *Globe and Mail*) might have proved to be helpful:

- As an aside, does anyone in Canada remember Brazil's outrage over Canada's ban on importing Brazilian beef products due to alleged BSE risk? (Our embargo was imposed on 2 February 2001 and not lifted until a full year later.[13]) This ban was imposed even though Brazil has never had a single case of BSE, up to the present day – curious, no?
- As of July 2003, Canada had import bans – to control BSE risk – against beef from twenty-two countries.[14]
- None of our outraged politicians and editorialists had the courtesy to mention that Japan had been complaining about a *de facto* Canadian ban on beef imported from Japan.[15]
- At no time in the entire controversy over Canada's first case of BSE have Canadian officials discussed with the public why Canada should be dealt with differently from the way we treat other countries who are in the same boat.

Now, let's look systematically at a number of key issues.

Table 10.1
Countries with BSE cases

Austria	1 (2001)	Italy	113 (2001–03)
Belgium	123 (1997–2004)	Japan	11 (2001–04)
Canada	1 (2003)	Liechtenstein	2 (1998)
Czech Republic	9 (2002–04)	Luxembourg	2 (1997–2002)
Denmark	12 (2000–03)	Netherlands	73 (1997–2004)
Finland	1 (2001)	Poland	11 (2002–04)
France	890 (1991–2003)	Portugal	868 (1994–2004)
Germany	299 (2000–04)	Slovakia	14 (2001–04)
Greece	1 (2001)	Slovenia	3 (2001–03, 1 per year)
Ireland	1,378 (1989–2004)	Spain	407 (2000–04)
Israel	1 (2002)	Switzerland	453 (1990–2003)

Special Case
United Kingdom: 183,803 cases (1987–2003), peaking in 1992 (37,280 in that year), including 612 in 2003

What Is Canada's Policy on Beef Imports from Other Countries?

As of summer 2003, the only countries recognized by Canada as being free of BSE were: Argentina, Chile, Australia, Brazil (subject to special conditions), New Zealand, Uruguay, and the U.S.[16] For another twenty-two countries where BSE cases had been reported – *including four countries other than Canada that have reported only a single case* – Canada had been maintaining an import ban on beef products.[17] Here is Canada's policy: "A country is considered by Canada to be free from BSE if ... for the preceding seven (7) years, the country of origin must have reported no reported [sic] clinical cases of BSE in indigenous bovines."[18] Has any Canadian politician or media commentator been heard to mention these awkward "facts"?

Table 10.1 gives the complete list of the twenty-three countries and the total number of cases reported as of 30 March 2004, from the website of OIE (*l'Office international des épizooties*), the international agency responsible for animal health issues.[19]

The other relevant statistics are the *annual incidence rates for bovines aged over twenty-four months*, which takes into account the size of a nation's herd (and thus represents the proportion of diseased animals in it as reported each year); this, of course, varies greatly among the nations listed above.[20] As of 2002, the last year for which the full calculations are available, the figures for the U.K. itself remain far higher than in any other country: 228.4 cases per million head of cattle aged over twenty-four months. The two countries with the next-highest rates were Portugal (107.80 per million head) and Ireland

(88.39); by comparison, Japan was at 0.97. France, with the third-highest absolute number of cases (after England and Ireland) among all countries, was at 20.96 per million head.

Clearly, this terrible disease in cattle and other animals is still a matter of major international concern, and many nations – including Canada – have invoked the "precautionary principle" in responding to it. The orientation of Canada's own established policy on this matter is crystal clear: The incidence rate doesn't matter. *Every country reporting even a single indigenous case of* BSE *(that is, a case not imported from another country) will have its beef exports proscribed for an indefinite period of time.* Period. No exceptions.

It doesn't matter whether you are the U.K., with an incidence rate in 2002 of 228 cases per million head, or Japan, with 1 case per million. It doesn't matter whether you are a country with only a single confirmed case in total, such as Austria, Finland, or Greece, where the first and so far only reported cases occurred in 2001, with none thereafter. It doesn't matter whether you have only one case per year, as Slovenia does. All of these countries continue to remain on Canada's list of countries "not known to be free of BSE," to use the CFIA's careful bureaucratic language.

In view of these "facts," it would be interesting if some Canadian politician would care to explain to the public why Canada should be treated differently from all other countries that have had no more than one confirmed case. Just why does Canada think that it has the right to be asking for special treatment for itself – in violation of its very own policy on BSE risk?

What Is Canada's Policy on Importing Beef from Japan?

Canada's crafty silence about its policy on Japanese beef imports was broken on 14 July 2003, when the Japanese embassy in Ottawa released a short paper entitled "Fact Sheet: Japan's Policy on BSE."[21] We read there:

Since the index [i.e., first] case of BSE was detected in Japan in September 2001, Japanese citizens have become increasingly aware of food safety, and accordingly the government of Japan has taken thorough measures. In the wake of the index case in Japan in 2001, the U.S., Australia, Canada, and other countries suspended the imports of Japanese beef.

Then two enterprising CanWest reporters, the *Edmonton Journal*'s Renata D'Aliesio and Michelle Lang of the *Calgary Herald*, pursued the story:[22]

BSE has been found in seven Japanese cows. The government has adopted sweeping changes, banning the use of rendered beef in feed and testing every slaughtered cow destined for human consumption for the disease. Despite the measures, Canada has not lifted its ban on Japanese cattle and beef, introduced after the United States announced a ban. Ottawa's ban, which includes shipments of highly prized Japanese Kobe beef, could be a factor in Japan's reluctance to reopen borders to Canadian cattle, export officials said. "As a principle, they are wondering why Canada and other countries would want access to their market before they get access to our markets," said Ted Haney, president of the Canada Beef Export Federation.

So far as I can tell, there is no discussion of Canadian policy towards Japan's beef on the CFIA website. In fact, in extensive searches on the web, the only mention of Canadian action I found was an assertion in 2001 by a CFIA official that Canada would *not* enact a ban:[23]

Last week, the U.S. banned all cattle and beef imports from Japan following reports of the suspected case of mad cow disease, or bovine spongiform encephalopathy. [CFIA official Claude] Lavigne said Canada will not follow the U.S. lead ... *Lavigne said Canada has never recognized Japan as free of mad cow disease, even though there was no evidence of the disease there until now* [emphasis added – W.L.].[24]

I could find no other information on this issue. Then Renata D'Aliesio published a follow-up piece in the *Edmonton Journal* on 17 July, "No ban keeping out Japanese beef." She wrote: "But there's really no beef ban [against Japan], officials with Agriculture Canada and the Canadian Food Inspection Agency said Wednesday. They said Japan is free to send us beef in cuts of under 20 kilograms – just no live cattle." The officials further explained that, because Japan has not signed a "meat inspection protocol" with Canada, Japanese beef requires a special permit to be imported. (Just 263 kg were imported into Canada in 2000, before Japan's first case of BSE.)

What is truly odd about these stories is that two senior Canadian officials, one from the Department of Foreign Affairs and International Trade, and one from the Canada Beef Export Corporation, *assumed that Canada did in fact have a ban on importing Japanese beef in place* when they were contacted by reporters on 16 July.[25] And there is the clear statement from the Embassy of Japan in Ottawa: "In the wake of the index case in Japan in 2001, U.S., Australia, Canada and other countries suspended the imports of Japanese beef." Curiouser and curiouser.

Canada's Risk Estimation for BSE (Part A)

The following is a summary of the CFIA's quantitative risk estimation, dated 2003-05-01 (that is, about three weeks prior to the belated discovery of the first Canadian case):

- quantitative risk estimate of the likelihood of at least 1 infection of BSE occurring in Canada prior to 1997 is very low (7.3×10^{-3});
- therefore the likelihood of BSE becoming established is negligible;
- risk is further reduced by the mitigating measures that have been in place since 1997.

The full document from which the number comes is: "Risk Assessment on Bovine Spongiform Encephalopathy in Cattle in Canada, Part C: Risk Estimation."[26] The CFIA's pre-1998 quantitative risk assessment (QRA) displays some fancy mathematics indeed; yet no similarly calculated QRA at all is given for the period after 1997.

The expression 7.3×10^{-3} refers to a situation with little more than seven chances out of one thousand that something very undesirable might happen, namely, in this case, finding "at least one [BSE] infection" in the entire Canadian cattle herd for all of the period prior to 1997. Note, however, that the *qualitative* descriptor changes, without explanation, from "very low" in point 1 to "negligible" in point 2, even though nothing else has changed. With the benefit of hindsight, of course, we can see that we Canadians were either just plain unlucky (only seven chances in a thousand, and yet it happened to us), or that the estimation protocol was blind to certain factors that caused the risk to be underestimated.[27] However, I want to focus here not on the possible deficiencies in the risk analysis, but rather on the qualitative terminology used by the CFIA to characterize the risk level, since that is what most non-expert people would look to in order to grasp the "bottom line" in the risk estimation.

What is referred to above in the expression 7.3×10^{-3} is the frequency, likelihood, or *probability* of an adverse occurrence of some kind. This is, however, only one side of risk; the other is *consequence*. The standard formula for risk estimation is $R = P \times C$ (risk = probability times consequences). I shall try to show that the CFIA, although recognizing the consequences side, then proceeded to ignore them in its overall calculation of risk level; as a result, the CFIA procedure violates a fundamental principle of risk assessment. To see how this happened we have to look at each of these two sides of risk separately, and then combine them.

First, how do we turn the quantitative expression of frequency (about 7 chances in a thousand) into some kind of qualitative measure? In 1996 the chief medical officer of health in Great Britain, Sir Kenneth Calman, proposed a five-point risk classification scheme that received much attention:

Moderate risk = less than 1:100 but greater than 1:1,000, e.g., smoking 10 cigarettes a day, parachuting
Low risk = less than 1:1,000 but greater than 1:10,000, e.g., influenza, road accident
Very Low risk = less than 1:10,000 but greater than 1:100,000, e.g., leukaemia, playing soccer, accident at work, murder
Minimal risk = less than 1:100,000 but greater than 1:1,000,000, e.g., railway accident, horse riding, fishing
Negligible risk = less than 1:1,000,000, e.g., hit by lightning or radiation leak from nuclear power station[28]

Additional support for placing "negligible risk" at the bottom of this scale comes from the extensive discussion of this term in the United States during the 1990s, in the context of the Environmental Protection Agency's re-evaluation of cancer risk associated with pesticides. Following advice from the National Research Council, the agency began to use the phrase "negligible risk" instead of the older "zero risk" as its threshold level of risk, defining it as "an estimated [lifetime] cancer risk of one additional case of cancer for every million people exposed."[29] This agrees with Calman's scheme.

So, considering only frequency for the moment, one notices immediately that the CFIA's qualitative terminology is far out of line with the usages of government agencies in Britain and the U.S. (One is free to choose to be idiosyncratic, of course, but the choice should be accompanied by a decent explanation, which we never get from the CFIA.) *Seven chances in a thousand is neither "very low" nor "negligible"*; on Calman's scale it is "moderate" (or close to "low") risk – and as we have already seen, this is *exactly* the qualitative descriptor that other government authorities (including Health Canada) used to describe Canada's BSE risk in this same period.

The second deficiency is even more serious. Frequency is one side of the coin; in estimating risk, looking closely at possible consequences is a fundamental part of the entire exercise, as the CFIA acknowledges ("Risk Estimation," sect. 6): "Risk estimation consists of integrating the results of the release, exposure, and consequence assessments to produce measures of the risk." Consequences may be arrayed in terms of deaths and injuries, for example, or in terms of monetary losses, or both. As explained later, BSE risk has three different dimensions – animal health, human health, and economics. In a published paper based on its risk assessment, CFIA officials looked briefly at all three, and in the "consequence assessment" they wrote:

The impact of the introduction and establishment of BSE in Canada would be extreme, based on the animal and human health impacts, impact on industry and the cost of eradication as exemplified in other countries ... The occurrence of BSE in Canada would affect many sectors of the cattle industry, including farmers, meat processing, rendering, transportation and distribution, and retail, among others. It could result in a substantial decline in the consumption of beef and beef products due to a perception of risk to human health and safety.[30]

They were right: costs of over $5 billion have been racked up, even without the feared decline in beef consumption (which occurred elsewhere under similar circumstances, for example in Japan). So the consequences were at least described qualitatively by the CFIA, with a single, short, devastating, statement – "the consequences would be extreme." No effort was made to quantify the consequences, however, which is a bit curious, given the exhaustive quantitative manipulations carried out on the frequency side of the equation in the CFIA's risk estimation.

In risk literature, this type of case would be instantly recognizable as what is referred to as a "low-probability, high-consequence" event – other examples are severe earthquakes in populated areas and terrorism attacks. In risk domains that are unusually sensitive, as food risks are, regulators sometimes demand that substantial resources be devoted to lowering such risks. A comparable case is nuclear power, also a highly sensitive risk domain of this type. In 2003 the U.S. Nuclear Regulatory Commission reviewed the risk of core-melt episodes in a group of eleven reactors; in four of them the probability of core-melt was estimated as $3 \times 10^{-4}/\text{RY}$, that is, three chances in ten thousand for each year of operation (RY = reactor year).[31] This was deemed to be too high, given the public sensitivity to nuclear power risk, and a risk reduction strategy, costed at U.S. $83 million, was chosen, with the objective of lowering the probability of such an occurrence to $1 \times 10^{-4}/\text{RY}$.

In the case of BSE risk in Canada, as we have seen, the probability should be described as "low" at best (not "very low" or "negligible") – but the consequences of an event, in the CFIA's own words, would be "extreme," that is, extremely *high* (conventionally, the term

Table 10.2
Example of risk ranking

Frequency	Consequence			
	Catastrophic	Critical	Marginal	Negligible
Frequent	I	I	I	II
Probable	I	I	II	III
Occasional	I	II	III	III
Remote	II	III	III	IV
Improbable	III	III	IV	IV
Incredible	IV	IV	IV	IV

"catastrophic" is used). The formula R = P × C is used to generate a formal matrix, where consideration of the *combined* impact of frequency and severity (consequence) generates a "risk ranking," as in table 10.2, an example from an engineering services firm.

The roman numerals refer to a series of classes of risk: Class I (intolerable risk), Class II (undesirable risk), Class III (tolerable risk), and Class IV (negligible risk).[32]

In every low-probability, high-consequence setting, the latter element drives the final risk estimation. For the situation in which Canada found itself, the trade policy framework – "one case and you're out for seven years" – turned out to be the single most important factor in the consequence assessment, because (as the CFIA knew) almost all of the economic damage from a single case of BSE would be caused by the shutting of borders. This is the basis for the use of the word "extreme" in this context. A loss of public confidence in the safety of beef, as happened in Japan and other countries, depressing the domestic market, also might have occurred, as the CFIA recognized, but in Canada it did not.

Now we can see why it is so important to complete the risk assessment using the formula R = P × C. Depending on the specific circumstances, either one or the other of the two sides may be the most important one. BSE risk in Canada was and remains a classic case of low-probability, high-consequence risk, and in all cases of this type, the final risk estimation is determined almost entirely by consequence, not by frequency. In other words, within certain boundaries, in such cases it doesn't really matter much what the frequency is thought to be. Whether it is seven chances in a thousand, or nine, or five, or three, the result (R = P × C) would be exactly the same, because the final result is overwhelmingly determined by consequence. (Only what is called an "order of magnitude" difference – that is, only if we were talking about seven chances in a hundred, or alternatively seven chances in ten thousand – would cause the result to be more strongly affected by the frequency dimension.) The tragedy here is that CFIA officials expended a huge effort on putting a number to the frequency estimation – the calculations and statistical manipulations in the risk estimation for this dimension are staggering in their complexity – but inexplicably, they stopped there, and did not complete the process by seeking to quantify consequences with comparable thoroughness. In effect, the expression 7.3×10^{-3} reflects R = P, and because C has not been factored in, the result is meaningless. Nowhere in the CFIA's risk estimation is C ever estimated; the calculation P × C is never done, because no quantitative expression is given for C; therefore there is no risk estimation, only a frequency estimation.

The importance of actually *including* C in the risk estimation – as opposed to just mentioning it in passing – can be appreciated if we compare the situations in Canada and the United States. Let's assume that both the index case and one or more additional cases had been discovered in the U.S. herd. Let's also assume, for the sake of argument, that the public reaction there would have been pretty much the same as it turned out to be in Canada: beef consumption remained stable or even increased slightly. Now the trade policy framework kicks in, however, and Canada, along with Japan and about thirty other beef-importing countries, immediately shut their borders to U.S. beef exports. The consequences would have been far less devastating. Why? Because the U.S. was exporting only 10 per cent of its beef, not 70–75 per cent as in Canada. Assuming stability in the domestic market, the loss of this relatively small export market would not have had very much of an impact; therefore, one can say that, in the period before the BSE cases appeared, U.S. beef farmers faced a far lower risk than did their Canadian counterparts. This is what is concealed because of the CFIA's failure to perform an adequate risk assessment. Although an integrated North American beef industry had been developing for some time, Canadian producers faced nothing less than a catastrophic risk, should even one case of BSE emerge, whereas U.S. producers faced no such risk. Canadian farmers should have been told. They were not told.

A comparison with Japan yields another result. Japan exports beef, but not a lot of it – mostly its prized and very expensive Kobe beef. But, in contrast to both the U.S. and Canada, the Japanese public is hypersensitive about food safety. Therefore it would have been possible to predict that, if and when one or more cases of BSE surfaced in Japan, domestic consumption of beef would decline sharply, at least for a while. Thus the chief determinant of consequences in this case would be the predicted scale and duration of the decline in domestic consumption; loss of Japan's export markets would have only a slight economic impact.

Table 10.3
Risk matrix for BSE in Canada

Frequency	Consequence			
	Catastrophic	Critical	Marginal	Negligible
Moderate				
Low	BSE: Class II (or I)			
Very Low				
Minimal				
Negligible				

We can now construct a risk matrix for BSE in Canada (table 10.3), using Calman's terminology for frequency and the four-part classification for consequences given above.

Had R = P × C been appropriately estimated for Canada, as it should have been, the risk rating scheme outlined above would have classified BSE risk in this country as *not lower than* Class II: "undesirable risk and tolerable only if risk reduction is impracticable or if the costs are grossly disproportionate to the improvements gained." An argument could even be made for putting BSE risk into Class I, depending on how one thinks the frequency categories "occasional" and "remote," used in the first matrix, line up with "very low" and "low," used in the second.

The main point here is that frank discussions of the dimensions of the serious (catastrophic) problem Canada faced, potentially, were cut off, before they could even begin, by the truncated risk estimation. What should have happened was for the regulator to hold frequent and intensive sessions with farmers, the beef industry, and provincial governments, beginning as far back as 1998, with the full estimation on the table, to determine what measures might have been taken, at what cost, to reduce the risk to more tolerable dimensions. Those other parties, faced with these realities, might have decided not to take those measures or incur any costs, but at least they would have known the true dimensions of the potential catastrophe that was staring them in the face. They never got the chance to make those choices, and this is what is wrong and unacceptable about the strategy of "see no evil" adopted by the CFIA.

Science or Policy? (Part A)

The newspaper coverage of Canada's BSE case is littered with references to "science" as the basis for Canada's position that all countries – but primarily the U.S. and Japan – should now re-open their markets to Canadian beef exports. The following examples are drawn from countless statements by Canadian politicians since 20 May 2003:

It's frustrating to see an industry suffer the way the beef industry is suffering now and nations being so stubborn as to not accept the scientific evidence that says all is clear. (Ralph Klein)

Some of the things they [Japan] are doing are ... not required by science. They may have done them for internal political consumer concerns but there is absolutely no justification for them whatsoever. And: I'm frustrated that scientific data isn't getting through to the world. (Lyle Vanclief)

The Prime Minister put emphasis on the importance of using scientific evidence to put a ban on or to lift it off. (Spokesperson for Jean Chrétien)

The information provided above, on Canada's own policy on banning beef from other countries, helps us to put these statements in their proper light.

The "science" referred to repeatedly (but rarely specifically) by Canadian politicians is – presumably – the evidence from the culling and tracking investigation mounted after 20 May. It is also the evidence from the subsequent slaughter and examination of about 3,000 head of cattle, as a result of which no other cases of BSE infection were found. This is the intensive investigation that was praised, quite justifiably, for its thoroughness by the foreign-expert team retained by the CFIA, when they delivered their 26 June 2003 report.[33]

But the decision by Japan to maintain its ban on importing Canada's beef is a policy choice, not a scientific judgment – exactly the same kind of policy choice that Canada has made on beef imports for many years. In *both* cases that choice is based not on scientific evidence *per se*, but rather on a risk assessment, which takes such evidence into account and then tries to estimate the probabilities of encountering future problems. The risk assessment is an expert judgment that is supposed to tell you, for example, what the probability is that, if one case is found, there will be others. Here is the expert judgment on that point from the leader of the team retained by the CFIA, Switzerland's former chief veterinary officer, Dr Ulrich Kihm: "The risk is there that [having found an index case] you will find a second or third case, or even more. I'm estimating that there will be other cases in this part of the world [i.e., North America] ... You have to implement a proper surveillance system in order to detect that."[34] Canada has not done so, in the opinion of the experts hired by the CFIA. Subsequent events have proved that Dr Kihm knows whereof he speaks.

Canadian politicians' appeal to science is a rhetorical device, representing "science" as a kind of trump card to be used when nations disagree about food safety. This rhetorical move carries the implicit notion that our own side follows faithfully the rational guide of scientific discovery, whereas our opponents are being irrational. Indeed, none other than Premier Klein uncovered the implication and made it public: "[Japan] is a race of people who are highly intelligent ... yet they are consumed by this unwarranted fear that this one cow that has been taken out of the food chain will somehow infect their population."[35] But this dispute has nothing to do with whether the Japanese people are more or less rational than Canadian politicians are. It is not about science, but about risk management.

"Science" is, for example, what tells you that a connection exists between BSE in beef and new-variant CJD in humans. Science is what tells you that it is probably an unfortunate genetic anomaly that puts some people who eat infected beef at higher risk of contracting the human disease than others are.[36] The science of prion diseases is also, of course, one of the bases of the risk assessment for BSE in a nation's cattle herd. But the risk assessment also includes many other factors that are not strictly scientific – for example, an estimation of the probability that animal feed infected with BSE will enter the cattle feed chain even though our country and others prohibit this practice (i.e., the compliance issue).

For example, FDA regulations in the U.S., similar to Canada's, require that animal feed products containing rendered ruminant (cattle) parts be labelled, "do not feed to ruminants." In 2001 FDA inspectors found that 20 per cent of such products sold by feed mills to farmers did not carry the required warning label, and as of July 2003 the FDA reported new actions taken against a Seattle-based animal feed producer found to be in violation of these regulations.[37] A proper risk assessment must make realistic assumptions about such factors.

The risk assessment also tells you how likely it is that you will find a case of BSE in your nation's cattle herd, based on what percentage of heads from slaughtered cattle are examined in a laboratory for evidence of the brain-wasting disease. This is called the surveillance program. As noted above, the Swiss expert who headed Canada's international review panel was quoted as saying that if you find one case you probably have more.

To date Canada – and the United States – have operated what can be described as a passive or minimalist surveillance program (see below). This is the real crux of the continuing stand-off between Japan and Canada: Japan simply does not trust our surveillance program. Remember Minister Vanclief's assertion that Japan hasn't been clear about its concerns? Rubbish. Here is what Japan's agriculture minister Yoshiyuki Kamei said to Vanclief directly: "'I asked that Canada set up a strict system of inspection as in Japan,' Kamei told reporters, indicating he asked Vanclief that all cows in Canada be inspected."[38] Unfortunately, that quotation can only be found in a Japanese news agency source. It is nowhere to be found in any of the dozens of Canadian press reports I have examined.

Canadian Risk Management for BSE – Surveillance, Animal Feed (Part A)

Trouble has been brewing for Canada's beef industry for many years, during which both political and industry leaders followed the well-known three monkeys' routine (hear no evil ...). The bottom line is that Canada – with what was once a $30 billion annual beef industry to protect – has been appallingly lax in its policies designed to minimize BSE risk. In more technical language, we have been insufficiently precautionary, by a wide margin, in response to the *economic risk* represented by BSE. The economic risk is the scope of the potential economic damage to Canada that could occur in the event of the index case being discovered, as it was in May 2003, in the context of an international regime – fully supported by Canada – where the discovery of one case means shutting all major export markets.[39]

Ironically, on 20 February of last year Peter Comrie, chair of the technical committee of the Canada Beef Export Federation, warned his members at their annual meeting that "the EU considers Canada a risk for mad cow disease and is expected to add more import restrictions."[40] The reasons for this are twofold: in two key dimensions – animal feed and surveillance – Canada's policies to control BSE risk have been seriously deficient. Abundant warnings were given on this score, all ignored. Now the international expert panel has told Canada to change these policies, and the federal minister has said that he will comply. Too late. Also, he hasn't said when.[41] That's another complaint from Japan: "The Japanese government has not received the details of the measures for BSE, and when the Canadian government will take the measures," said Yutaka Kawano, the agriculture officer at Japan's embassy in Ottawa on 15 July.[42]

Animal-feed policy. Like the U.S., Canada chose in 1997 to adopt a limited ban on rendered ruminant material in animal feed products: such material (except for blood, milk, and fat) could not be used in animal feeds for ruminants, but could be included in other animal feeds, such as those for poultry and pigs. Over the intervening years many warnings have been issued about the inadequacy of the North American policy. The excessive risk represented in this policy choice was summed up recently by another Swiss expert:

There is no other known route of transmission [other than animal feed]. Ruminant feed can still end up in other cattle feed even if it is not on purpose. It's accidental contamination that cannot be prevented if it's produced in the same feed mill. If your first batch is non-cattle and you have meat and bone meal in there, in the beginning of the next batch you will have cross-contamination. You end up with ruminant protein in the ruminant batches even if it was not intended.[43]

The availability of this feed leads to other risks: faulty labelling by producers, as noted earlier; accidental misuse of feed on farms; and intentional (knowing) misuse on farms, for example, because of cost considerations. What this all means is that Canada's policy of permitting continued use of ruminant material in some animal feeds *substantially increased the risk* of cattle being fed this material – the only known route of transmission for BSE. The inadequate risk assessment performed by the CFIA for the post-1997 period does not try to estimate this risk.[44] As other commentators have argued, our regulatory officials and our industry have been far too complacent about BSE risk.[45] That will change now, but the price our beef industry and the Canadian economy will pay for that complacency will be very steep indeed.

Surveillance. This whole aspect of the matter started badly for Canada, when it was revealed that Alberta's provincial laboratory took almost four months to deliver results for the head from the slaughtered cow that ultimately tested positive for BSE.[46] But as it turns out, this was not the worst of our problems. The perspective from Europe was summed up as follows: "The U.S. and Canada test so few animals that low levels of BSE infection would not be detected."[47]

In 2002 Canada slaughtered 3.6 million cattle and tested 3,377 for BSE, a surveillance rate of under .001 (one per thousand).[48] Japan currently tests *every* slaughtered cow destined for human consumption. Why do more tests? The E.U. concluded some years ago that, in every country where more active surveillance programs were introduced, more cases of BSE were found, without exception. The Swiss expert Marcus Doherr put it bluntly: "There must be more cases [in Canada]. For every case we detect, we estimate there were three to five animals exposed."[49]

Canada's entirely inadequate passive surveillance program has over the years *substantially increased the risk* that we have missed other cases of BSE in our cattle herd – as the E.U.'s risk assessment concluded. That's why the E.U. categorized us as a Category II country for BSE risk in July 2000, one where "it is unlikely but cannot be excluded that domestic cattle are (clinically or pre-clinically) infected with the BSE-agent."[50]

The Last Word

At the very outset of Canada's BSE troubles columnist Don Martin wrote in the *Calgary Herald*: "It's not that solitary mad cow that has put Alberta's beef industry at stake ... The chances of just one cow becoming uniquely infected by the disease from one feeding trough, or arriving in Alberta as a single-case import from somewhere else, are laughingly [sic], alarmingly remote."[51] That's still a pretty good summary of the informal risk assessment for BSE in Canada, as the episode of the first cow drew to a close.

At this point in the story, as of fall 2003, as Canadian beef farmers were anxiously awaiting the reopening of the U.S. border – something that both provincial and federal politicians were promising them was just around the corner – three conclusions could be drawn from what had transpired since the previous May:

First – The only known route of transmission for BSE is through the animal feed chain. Our "index case," which occurred in northern Alberta, was a cow born before the 1997 feed ban came into effect (as was the second case); it was given infected bovine material at some point in its life. Had the CFIA done a proper post-1997 risk assessment, as others had done, it would have highlighted the risk posed by this cohort of cattle within the national herd. By any reasonable standard of risk assessment, the threat posed by this cohort could not have been described as "negligible." The CFIA failed to communicate to Canadian beef farmers the true risk they faced.

Second – Canada's surveillance program for BSE has been seriously deficient from the get-go. As a result, this country had, as of summer 2003, no basis for assuring the world that we have had but "one stinking cow" with BSE – as our politicians were loudly proclaiming. Independent experts, quoted above, suggested in summer 2003 that, under the conditions prevailing in Canada since 1997 (namely, our deficient surveillance policies), it was highly likely that there were then or had been some additional cases. Subsequent events proved them right.

Third – Whatever the actual BSE risk is in Canada, it is Canada's own policy to exclude all imports of beef from countries "not known to be free of BSE." Canada excludes beef from some countries that have had only one reported case of BSE. Therefore we have no basis for arguing that other countries should now re-open their borders to Canadian beef.

The fact that since 1997 Canada has been far less precautionary than it should have been in protecting its beef industry is a hard lesson for all of us. Among other things, we failed to recognize that not one, but three, quite different risks were associated with BSE in cattle, risks that we were required to manage. The first is the *animal health risk*: countries with large cattle herds must take steps to ensure that they are not struck, as Britain was, by an epidemic of BSE in their herds. The second is the *human health risk*: here, it is reasonable to say that Canadians should have no concern about risks to their own health from consuming Canadian beef. (Many Canadians might wish that Premier Klein had extended his $10 billion wager to them!) Even if a few more cases have gone undetected, as the Swiss experts have conjectured, there would still be no cause for concern on this score. There just aren't enough infected animals in our system to raise the probability of a Canadian case of new-variant CJD above the level of truly negligible risk.

But the third risk, representing another type of risk altogether, that we neither recognized nor managed at all, is the *economic risk* to our beef industry and to the larger economy, which was concealed in the policy decisions taken in 1997. Canada's own policy of embargoing beef from countries with even one reported case of BSE should have tipped us off to the great risk we were running on this score. The tragedies to Canadian families and businesses now unfolding will take a high toll, especially on farm families, who have been battered over recent years with difficult challenges issued both by nature and by our trading partners.[52] The embargoing of Canadian beef is another blow.

What can we do? First, the undignified whining and pleading has to stop. We are not going to receive special treatment from our trading partners, nor do we deserve it. Our only recourse is to seek a new international consensus on collective action – but we must recognize that it will take years to achieve this, if it can be done at all. Canada will have to go to the OIE and other international bodies and request a period of negotiation, leading towards a new policy for all countries importing beef.[53]

This policy would cover *all* beef-exporting countries that have reported small numbers of indigenous BSE cases and have then implemented a series of specified measures designed to reduce – to negligible levels – the risk that further cases will occur. An international inspection routine will have to be established, for verification and certification that the measures have been implemented appropriately. The agreement would specify that, once a country has fully complied with the requirements of these measures, its beef exports would again be welcomed on world markets.

THE SECOND COW

We probably have to do something to reassure people that this province, anyway – notwithstanding what the federal government might or might not do – is willing to put in the highest of protocols relative to testing. They've done that in Japan.

Premier Ralph Klein, 7 January 2004,
announcing his government's consideration of a plan to test
for BSE in every cow slaughtered in a provincial facility[54]

The usual suspects were rounded up after the discovery of a second case of BSE in North America on 23 December 2003, to whistle again the tunes of complacency and inaction. Once again "science" was used to justify foot-dragging and to obscure major failures in risk management and risk-based policy choices. These failures include unacceptable defects in risk assessment, sloppy surveillance programs for animal disease control, and a stubborn refusal to impose a total ban on recycling ruminant protein in animal feed. It all boils down to idiot economics where, billions of dollars in losses later, Canadians are still told we can't afford to spend on necessary and cost-effective tests to restore confidence in our animal health programs.

Apart from the Premier's bold statement quoted above, confusion still reigns. The federal announcement, made on the eve of the new federal agriculture minister's futile trip to the Far East in January 2004, promised an increase of testing – over a five-year period – to 30,000 animals per year. This might appear to be a bold move (except to the Japanese, of course), were it not for the fact that, about six months earlier, the same officials were promising to ramp up Canada's testing to 80,000. What happened in the meantime, other than the discovery of the second Canadian BSE case? Would it not be logical to respond to the second case with a promise of more testing, not less? Apparently not in Canada. The plain fact is that spending the promised $90 million of new federal money over the coming five years to increase our BSE testing to 30,000 animals in 2009 may be pointless, because it's likely we won't have a major beef export industry by then – unless we take a series of bolder steps, as outlined below.

The Way Forward

Demonstrating to our export markets that we are serious about controlling BSE risk in Canada requires a systematic approach, which to date we have not taken. A number of sequential steps should be undertaken, as follows:

- Complete a current, quantitative risk assessment of the estimated (hypothetical) numerical prevalence of BSE in the Canadian herd, taking into account the discovery of the two cases in 2003;
- At the same time, choose a surveillance program that is sufficiently robust in terms of current expectations around the world, rather than one based on arbitrary assumptions and justified by a rhetorical and misleading appeal to "science";
- Use the currently available array of testing methods to screen large numbers of slaughtered animals for BSE, as is done in Europe and Japan;
- Correct the remaining serious flaws in the ruminant feed ban and rendering processes.

After our governments have made a firm commitment to such a program, we should announce it to the world. We should be able to expect that, once others are convinced of our seriousness, they will begin to look to Canada again as a preferred supplier of beef in the export markets.

Canada's Risk Estimation for BSE (Part B)

The U.S. Department of Agriculture commissioned two risk assessments of BSE from the Harvard Center for Risk Analysis (HCRA), the first issued in 2001 and the second in 2003.[55] The second report, interestingly enough, attributes the potential risk of BSE in the United States solely to importation of either infected animals or infected feed from Canada. In the abstract we read: "In the most pessimistic case (introduction of contaminated feed into the U.S. in 1990), the prevalence of infected animals peaks at 600, with 24 animals showing clinical signs (median simulation predictions)."

The purpose of this type of quantitative risk assessment is to estimate the hypothetical numerical prevalence of BSE in a nation's herd. (Hypothetical refers to the initial assumptions about what *might* have happened over a certain time frame.) Such an estimate is one of the necessary preliminary steps to making an informed decision about an appropriate surveillance program – in which one has a reasonable chance of finding any actual cases. As pointed out earlier, Canada has not bothered to do a comparable study. Instead, our officials simply made the arbitrary judgment that Canada was at "negligible risk" for a case of BSE in its herds. Of course, since then we have found out, the hard way, that this was an unfounded assumption.

Now we refer to ourselves as a country "at minimal risk" of BSE, although no one at the CFIA thinks it's necessary to explain what the agency thinks is the difference is between "negligible" and "minimal" risk.[56] And we continue to use different terminology when referring to other countries. Our "Canadian Bovine Spongiform Encephalopathy (BSE) Import Policies" statement lists no fewer than ten conditions, the first of which is: "For the preceding seven (7) years, the country of origin must have reported no reported clinical cases of BSE in indigenous bovines." All of the ten conditions must be met before a country may be classified as being "free of BSE." Only seven countries meet those conditions: Argentina, Australia, Brazil (special conditions apply), Chile, New Zealand, United States, and Uruguay.[57] Canada bans the importation of both "live ruminants" and meat and meat products from all countries "not known to be free of BSE." In other words, Canada does not meet *its own conditions* for allowing beef exports to take place, and yet we continue to send our politicians hither and thither around the world, whining about the borders closed to us and pleading for special consideration. This is undignified, to say the least.

If we wish to be regarded, elsewhere in the world, as a responsible actor in controlling BSE risk, we have an obligation to undertake a current, quantitative risk assessment, which would build its working assumptions around the discovery of the two cases in 2003.

Science or Policy? (Part B)

Ever since the BSE crisis erupted in May 2003, politicians on both sides of the Canada–United States border have used a common theme in their speeches: Our policies on matters of beef are based on "science." This rhetorical appeal to science reached its apex recently when a senior Canadian political leader said that science "dictates" that international borders be re-opened to Canadian beef. Both sides use the same language, and the border remains closed despite repeated Canadian entreaties to open it – surely a clue that either science or language is being misused. Another clue suggesting something is amiss is that none of those telling the public what science supposedly dictates is actually a scientist. In the sections that follow, a number of abuses related to the rhetorical appeal to science are detailed.

Canadian Risk Management for BSE – Surveillance, Animal Feed (Part B)

Surveillance. The purpose of a surveillance strategy is to decide how many animals should be tested, to find and remove infected animals from the food supply, and to provide empirical evidence about the prevalence of BSE in the herd. Ever since Canada's first case of BSE was discovered in May 2003, a chorus of loud voices has been heard from Canadian officials, arguing that our surveillance strategy was perfectly adequate because it was based on "science." The same voices are still heard, but the message gets odder and odder: now we are going to do more testing, but, it is said, only what science "dictates." Yet, if our strategy before May 2003 was as scientifically rigorous as we claimed at the time, why are we now going to include more animals in our surveillance? "Science," apparently, justifies whatever we Canadians think we ought to do – but not what other countries demand, of course.[58]

A surveillance strategy is (or should be) a reasoned choice, but it is still a *choice* – specifically, a *policy* choice – and, moreover, a choice based on certain working *assumptions*. Science does not "dictate" anything at all in this regard. Rather, the body of relevant science – in this case, on animal disease surveillance – is (or should be) the primary guide in the making of appropriate assumptions. But reasonable people can and do differ on what assumptions are or should be regarded as being reasonable under a given set of circumstances.

Following the discovery of BSE cases in Japan, now totalling eleven, and the confession of its own inadequate risk management of BSE, the Japanese government made a simple choice: To restore consumer confidence, every cow destined for human consumption would be tested for BSE. Following the discovery of BSE cases everywhere in European nations, the E.U. made a less stringent, but still dramatic choice: to test a significant portion of the population of healthy animals. In the first eleven months of 2003, E.U. countries did BSE tests on 8 million healthy animals.[59]

The most important single choice about a surveillance strategy has to do with *which* animals are sampled. Unless this is clearly realized, the nature of the policy choices being made by officials is not understandable. The strategy adopted by both Japan and the E.U. is based on sampling the entire population of animals, all of which are apparently healthy, i.e., showing no overt signs of disease, especially neurological disease. The reason for this choice is the reasonable assumption that, as a disease with a lengthy incubation period, BSE could very well be developing in animals that are apparently healthy at the time of slaughter.

In a system of massive testing, the animal carcasses are held overnight in refrigerated warehouses until the test results are returned.[60] Cases of "false positives" may well appear in the test results, but this is not in itself a reason to avoid large-scale testing. Secondary screening (a different test) can be used to deal with false positives. Many people will be familiar with such procedures at airport screening locations.[61]

In North America to date, both Canada and the United States have made a different policy choice for their surveillance programs – namely, to examine only animals with some obvious health impairment, usually called "downers." Officials in both countries assert that their surveillance strategy is designed to detect the incidence of BSE at the level of one-in-a-million cases; however, this strategy is based on the assumption that apparently healthy animals do not need to be tested. The USDA has provided a full explanation for its approach (so far as I can determine, the CFIA has made no comparable explanation):

Given that the United States has an adult cattle population of approximately 45 million, if we did have BSE in this country at the one in a million level, we could assume that we would have 45 infected animals. To achieve a 95 percent confidence level in the accuracy of a random sample of adult cattle, we would have to sample and test some 3 million animals.

However ... USDA's program instead focused on the higher risk population of cattle: adult cattle with central nervous system clinical signs and nonambulatory cattle [estimated 195,000 cases per year] ... *An assumption is made that the 45 potential cases of BSE would all be found in the high-risk cattle population* [my italics]. Dividing the potential cases into the high-risk population (45/195,000) gives a prevalence of 0.023 percent. This is the level of the disease that has to be detected in the high-risk population ... [and] it is determined that, nationally, a sample size of 12,500 is needed.[62]

Here is the most recent explanation of Canada's policy from the CFIA:

The Canadian Food Inspection Agency will aim to test a minimum of 8,000 animals over the next twelve months, and then continue to progressively increase the level [to a maximum of 30,000] ... Testing will focus on those animals most at risk of BSE. These include animals demonstrating clinical signs consistent with BSE, so called "downer" animals – those unable to stand, as well as animals that have died on farm, are diseased or must be destroyed because of serious illness. A sample of healthy older animals will also be tested.[63]

These quotations enable us to see more clearly the nature of the current dispute between Canada and countries that used to import Canadian beef. Canada and the United States have similar surveillance policies, so this is not the issue as far as the cross-border movement of beef is concerned. Rather, the U.S. has a strict policy: *any* country reporting even a single case, or suspected of having unreported cases of BSE, will have its imports cut off.[64] There are thirty-four such countries, including Canada.

The issue is different with countries such as Japan and South Korea. Those countries do not believe that our surveillance and testing strategy is adequate to the task of accurately assessing the prevalence of BSE in the Canadian herd. It is against such countries that Canadian politicians launch their tirades about lack of respect for "science." Such pronouncements are nonsensical, and we really ought to stop issuing them. The dispute is not about the science of animal health; rather, it is about *the reasonableness of the assumptions on which our surveillance strategy is based* – in particular, our focus on testing sick animals.

Reasonable people can disagree on this point. The position taken by Canada and the United States is not unreasonable in itself.[65] However, it is by no means the only position one can take that is justified by a scientific approach. It is just as reasonable, and just as "scientific," to argue, as the Japanese do, that since we Canadians have no idea about the real prevalence of BSE in our herd, we should do substantially more testing – especially testing of apparently healthy animals.

Canada should stop trying to impose on its former trading partners a *unilaterally determined* and *arbitrary* surveillance strategy. Rather, we should negotiate in good faith a mutually determined, enhanced surveillance and testing regime. Whether or not this will require testing every cow sent to slaughter is an open question.[66] The main point is that we have no right to impose our own definition of the situation on others – not if we wish to have any hope of regaining our export markets. Premier Klein's recent statement contains the heart of the only approach that is likely to succeed: so far as testing is concerned, we will do whatever is necessary to restore others' confidence in our product.

A NOTE ON BSE TESTING METHODS

Canada's second case of BSE has stimulated an increased discussion about the range of post-mortem tests for the disease, which cannot be detected, not yet at least, in live animals.[67] For example, using the luminescence immuno-assay, manufactured by Prionics AG of Switzerland, a lab worker can screen 200 samples in three hours.[68] Recently the CFIA announced that it was "adding the Prionics Check-Western rapid test as a routine screening tool to further support the national BSE surveillance program" and that it is evaluating other such tests. However, the governments of both Canada and the U.S. – supported by the major industry lobbyists – refuse to allow individual beef producers to make their own decisions on testing, even when the producers are prepared to absorb all of the associated costs.[69] (Both countries have legislation in place that gives officials the sole authority to carry out animal health testing.) For example, some producers of high-end products, such as Angus beef, hope that by testing every cow slaughtered in their operations, they could persuade their target export market (Japan) to accept their products. Government officials justify their refusal to allow this by saying that these tests are designed for "surveillance" and do not provide a measure of "safety."

This is another blatant example of the government obfuscation practised by Canada and the u.s. – all under the banner of "sound science," of course. These tests are designed for the specific purpose of detecting the presence of the infectious prion, which is, after all, the whole point of doing any testing. Japan, for example, uses these selfsame tests (on every slaughtered cow) for exactly that reason – namely, to reassure their consumers that, if additional cases of BSE occur in their own herd, they will be found before the meat goes to market. One just cannot resist the suspicion that neither governments nor the dominant industry associations in North America want to find any more cases of BSE in their herds.

Animal Feed and Rendering

The last area of policy choices related to a new strategy for Canada has to do with the use of ruminant (cattle) protein in animal feed. I argued earlier that Canada's policies in this regard are insufficiently precautionary. The two key issues are inadequate procedures at animal feed-processing mills and the use of ruminant blood in the feeding of calves.

Feed mills – I have already referred to a USFDA audit in 2001, reporting a number of cases of lack of compliance with the ruminant feed ban, including cases where feed bags supposed to be labelled "do not feed to ruminants" were not so labelled.[70] We now have some evidence of similar problems in Canada at an Edmonton feed plant, which might be a source of infected feed.[71] Taken together, enough evidence already exists to suggest that practices in the North American feed industry are almost certainly contributing to the endless recycling of some amounts of near-indestructible prions in animal protein.[72]

Use of ruminant blood – Fully *six years ago*, an expert group at Health Canada "warned CFIA that Canada's policy of allowing animal blood to be rendered back into animal feed could not be considered safe." The CFIA refused to take that advice. In August 2003 CFIA's chief vet, Brian Evans, would only say that a ban on this practice is "under active consideration" – *five years* after Health Canada's advice was given![73] Stanley Prusiner, the scientist who discovered the prion particle, has referred to this practice as "a really stupid idea."

On 26 January 2004 the U.S. Department of Health and Human Services announced that the USFDA would implement a series of new rules, including a ban on feeding mammalian blood to ruminants as a food source, stating: "Recent scientific evidence suggests that blood can carry infectivity for BSE." In addition, the new rules "will further minimize the possibility of cross-contamination of ruminant and non-ruminant animal feed by requiring equipment, facilities, or production lines to be dedicated to non-ruminant animal feeds if they use protein that is prohibited in animal feed."[74] When the CFIA will follow suit is anybody's guess.

Canada should ban all recycling of ruminant protein in animal feed, effective immediately. High-temperature incineration, or some other method for destroying the prion particles, should be used to dispose of this material. And Canada should commission a comprehensive, *independent* audit of its animal feed mills, making the audit report publicly available.

CONCLUSIONS

At present it is impossible to say whether Canada will ever have a significant beef export industry in the future. The second case of BSE has intensified the crisis afflicting the Canadian beef industry, especially farmers in Alberta, where 70 per cent of the industry is located. One wonders at the wisdom of rebuilding a food industry that is designed to export three-quarters of what it grows, which, as we have seen, makes us extremely vulnerable to the closing of borders to our exports. By way of contrast, the U.S. exports only 10 per cent of what it produces, so the closing of most of its export markets by other countries (including Canada) after 20 December 2003, when the second North American case was discovered in the state of Washington, has had comparatively little economic impact.

Animal-health issues can only be expected to be more, not less, troubling in the years ahead. For example, it may be only a matter of time before one of the worst scourges, foot and mouth disease, returns to North America.[75] And at the time of writing (April 2004), the avian flu epidemic is causing millions of birds to be slaughtered in British Columbia; perhaps a necessary move, but not one that will guarantee the eradication of the virus, raising the prospect that another round could re-ignite at any time.

Because animal protein from domesticated species is a very important part of our food supply, animal health issues are highly sensitive. This sensitivity can be expressed as a high level of economic risk – for the producers; for the governments who will always be called on to bail them out with billions of dollars in compensation payments when these disasters strike; and for the public, which foots the bills in the end. All of the affected parties – producers, governments, and the public – need clear communications about risk assessment and risk management options, to make well-informed policy choices in these domains. This has not been supplied in the BSE case in Canada. Rather, the key risk communications have been inaccurate and misleading, and they have also been surrounded by obfuscating clouds of rhetoric in what can only be described as a deliberate effort to prevent the public from grasping the nature of the failures to date. Two examples follow.

The CFIA used to describe Canada as a county at "negligible" risk of BSE; that has been changed, and now we are said to be a country at "minimal" risk of BSE. What is the difference represented by these two terms? No one at the CFIA will say. Even worse, the current description is an artful stretching of standard international terminology in this area. OIE, the Paris-based international agency responsible for coordinating animal health issues, has established a set of categories. Category 3 ("minimal BSE risk") applies to countries where:

the last indigenous *case* of BSE has been reported less than 7 years ago, and the BSE incidence rate, calculated on the basis of indigenous *cases*, has been less than one case per million during each of the last four consecutive 12-month periods within the cattle population over 24 months of age in the country or zone ... and: i) the ban on feeding ruminants with *meat-and-bone meal* and *greaves* derived from ruminants has been effectively enforced for at least 8 years. (article 2.3.13.5)

The CFIA loses no opportunity to proclaim loudly that Canada follows OIE guidelines in animal health matters. However, our country does not qualify under the last of the three criteria in this extract for inclusion in category 3. And still the CFIA goes merrily on, making up its own rules for such things and using characterizations (minimal risk) that it knows full well are potentially misleading.

The other chief instance of terminological abuse is the frequent reference to "science." Federal officials insist that all of their policy decisions – such as those on which surveillance and testing policies are based – are "scientific" in nature; moreover, if other countries (such as Japan) disagree, this constitutes *prima facie* proof that those others are being "unscientific." This is nothing less than a long-running charade being staged both in Canada and the United States.[76] Officials strenuously defend existing policies as being based on sound science, e.g., how many cows should be tested; then they change the policy, and announce that the new policy is based strictly on sound science! This would be acceptable if some scientific knowledge relevant to the policy choices had changed, but such is not the case (nor do the officials claim that it is the case). Again, some explanation must be offered for these absurdities. What comes to mind is that hiding behind the skirts of science is an attempt to truncate debate on those policy choices and the real reasons why they were made, or not made, at a particular time.

For years the United States and Canada (that is, the CFIA) insisted that there was no scientific basis for banning the use of ruminant blood in calf supplements – even though Health Canada told the CFIA in no uncertain terms, six years ago, that a scientifically based risk assessment would lead to a ban on this practice. Then, out of the blue, on 26 January 2004 the USFDA announced that it would "eliminate the present exemption in the feed rule that allows mammalian blood and blood products to be fed to other ruminants as a protein source. Recent scientific evidence suggests that blood can carry some infectivity for BSE."[77] No new evidence was in fact adduced – the scientific arguments against this practice had been around for years. As of this time, the CFIA has refused to follow suit. Apparently, the appeal to science serves as little more than an excuse to do whatever you want.

The truth is that bad policy choices about the risk management of BSE have been made. But the use of misleading terminology by officials in defending those policies has made it impossible for the public to get a clear idea of what the alternative policy choices might be, or why it might be reasonable to prefer them to the prevailing ones. This has been going on for quite some time now, and we are all paying the costs. But there is no sign that anything is likely to change.

11 A Night at the Climate Casino: Canada and the Kyoto Quagmire

STEPHEN HILL AND WILLIAM LEISS

"WHAT, ME WORRY?"

Climate change is a devilishly complex business. The average citizen who sought to follow the political wrangling surrounding the federal government's ratification of the Kyoto Protocol in 2002, over the anguished complaints of some provincial and industry leaders, could be excused if he or she decided that, like the legendary sage Alfred E. Newman, it would be preferable to stick one's head in the sand rather than try to make sense of climate policy.

Climate change is complicated, but the reasons why Canada and others should take action on climate change are not. Developing climate change policy is essentially a risk management decision. In this chapter we argue that Canadians can and should react to climate change risk, in just the same way as we have learned to do for a whole range of other health and environmental risks. By definition, risks carry inherent uncertainties about outcomes, and yet, both governments and industry manage many such risks on behalf of citizens all the time, by incurring costs to reduce them to a level that is regarded as acceptable.

This is done by first estimating risks, a process that is a kind of forecasting of possible harm. It is impossible to get direct evidence of harm for a simple reason: we do not intentionally conduct experiments on humans by exposing them to various doses of possibly harmful substances to see what happens. Instead, we devise indirect techniques, such as experimenting on laboratory animals, and then use models to predict likely human effects. This is the way we set standards or limits for human exposure to thousands of potentially dangerous (but often very useful) substances, whether they are chemicals, metals, minerals, or gases.

Second, enforcing the limits to exposure for all of those substances is done by incurring real costs; for example, by installing pollution-control equipment, changing technology, or providing safety gear. For many substances we cannot know for certain where the exact limit of safe exposure is (it also varies among individuals), so safety factors are used to provide some margin for error. This, too, costs money. In the end, this is just the application of a straightforward precautionary approach, which is done routinely across a wide range of activities every day.

Today almost no one proposes to scrap all of that busy precautionary activity in favour of an alternative that would, for example, have us find out where the limits of safe exposure are by waiting until the bodies fall and then counting them.

In this chapter, we argue that the risks of climate change are sufficiently well described to warrant immediate precautionary action. We examine the costs of reducing greenhouse gases initially in line with the Kyoto targets and argue that these costs are acceptable given the nature of climate risk. We argue that Canada's best strategy for managing the risk of climate change is to demonstrate strong leadership to the international community; for the time being, this would take the form of making sure that we can live up to our commitments under the Kyoto Protocol. We should expect and be prepared to change our actions as the international context changes and as our understanding of climate risk improves.

THE RISK OF INACTION

Some participants in the climate policy debate leave the impression with the public that substantial doubts vex climate science, so much so that any predictions of future trends and impacts are unreliable, and therefore any action now is ridiculous.

There is a charming naïveté in the gushing enthusiasm of some newspaper columnists for the alternative theories of climate change they offer up to the hapless citizen: our climate is not really warming at all, we're told, there's no evidence of such a trend; or, different measurements of temperature disagree, so we're not sure if it's warming or not; on the other hand, if the climate is warming, that's actually a good thing, because our population is aging and warmer is better for them; besides, our plants will be happier with more carbon in the atmosphere. But remember, if the climate is warming, it's certainly not our doing! Blame it on the sun's cycles, not on our greenhouse gas emissions. Clearly this is all part of Mother Nature's doing, because She thinks it's more interesting for us to have a variable climate, rather than one that stays the same all the time.

Are these assertions accurate? The plain answer is: No. Our citizens would do well to take claims such as these with a grain of salt. Yes, the future always contains an element of unpredictability, and yes, the climate forecasts contain a range of outcomes. During the recent debate over Canada's ratification of the Kyoto Protocol, there was little fair or adequate representation of what the Third Assessment Report (TAR), produced by the Intergovernmental Panel on Climate Change (IPCC), actually contained.[1] Nor was there any hint as to why so many distinguished climate scientists regard the results of this vast consensus project as highly credible.[2]

Of course, some legitimate disagreement occurs among reputable climate scientists over detailed aspects of their work, as always in every branch of science. In addition, the views of those few reputable scientists who are on the outer edges of the distribution of viewpoints are not reflected in the IPCC consensus positions.

As citizens we all rely on the consensus of professional, expert opinion in our lives. We all need to learn how to decide whose judgment to trust when we visit our doctor, engage a contractor, or hire a babysitter. So it is with public policy decisions, when those decisions turn on what to believe about what our scientists are telling us. It is no exaggeration to say that our lives and those of our children depend on learning who to trust when it comes to the contest of opinion. Certainly we cannot rely on averaging out the opinions that appear in newspaper coverage or on Internet websites for such matters.

On matters of climate change or any other type of risk, both governments and industry need to be able to rely on "consensus science" to make robust risk management decisions. "Consensus science" is, simply, the current "weight of evidence" on an issue as reflected in the total of peer-reviewed, published research. This does not mean that no disagreements exist within the collection of reputable scientists. On the contrary, some disagreements occur in every area of research – it isn't surprising that it's true of the science of climate change as well. These caveats ought not to obscure the essential point, namely, that a strong consensus exists among reputable climate scientists on all matters directly relevant to the need for action on climate change.

Clearly, the scientific method – a measured and systematic process for observing, developing hypotheses, testing, and submitting the methods and results to others for peer review – is critical in assessing the merits of a scientific claim. The process is slow and requires researchers to be manifestly skeptical of others' work and claims. A good summary definition comes from the Society of Environmental Toxicology and Chemistry (SETAC): The scientific process consists of "organized investigations and observations conducted by qualified personnel using documented methods and leading to verifiable results and conclusions."[3]

But humans carry out science: choosing methods, data sampling strategies, and peer reviewers; deciding on the acceptability of findings (e.g., is something significant at 95 or 99 per cent?); and so on. Human judgment is obviously integral to the scientific method. According to John Ziman, the goal of science is a consensus of rational opinion over the widest possible field.[4] If we accept this assertion, then sound science is the consensus position of scientists actively working in a field regarding knowledge acquired through the scientific method, including what knowledge is agreed upon and what remains in dispute. Consensus on scientific matters ideally emerges only after critical, transparent, and skeptical debate of the issue at hand.[5]

Focusing on the consensus science position is an extremely important issue, especially for major Canadian industry sectors. These sectors have spent the past decade seeking to persuade governments and other stakeholders to adopt a risk-based approach to decision making, an approach that includes the notion that "sound science" should form the cornerstone of all decisions. To illustrate: Bob Peterson, former CEO of Imperial Oil and a well-known opponent of the Kyoto Protocol, makes this call for sound science: "We believe the development and implementation of public policy should be based on sound science and sound economics. This is particularly true as society addresses potential climate change."[6] Thus, what we witnessed in the Kyoto debate – where some industry representatives ignored the consensus expert view and instead promoted the views of a minority of scientists who seek to undermine the credibility of the IPCC consensus – calls into question the fundamental principles of risk-based decision making.

Why should Canadians trust the work of the IPCC? Despite claims that it is a biased international organization working on unfounded scientific assessments,[7] we argue that the only rational policy choice is to accept the findings of the IPCC. To do otherwise would be an irresponsible rejection of sound science in policy. The IPCC represents the single most comprehensive and exhaustive effort in history to translate scientific information into policy-relevant information.[8]

Canadian governments may decide to supplement the work of the IPCC with some form of national expert assessment (for example, under the auspices of the Royal Society of Canada[9]) as the U.S. White House did in 2001.[10] This could provide a useful second opinion to support the IPCC. In the absence of a national assessment, Canadians might decide to look around for a few independent Canadian scientists of international reputation who have taken the trouble to prepare an overview of current climate science. Just such an assessment, published in December 2001,[11] was co-authored by three Canadian scientists of international repute: Professors Gordon McBean, Andrew Weaver, and Nigel Roulet, of the University of Western Ontario, University of Victoria, and McGill University, respectively.

We suggest the following propositions represent a sufficient basis for deciding that action on climate change is required:

- Greenhouse gases (GHGs) play an important role in the planetary energy balance and, therefore, in regulating the global climate.
- Their concentrations have been increasing steadily for the past 100 years due to human activities (i.e., burning fossil fuels, land-use changes).[12]
- Greenhouse gas concentrations are at levels higher than at any point in at least 420,000 years[13] and are projected to at least double within the next century.[14]
- The climate system appears to be sensitive to changes in greenhouse gas concentrations and their radiative forcing of the planetary energy balance.[15] A long time delay exists before there is an equilibrium climate response to concentration changes.

The bottom line is summed up in this three-part proposition:

- Greenhouse gas concentrations influence climate;
- Human actions now influence greenhouse gas concentrations;
- Therefore human actions may influence the climate. In the language of risk, increased concentrations increase our exposure to the hazard and the probability of adverse consequences, whatever they might be.

Certainly one of the major findings of climate science, which every expert accepts, is that the climate record shows natural variations (including greenhouse gas concentrations and global mean temperature). Every expert also assumes that these natural processes are still at work. There is no dispute here. What is at issue is whether the incremental impact of human activity since the beginning of industrialization is of any significance – specifically, whether or not this impact is of enough significance to become an important variable in climate forcing. The only sane answer to this question is "probably yes."

Agreeing that climate change is a serious risk is a matter of common sense. Is it reasonable to believe, knowing the strong relation between greenhouse gases and climate, that the addition of massive quantities of carbon dioxide and methane to the atmosphere, at an accelerating rate over merely a few hundred years (a brief episode in climate history), would have no impact on climate patterns? This is so convenient a belief, in terms of our naked self-interest as a species, that we should be immediately suspicious of it. Current human emissions of greenhouse gases around the planet total about nine gigatonnes (that is, nine billion tonnes) annually of carbon equivalent. This figure is rising and, according to some projections, is unlikely to level off at less than fifteen gigatonnes annual carbon equivalent, every year, unless action is taken to limit and reduce it.

From a common-sense perspective, is it reasonable to believe we can continue this pattern and claim our actions have no consequences for climate change? We think not. On the contrary, this should be regarded as an incautious belief, inconsistent with the way we manage our exposure to all kinds of other risks.

Whatever else we choose to believe, there are solid reasons to believe that humans are influencing the global climate.

LIFE AT THE CLIMATE CASINO: HOW LUCKY DO WE FEEL?

How should we decide what to do about climate change? It all comes down to what kind of risk-takers we are, collectively. Climate policy requires us to trade off the downside risks associated with climate change (the risks of inaction) with the costs and risks of action. Let's see whether using Pascal's wager can help us.[16] The famous seventeenth-century French mathematician offered his wager as a way of deciding whether to believe in God, and this was the first time probability and decision theory had been used for this purpose. For Pascal's question we substitute this one: Are humans today responsible in significant part for climate forcing? Pascal admitted we can never know for certain whether God exists until it is too late to matter (after we die), just as we concede we may not know for sure the answer to our climate-forcing question until after it is too late to take remedial action. Pascal says the way to answer our respective questions is to array the consequences of our beliefs in the form of a decision matrix with four possible outcomes:

A. Suppose human actions ARE now significant for climate forcing:

   1. If we believe this (and if it turns out to be a true proposition), and if we act accordingly in time, we can *possibly* avoid some serious adverse consequences in the future (it's a gamble, remember – there is no certain outcome, no matter what we believe or do).

   2. If we do not believe this (and it turns out to be a true proposition), and take no action to forestall it, we may *possibly* contribute to great adversity for human civilization in the future.

Table 11.1
Pascal's wager applied to the problem of climate change

	Action taken	
	---	---
Climate Outcome	Act	Don't Act
Humans DO affect climate	A1: climate change mitigated?	A2: irreversible climate changes?
Humans DO NOT affect climate	B1: waste resources	B2: money saved, no climate change

B. Suppose human actions ARE NOT significant for climate forcing:
   1. If we believe this (and it turns out to be a true proposition), and act accordingly, we will save ourselves any economic costs of taking action against climate forcing.
   2. If we do not believe this (and it turns out to be a true proposition), and act accordingly, we will waste any resources we have devoted to adjusting our economy to reduce climate change risk.

Pascal suggests we just compare the two downside risks (A2, B1) and ignore everything else. The downside risks – the bad things that may happen as a result of our choices – are represented by outcomes A2 (contribute to serious adversity) and B1 (waste some economic resources). We contend that, given the possible range of economic costs (discussed later in this chapter), A2 represents a significantly worse outcome than B1, and therefore taking action now is a sensible thing to do (see table 11.1).

Climate change is a risk scenario, that is, a matter of probabilities or chances. We use risk scenarios (or risk estimates) every day to forecast possible harms from many sources and to allocate resources to reducing those risks even though we do not know with complete certainty that the harms will occur, or to whom, or with what degree of severity.

Our argument does not depend on making *specific* predictions about adverse impacts from future climate change. The risk-based perspective on climate change runs something like this: The global climate system is a unified process involving massive energy transfers throughout the subsystems of oceans, land masses, and atmosphere, driven by the sun's energy and variation in the Earth's orbit, as well as by other natural and human-originated developments. Because it is based on such a massive and complex energy-transfer system, global climate can be expected to have a great deal of inertia, so that it is not amenable to short-term manipulations involving any of its individual drivers. At certain points climate changes may become, for all intents and purposes, irreversible in time frames meaningful to humans.

Paradoxically, geological ices provide evidence of sudden, abrupt episodes of warming and cooling, suggesting elements of instability in the climate system. The possibility of abrupt climate changes,[17] such as a reversal of the Atlantic gulf stream that warms much of Europe or rapid deglaciation with accompanying sea-level rise,[18] while seemingly remote, should be a concern because of our collective vulnerability to dramatic changes in climatic patterns. The preceding 10,000 years of climate history (the period within which human civilization has arisen) has been a period of relative climate stability. From a common-sense standpoint, citizens are well aware that our mode of life is closely adapted to what we have come to regard as normal climate and weather patterns. Some of our important economic sectors, such as agriculture, forestry, recreation, and tourism depend on the continuation of established patterns, as they relate to rainfall and snowfall, heat and forest fires, and insect pest populations. Our urban settlements are at risk from major disruptions in the established patterns of floods and drought, extreme weather, high summer heat, and other factors. We have an obvious self-interest in maintaining a predictable climate; therefore it is very much in our interest to take steps to do so. A program of risk reduction is a way of seeking to protect ourselves.

Yes, such eventualities are all uncertain. This is, admittedly, a nasty dilemma. One way of trying to avoid it is to say: Couldn't we just take a little more time to see whether, according to the further development of climate science, we really have to make these emissions reductions? Taking more time to decide is sometimes a legitimate response to uncertainty. But is it the right thing to do in this case? We suggest it is not, for specific reasons:

- Greenhouse gas emissions around the globe are not stable, but rather are increasing, which means we cannot hope to achieve the key policy objective (stable or declining concentrations) without much further effort.
- The delayed effects between emissions and ultimate climate responses occur over such a long time (more than a century) that the effects of our actions, taken now or in the near future, cannot make a difference for some considerable period (so we should act sooner rather than later).
- The result of the first two points is to build a large element of de facto irreversibility into future possible climate change and the potential major adverse impacts on us that would result if the risk scenarios that predict these outcomes are ultimately borne out.
- There is a low probability that the essential climate science propositions listed above, which encourage us to act now, will be modified by future science to suggest we should not have acted earlier.

Therefore, we cannot improve matters by waiting longer. Common sense tells us we should act in a precautionary way. And we need to act now.

THE KYOTO DILEMMA

So far, we have made the simple contention that taking precautionary action to reduce the risk of climate change is eminently sensible. We have said little about the nature or cost of this action. If we agree that something should be done now, what should that be? More specifically, is the Kyoto Protocol the right path for Canada? To answer this, we need to examine two issues:

• the cost of meeting Canada's commitments under Kyoto; and
• whether there is some preferable alternative to Kyoto.

Making the right choice requires us to compare the risks associated with a set of actions and ask which set of uncertainties could do our descendants and us the most harm. This approach asks us to compare the downside risks of competing scenarios that have different types of uncertainty attached to them.

What Is the Kyoto Protocol?

Before we go further, a brief background to the Kyoto Protocol is in order. Negotiations for the 1992 United Nations Framework Convention on Climate Change (UNFCCC) led to an agreement that "the ultimate objective of this Convention ... is to achieve ... stabilization of greenhouse gas concentrations[19] in the atmosphere at a level that would prevent dangerous anthropogenic interference with the climate system. Such a level should be achieved within a time-frame sufficient to allow ecosystems to adapt naturally to climate change, to ensure that food production is not threatened and to enable economic development to proceed in a sustainable manner."

Parties (i.e., countries) that signed this convention have met nine times since its inception to promote and review implementation of the agreement. The third Conference of the Parties (COP) held in Kyoto in December 1997 negotiated specific targets for greenhouse gas reductions within the richer nations of the world (Annex B nations). For instance, Canada agreed to average reductions of 6 per cent, using 1990 as the base year, by 2008–2012. Because our emissions have risen steadily since 1990, this works out roughly to a 30 per cent reduction from the so-called "business-as-usual" scenario, or approximately 240 megatonnes (Mt) of greenhouse gases (measured in carbon dioxide equivalence, CO_2e).[20] The emission-reduction targets set in the Kyoto Protocol represent a first step toward the long-term reductions required to stabilize atmospheric concentrations of carbon dioxide. Robert Watson, chairman of the IPCC when the Third Assessment Report was completed, has said: "If one wants to meet the ultimate goal of the convention – that is, stabilization of greenhouse gas concentrations – it would require far more than Kyoto. It would require emissions reductions not only in industrialized countries but also in developing countries."[21]

The IPCC Second Assessment Report estimated that stabilization of greenhouse gas concentrations at about double pre-industrial levels (550 ppm) would require average per capita emissions of approximately five tonnes per year for this century. Current average North American emissions are twenty tonnes per person, while average African emissions are less than one tonne per person.[22] Significant reductions are required, but even the initial targets of the Kyoto Protocol are proving difficult to meet. In Canada, 1990 emissions were 607 megatonnes of carbon dioxide equivalent (Mt CO_2e), making our Kyoto target 571 Mt CO_2e. By 1999 emissions were 15 per cent above 1990 levels (699 Mt CO_2e) and by 2010, emissions in Canada are predicted to be 770 if we continue business-as-usual.[23]

The Kyoto Protocol includes flexibility mechanisms – for which specific rules were finally agreed to in the November 2001 Marrakesh Accord – by which Annex B countries can reduce the costs of meeting emission targets. These include emissions trading between Annex B countries; joint implementation, where Annex B countries undertake emission reduction projects in other Annex B countries for credit against their national targets; and the Clean Development Mechanism, where Annex B countries receive credit for projects undertaken in non-Annex B countries. The Kyoto Protocol would come into force as a legally binding agreement, however, only once fifty-five countries, representing at least 55 per cent of the emissions of the Annex B countries, have ratified it.[24]

The Canadian government agreed to ratify the Kyoto Protocol in Bonn, Germany (COP6) in 2000 and then agreed to the detailed rules for implementing Kyoto contained within the legal text of the Marrakesh Accord (COP7) in November 2001. According to the government press release after the Marrakesh meetings, Prime Minister Chrétien indicated the federal government's intent to ratify the Kyoto Protocol in 2002, after consultation with stakeholders and the public.[25] After votes in the House of Commons and Senate, and a great deal of acrimonious debate, the federal government ratified the Kyoto Protocol on 17 December 2002.

The federal government released the *Climate Change Plan for Canada* in November 2002.[26] The plan includes policy tools such as a domestic emissions trading program for large industrial emitters;[27] targeted measures to encourage public transit; incentives for ethanol fuel, residential energy efficiency, and alternative energy; and the purchase of at least some credits from the international market. This plan builds on earlier efforts, including the 1995 *National Action Plan on Climate Change* (NAPCC) and *Action Plan 2000*. The federal government provided C$1.3 billion for *Action Plan 2000* and identified C$2 billion for the *Climate Change Plan for Canada* in the 2003 budget. The *Climate Change Plan for Canada* estimates that approximately 100 Mt of greenhouse gases emissions will be prevented as a result of the planned initiatives, while about 80 Mt of reductions stem from actions already underway, including about 50–60 Mt from *Action Plan 2000*. This leaves about another 60 Mt still to be accounted for before the government can reduce emissions 240 Mt below business-as-usual.

The Large Final Emitters Group (LFEG) – arguably the centrepiece of the federal climate policy – is predicted to yield 55 Mt of reductions in total. The program revolves around an emissions trading scheme where emissions reduction targets are negotiated between the federal government and each industry sector (to achieve an average of 15 per cent *intensity* improvement; in other words a reduction of 15 per cent from emissions growth under business-as-usual). The government has guaranteed that the emissions trading market will have a price cap of C$15 per tonne of greenhouse gas equivalent, agreeing to pay from federal coffers any difference between this and the actual price. The program and accompanying legislation are currently being developed but will likely not take effect until at least 2005. Some environmentalists feel that agreeing to intensity rather than absolute targets and assuring industry of a cap on the price of emissions was too high a price to pay to bring industry on board, but the emergence of a domestic market for carbon can only be considered a step forward.[28]

Many commentators feel that, even excluding the 60 Mt that remains unaccounted for in the *Climate Change Plan for Canada*, the plan as outlined lacks sufficient detail and is unlikely to meet the Kyoto targets without significant purchase of international credits. For example, John Drexhage of the International Institute for Sustainable Development and a former federal climate change official, writes, "even if we were to accept the government's calculations (and the vast majority of stakeholders in industry and the environmental community do not) the current plan only closes the gap to around 174 Mt, leaving a shortfall of at least 66 Mt." Furthermore, the *Toronto Star* has reported that an unreleased government review of *Action Plan 2000* points to a significant overestimate of the plan's effectiveness. "'We seriously underestimated the difficulty of getting reductions and overestimated the payoff from new technologies,' said a senior official working on climate change."[29]

Won't Kyoto Cost Too Much? The "Carbonomics" View

How much might it cost to deal with climate change? There appears to be a choice between two competing sets of uncertainties: economic costs of action on the one hand and the environmental impacts of inaction on the other.

Earlier, we argued that the scientific basis for climate change is sufficient to justify initial precautionary action, first in the form of emission reductions in line with Kyoto, and, thereafter, further actions as circumstances warrant. Our application of Pascal's wager to climate change makes sense only if the downside risks of action (i.e., the cost of reducing greenhouse gas emissions, initially in line with our Kyoto targets) are not worse than the downside risks of inaction (i.e., the risk of climate change, whatever it might be). If there is a possibility that the Kyoto Protocol will create *catastrophic* economic and social hardship, then ratification makes little sense.

Here we want to ask: Does the climate risk analysis provide an adequate basis for the policy choice that Canada should ratify the Kyoto Protocol? Is that set of propositions, by itself, enough to warrant our ratification and ongoing support of the Kyoto Protocol, because *whatever the other uncertainties about conclusions to be drawn from climate forecasting, the possible adverse impacts of future unconstrained growth in greenhouse gas emissions and concentrations are potentially so momentous that they outweigh the possible adverse economic impacts now?* This is the crux of the matter so far as Canada's Kyoto policy choice facing Canadians is concerned: how do we trade off the risks of climate change with the risk of economic impacts from reducing greenhouse gas emissions. The essence of our argument is this:

- Cost estimates are based on economic models and are uncertain, just as the predictions of climate impacts are uncertain.
- The cost estimates for meeting the Kyoto targets ignore the benefits of managing the risks of climate change, whatever these might be.
- The likely economic costs represent an acceptable course of action, when compared with the risks of climate change.

Estimates on how much it will cost to meet the Kyoto targets abound, and many are using these estimates as the reason to either ratify or reject the plan (see tables 11.2 and 11.3). Will Kyoto create an economic doomsday? Will it spur the economy to find innovative

Table 11.2
Comments regarding the costs of ratifying the Kyoto protocol

Perrin Beatty, President and CEO of Canadian Manufacturers and Exporters[30]	The government's economic analysis seriously underestimates the costs to meet Canada's Kyoto target. It does not consider the impact that higher costs would have on the competitiveness of Canadian industry or on investments in Canada, especially since our major trading partner, the United States, is not party to the Kyoto protocol … Our calculations show that, if Canada were to meet its Kyoto target, at least 450,000 jobs would be permanently lost in Canada's manufacturing sector by 2010 … Net job losses across our national economy would be even greater. Apart from these economic dislocations, all Canadians would have to drive less, drive smaller cars or take public transit that would, in turn, require massive infrastructure spending on the part of governments. We would have to re-insulate our homes, change our furnaces, windows and appliances, at an average expense of around $30,000 per household. We would pay up to 100% more for electricity, 60% more for natural gas and 80% more for gasoline, while paying more taxes, in part to finance the purchase of emission credits.
David Anderson, Federal Minister of the Environment[31]	The best evidence suggests we could have GDP levels that would be a full 99 and six-tenths of what we would have if we did not pursue our international commitments. It suggests that Canada could have almost 1.26 million new jobs by 2010, compared to just over 1.32 million in a business as usual scenario.
Michael Murphy, senior vice-president of policy, Canadian Chamber of Commerce[32]	Canada will have to "shut down pieces of the economy" if it ratifies the Kyoto protocol.
Pierre Alvarez, President, Canadian Association of Petroleum Producers[33,34]	We remain agnostic on the question of Kyoto per se. Governments are going to have to make a decision on whether they should proceed or not and whether Kyoto is the right mechanism. That's not for industry.

Our major competitors – Venezuela, Mexico, and OPEC – are not in the agreement. Yet they all supply into the United States market … To date it's been impossible to determine what the federal government's implementation strategy is going to be, in terms of: how are costs to be spread across the economy, across different sectors. |

Table 11.2 (continued)

Aldyen Donnelly, President, Greenhouse Emissions Management Consortium.[35]	If Canada signs on to it as it now stands, it will elicit trade sanctions for noncompliance that's going to make software lumber [disputes] look like kindergarten.
Bob Peterson, outgoing CEO of Imperial Oil[36]	Kyoto is an economic entity. It has nothing to do with the environment. It has to do with world trade ... This is a wealth-transfer scheme between developed and developing nations. And it's been couched and clothed in some kind of environmental movement. That's the dumbest-assed thing I've heard in a long time.
Ross McKitrick, University of Guelph economist[37]	The bottom line for Canada is that Kyoto will precipitate a recession that will cause a permanent reduction in employment, income and the size of our economy. And if global warming is going to happen, Kyoto will do nothing whatsoever to prevent it or even slow it down. Why are we still considering it?

Table 11.3
Various cost estimates for Kyoto ratification

Canadian Manufacturers and Exporters[38]	• $40 billion and 450,000 manufacturing sector jobs, with larger job losses for the economy as a whole. • We would have to: drive less, drive smaller cars, or take public transit that would, in turn, require massive infrastructure spending on the part of governments; • Re-insulate our homes, change our furnaces, windows and appliances; • Pay up to 100% more for electricity, 60% more for natural gas, and 80% more for gasoline; and • Pay more taxes, in part to finance Canada's purchase of emission credits.
Alberta Government[39]	• $2.9–5.5 billion annually for Alberta or 2–3 percent GDP. • $23–40 billion per year for Canada by 2010.
Canadian Chamber of Commerce[40]	• Up to 2.5% drop in GDP by 2010. • [T]his is equivalent to an average year of economic growth … It would mean $30 billion less in income for Canada … about $1,000 per person less than we would have to spend.… If we consider that total annual public spending on health care today is about $67 billion, then a 2.5 per cent decline in GDP would equal almost half of our current public health care budget.
Environment Canada[41]	• $500 million per year; or • 1.0% decline in GDP (or $10 billion) over the next eight years.
Industry Canada[42]	• Review of other studies showed a range of 0 to 2.3% GDP losses in 2010 from stabilizing energy-related emissions of greenhouse gases at 1990 levels. • [Even without international trading] the costs of [Kyoto] compliance are only likely to be modest if domestic implementation is achieved through a cost-effective scheme. That is to say, a scheme with limited sectoral exemptions. If exemptions are too broad, or poorly designed, the welfare cost of complying with Kyoto commitments is likely to be dramatically higher.
Dutch Report (RIVM)[43]	• 0.02% of GDP by 2010.

Table 11.3 (continued)

NCCP AMG[44]	• 0–3% reduction in GDP, depending on the assumptions. The worst case scenario, Canada achieving its reduction without any international help and no credits for sinks, could result in a 3 per cent drop in GDP over the next decade, that is the economy will grow by 27 percent instead of 30 percent, which is roughly $40 billion in lost economic output.
Diane Francis, The CEO Council, and Bob Peterson[45]	• To meet the emission cuts by 2010, all thermal power plants would have to be converted to nuclear plants. • A 6% reduction means eliminating 139 megatonnes of greenhouse gases by 2010. Stopping all economic growth between now and 2010 could save 120 Mt. • Another 27 Mt could be saved if Canada eliminated 50% of all automobiles from the road. • Alternatively, some 30 Mt could be saved if only one car per family was allowed. • Outlawing cars forever would save 45 Mt. • A total ban on exports from Canada's forestry, mining, oil and gas, chemical and cement business would cut 80 Mt.
Pembina Institute[46]	• The Institute developed a theoretical framework to argue that Canada's competitiveness would not suffer from policies to reduce greenhouse gas emissions consistent with Kyoto.
Suzuki Foundation/World Wildlife Fund study[47]	• The study developed a set of policies designed to achieve more than half of Canada's reduction target under the Kyoto Protocol. It found that measures would yield net economic benefits for Canada over and above the "business-as-usual" scenario including: – A cumulative net economic savings of $4 billion across the economy, reaching $1.6 billion per year or $47 per capita in 2012; – The net addition of an estimated 52,000 jobs in the economy generally, due to the redirection of consumer spending away from fuel and electricity and toward other goods, services, activities, and investments; – A $135 average annual gain in household income related to the creation of new jobs; and a $2 billion increase in the national GDP beyond that projected in the business as usual scenario.

and alternative energy systems? Those who wish we had rejected the accord, the anti-Kyoto chorus, suggest that the cost of compliance would be overly onerous and put Canada at a competitive disadvantage, particularly with the U.S. out of the agreement. Those who favour Kyoto believe that policies to meet the required greenhouse gas reductions would encourage innovative technologies and practices, and increase our energy productivity and economic competitiveness. How can the average citizen make sense of these seemingly polar views?

To understand how the costs of reducing greenhouse gases are estimated – what we call "carbonomics" (the economics of carbon) – one must recognize that costs reflect the relative value of scarce resources. By choosing to take action on climate change, we divert our efforts and attention from other, perhaps more appealing choices.[48] Costs reflect choices to divert resources away from priorities like health care and education to efforts to reduce greenhouse gas emissions.

Understanding the economic implications for Canada from ratification of the Kyoto Protocol is an attempt at predicting the future.[49] Predictions of costs rely on economic models, each with its own set of assumptions and notions of how the economy works. Depending on how the model operates, as well as on the input assumptions, the resulting costs can vary widely, from a small net benefit to a significant cost.

The Canadian Manufacturers and Exporters, an industry association that was quite vocal about the possible costs of Kyoto, makes these comments about economic models: "Different models have been employed by economists to assess the impacts of Kyoto compliance on the Canadian economy. But there is no consensus in the findings. And, regardless of the modelling methodology employed, there are still big gaps between the assumptions that they use and the reality of how the Canadian economy actually works. In short, the models are incomplete, their assumptions are often wrong and their findings are unreliable at best."[50] Most models examine the cost-effectiveness of meeting a pre-existing emissions target, such as Kyoto; they are not trying to balance the myriad costs of climate impacts with the costs of climate mitigation and adaptation in search of some optimal trade-off.

Those advocating a smaller economic burden will argue for less stringent targets and longer time frames to reach them; those advocating more effective climate protection would desire more stringent targets at greater cost. Cost-effectiveness models, however, can only provide some indication about the economic cost to reach whatever targets are established, either unilaterally or through some international negotiation.

Canada's framework for understanding how the Kyoto targets might be achieved and what it might mean to our lives and economy was developed under the auspices of the National Climate Change Process.[51] This process ran from 1998 to 2001 and included sixteen different tables, with representation from federal and provincial governments, industry, and environmental groups. Each table examined options to reduce greenhouse gases within their respective issue or sector. One of these groups was the Analysis and Modelling Group (AMG), which assessed the economic and social impacts of different paths to achieve the Kyoto targets.

The AMG "rolled up" much of the work from the other fifteen tables to conduct its economic analysis. The net result of the AMG analysis was an estimate of between zero and 3 per cent decline in GDP by 2010 if Kyoto were ratified, which implies, in the worst case (where Canada makes all the required reductions domestically and no one else participates in Kyoto), that the economy will grow by an estimated 27 per cent instead of 30 per cent by 2010.[52] Environment Canada has refined this cost to reflect the *Climate Change Plan for Canada*, as they envision it, and estimates the costs will be in the low end of the zero to 3 per cent range,[53] primarily because the cost of international credits may be lower than previously expected.

Where is the source of uncertainty in predicting the costs of reducing greenhouse gas emissions? John Weyant of Stanford University identifies four areas:

1 the nature of, and assumptions within, the model
2 the projected business-as-usual emissions, which indicate how much work is required to achieve the reduction targets
3 the economic efficiency surrounding the rules and policy regime for reductions
4 whether or not the ancillary health benefits of reducing greenhouse gases are included[54]

We shall examine each of these further.

SOURCES OF UNCERTAINTY

1 The structural nature of the model, including its representation of the ability of consumers and industry to find technological innovations and alternatives.

Numerous economic models to analyse the costs of mitigating climate change are available; we are aware of sixteen. Some examine the costs from a macroeconomic level (top-down models) while others (bottom-up models) examine microeconomic issues such as how existing and emerging technologies diffuse through the economy. Bottom-up models tend to provide more favourable estimates of the costs of climate mitigation policies.[55]

However, both top-down and bottom-up models have shortcomings. According to Simon Fraser University economist Mark Jaccard,[56] bottom-up models fail to recognize that some, perhaps many, innovative technologies are not perfect substitutes in the eyes of businesses and consumers; to switch to a low-greenhouse gas technology, some kind of inducement, penalty, or regulation may be required. The size of financial inducement needed reflects the extra value consumers and businesses attribute to existing technology. In contrast, top-down models incorporate these costs by using historical data on the elasticity of energy prices.

Jaccard also believes that the top-down approach can be criticized. Historically derived relationships between relative prices and consumption may not accurately indicate consumer preferences in the future, as new technologies with different characteristics become available. Furthermore, if historical price-consumption relationships of top-down models are not technology specific, but are instead aggregated for an entire sector or the whole economy, they are of little help to policy makers seeking to probe the effect of technology-specific policies.

To rectify these problems, some models strive to blend the best of both approaches in a hybrid model. In an effort to be robust and thorough, the AMG incorporated findings from two micro-models into a macro-model. It compared these results with a Department of Finance macroeconomic model.[57]

2 *The projected emissions under a business-as-usual scenario can vary*
   depending on assumptions. The higher the projected future emissions,
   the greater the effort and costs of reducing emissions to meet
   the Kyoto target.

In Canada, the official emissions projection is the Canada Emissions Outlook (CEO), first prepared in 1997 and updated in 1999 and 2002,[58] which projects reductions of 238 million tonnes of carbon dioxide equivalent ($MtCO_2e$) each year over Kyoto's first compliance period. Clearly, this reduction target could be higher or lower depending on how things unfold. John Drexhage of the International Institute for Sustainable Development suggests that, as of January 2004, "the word in the corridors around Ottawa is that it may actually be as high as 280 Mt."[59] The projection uses factors such as expected economic and population growth, expected technological and industrial sector development (the decommissioning of a nuclear plant in Ontario, the development of oil sands in Alberta), and the rate of energy-efficiency improvements without other policy incentives or price changes.[60]

Normally, it would seem prudent to develop a range of business-as-usual scenarios and then develop a range of costs to reflect these.[61] However, the AMG used the CEO projections as the single basis for cost projections. The government of Alberta has criticized this approach and has suggested that Canada's business-as-usual forecast underestimates the size of the "gap" between expected emissions and the Kyoto target.[62]

3 *What are the rules and the policy regime surrounding reductions, both domestically and internationally? Does the policy regime facilitate economic efficiency?*

At the international level, rules were established at the Conference of the Parties in Bonn and Marrakesh for three flexibility mechanisms: international trading of emissions reductions, joint implementation, and the clean development mechanism. It is widely recognized that market approaches – setting either a price via carbon taxes or an emissions ceiling with permit trading, and then allowing the market to find the most efficient reductions – are more economically efficient for meeting a specific environmental target. The potential and expected cost of international trading is a significant component in Canada's cost analysis: it is much cheaper if we can buy less-expensive international credits rather than find ways to reduce emissions domestically, particularly if we can buy the excess credits belonging to Russia at a reasonable price.

The withdrawal of the U.S. from the Kyoto Protocol has reduced the expected international demand for Russian credits, often referred to as "hot air." This reduced demand should in theory reduce the cost for international permits. But the way that Russia deals with these hot air credits remains a wildcard as does its very participation in the Kyoto Protocol.[63] If Russia does not ratify Kyoto or is not willing to sell all of the hot air on the international markets, then the price will not be as low as expected.[64] The worst-case economic scenario (a 3 per cent reduction in GDP by 2010) developed for the AMG models considered how Canada could meet the Kyoto targets without any international trading of emissions – all reductions would be met domestically. If Kyoto does not come into force, it remains unclear whether Canada would unilaterally move forward on its Kyoto targets. The Minister of Environment, David Anderson, stated that "Whether ratification takes place by Russia or not, Canada expects to continue to meet its minus six per cent target,"[65] which gives some indication that unilateral action is likely. On the other hand, some feel Canada might be hoping for a way out of its Kyoto commitment. A March 2004 twelve-page federal advertisement on climate change failed to mention Kyoto or the Kyoto targets.[66]

If Kyoto comes into force, the international trading rules established in Marrakesh should improve upon the 3 per cent decline in GDP, so any trading with Russia should reduce this cost.

The AMG examined possible domestic policy paths for achieving the Kyoto targets, primarily varying the extent that permit trading was allowed (either for large emitters only or for others as well). For example, economist Randall Wigle of Wilfrid Laurier University found in a study for Industry Canada that the more industry sectors are given exemptions from meeting reduction targets, the less economically efficient this would be for Canada as a whole. The *Climate Change Plan for Canada* calls for reductions of 55 Mt CO_2e from large industrial emitters.[67] Each industry sector of this so-called Large Final Emitters Group will negotiate covenants with the federal government and then trade credited reductions among firms with reduction obligations. The federal government assured industry that they would not have to pay more than C$15 per tonne of reductions and that 55 Mt was the most they would be expected to reduce (regardless of whether Canada's Kyoto gap was higher than 238 Mt). This shifting of the economic risk of reductions away from industry onto the public purse was the political price for getting industry to tacitly accept the Kyoto targets.

4   *What are the benefits of reducing greenhouse gas emissions and how are they considered, if at all, in the economic model? This includes so-called co-benefits, those health and environmental benefits that result from the improved air quality associated with climate policies, and the direct benefits that arise many years in the future from maintaining a stable climate.*

Estimates of the costs of reducing emissions often ignore the co-benefits associated with reductions. The AMG estimated $300–500 million a year in benefits associated with improved health from better air quality. In addition, some economists have attempted to put an economic value on the long-term impacts of climate change, an exercise fraught with uncertainty.

In sum, the cost predictions of meeting Canada's Kyoto obligations are uncertain, and vary according to the assumptions and types of models that create them.

We think it is plausible to guess that actions to meet the requirements of Kyoto will incur some costs to the Canadian economy, because reducing greenhouse gas emissions diverts attention and resources from other priorities. Without a doubt, creating the incentives to shift away from business-as-usual requires that the cost of carbon-intensive energy increase. This will affect the economy and change how we consume energy. It is important that we find fair and efficient means to manage this change. It is also in Canada's economic interest to promote international coordination on climate change and to increase the supply of greenhouse gas reductions available on the international market.

We agree that it is important to determine the economic costs of greenhouse gas reductions as accurately as possible, but it is also important to remember that uncertainty will always surround the predictions. We also suggest that it is a plausible supposition that the likely costs associated with greenhouse gas reductions in line with the Kyoto targets, while not insignificant, particularly given the competing policy priorities such as health care and education, do not place an unreasonable economic burden on Canadians, even in the worst case scenario of 3 per cent forgone growth of GDP by the year 2010,[68] when compared to the possible downside risks to Canadians of climate change.

BUT KYOTO DOESN'T COMPLETELY SOLVE THE PROBLEM, DOES IT?

If all or even most countries eventually agreed to reductions in line with Kyoto, the climate problem would remain. Despite Canada's ambitious target of 6 per cent below 1990 levels, or roughly 30 per cent reductions from business-as-usual, Kyoto does virtually nothing to solve the problem of climate change. The Kyoto emissions cuts are not big enough to come anywhere near what is required if we wish to stabilize greenhouse gas concentrations at some point in the future. Achieving Kyoto targets worldwide, and then doing nothing more, would merely delay the doubling of greenhouse gas concentrations for one decade. Thus if the only environmental benefit we seek is to stabilize greenhouse gas concentrations, we cannot derive this benefit from Kyoto compliance alone; further emissions reductions will be necessary.

So what we have with Kyoto is an international agreement that asks some countries to make significant efforts to reduce greenhouse gases, while allowing others to do nothing, yet doesn't seem to solve the problem. While this, at first inspection, seems to be a foolish plan, it turns out to be the best path forward for two reasons: one, the burden for reducing greenhouse gases will be with us for a long time and the sooner we get started the better; and two, global action is required and we need to show leadership to encourage and cajole others to act with us.

The risk of climate change will not be resolved in the short term, whether we ratify Kyoto or not. We will be dealing with climate risk for the rest of this century, at the very least. No quick fixes lie on the horizon. Three climate-related time lags makes us sure of this. First, the average molecule of carbon dioxide remains in the atmosphere for a long time – one to two hundred years – before it is naturally sequestered. (We've seen recently how this type of atmospheric residency can create problems with CFCs, notorious for destroying stratospheric ozone. Scientists are finding that ozone thinning is still worsening despite aggressive and global action to eliminate CFCs in the late 1980s and early 1990s under the Montreal Protocol.) The gases we put into the atmosphere, in effect, become our legacy. Second, carbon dioxide concentrations do not increase immediately with increasing emissions. Rather, there is a lag of some decades as the ocean's surface becomes saturated with aqueous forms of carbon dioxide, much like a giant buffering solution. Third, because of the thermal inertia of the oceans (they are slow to warm), the climate will take decades to centuries to completely respond to increases in greenhouse gas concentrations. Even after the climate has stabilized (within the bounds of natural variability), sea levels will continue to rise and ice sheets will continue to melt for centuries and millennia.

James Hansen of NASA estimates that "even in 100 years, the response may only be 60–90 percent complete ... It means that we can put in the pipeline climate change that will only emerge during the lives of our children and grandchildren."[69]

These time lags mean that properly managing the risk of climate change will require healthy doses of both adaptation and mitigation. We can expect the climate to continue changing even if we completely stopped putting greenhouse gases into the atmosphere tomorrow. And Canada, as a northern nation, is particularly vulnerable, since climate models predict greater warming in northern latitudes.[70]

The time lags in climate response mean that the sooner we start making reductions, the lower the long-term risk to the climate, whatever it might be. If we want to stabilize greenhouse gas concentrations – the necessary ultimate goal for mitigating climate risk – scientists estimate that we will need to reduce absolute global emissions somewhere on the order of 50 per cent in the coming decades. The sooner we get started and the faster we reduce emissions, the lower the ultimate concentration will be, and hence the less likely we will be to experience severe climatic disturbance. Unfortunately for policy makers, this magnitude of reductions is a tall challenge. Even more difficult for policy makers, the time lags in how climate responds to greenhouse gases mean that we will need to reduce emissions *without a priori*

knowing whether our actions have been too much or too little risk mitigation.
Even if we are able to make such dramatic reductions, we won't know
for decades and indeed centuries after concentrations eventually
stabilize exactly how the climate responds to the new concentrations.

So where does this leave Canada in trying to respond to the risk of
climate change? First, we should be putting a great deal of effort into
trying to anticipate and prepare for climate change. Canada in particular will need to learn how to adapt because northern regions are
predicted to warm more than the global average. In short, climate
change will likely have a big effect on us.

Second, because we are such a small emitter in the global scheme
(some 2 per cent of total world emissions), we should do everything
we can to encourage and cajole others to reduce their own emissions.
Our ratification of Kyoto and our sincere efforts to set in place the
necessary policies are important gestures in this regard. If Canada,
with all of our financial and intellectual resources, cannot find ways
to reduce our greenhouse gas emissions, how can we expect the
developing world to follow?

Is it really necessary to point out that, to achieve an ultimate goal,
one must start taking the initial steps that Kyoto requires? Is it really
necessary to point out that, if attaining the ultimate goal is likely to
entail making a long and arduous journey, over terrain that will not
remain stable but rather will get rougher with the passage of time, we
ought to get started now? If climate risk turns out to be more or less
serious than thought now, we will be able to adjust our actions accordingly. Suggesting that we shouldn't get started is disingenuous.

The genuinely serious problem in global greenhouse gas management revolves around the difficulty in achieving global coordination.
As a result of the incompleteness of the Kyoto Protocol, Canada would
be incurring costs to reduce emissions while other non-signing parties
such as China and India likely will be increasing theirs. These increases
by other parties are likely to be large enough to cause net increases
in total greenhouse gas emissions of human origin, as Canada struggles to comply with our Kyoto targets for the first commitment period,
2008–12.

Certainly for that period, and almost certainly for one or more
subsequent ones, that is what will happen. Unfortunately for the anti-
Kyoto elements, conceding this point does not grant even weak support to the position that there is no benefit from adherence to Kyoto
targets. Countries such as Canada can legitimately be called upon to
start reducing their emissions now, while it is equally appropriate for
others to be increasing their emissions for some time yet, for a very
simple reason: Canada and other nations of the industrialized West

are almost entirely responsible for creating the climate risk problem as it now exists. This follows from delayed effects: rising greenhouse gas concentrations occurring now and in the near future are primarily a result of the history of the West's industrialization – beginning in the nineteenth century, when the rest of the world remained locked into the premodern pattern of life – as well of the social changes initiated elsewhere by the West's colonial domination during the nineteenth and twentieth centuries. The anthropogenic share of current greenhouse gas concentrations is the condensed remainder of emissions that are largely our responsibility. That is why it is not only eminently fair, but also just, that we should take action for some time before others' responsibilities begin to kick in. Part of the very real benefit to Canadians and others that accrues from Kyoto ratification is the inducement it provides for others to follow suit later, as they must do if both we and they are to reduce climate change risk.

Considered purely from a practical standpoint, China and other countries without binding reduction targets are simply not going to take climate change risk reduction seriously unless they have seen the West demonstrate its willingness to act first. The benefit to us of acting now is to increase the likelihood others will act later. Those parallel responsibilities of others rightfully do not exist now but they will arise in the foreseeable future. Reducing the risk of climate change will be a labour spanning decades; to have any hope of stabilizing greenhouse gas concentrations, the larger industrializing nations such as China and India will have to be brought into the post-Kyoto process, through the setting of emissions control levels for all significant human sources, probably not later than 2020, preferably sooner.

This mission, the creation of a low-carbon industrial future for all nations of the world, including technology transfer gifts from West to East, represents an enormous task whose success is itself highly uncertain. Quite possibly, even if we and other countries start to get serious now about Kyoto compliance, in the full knowledge that this is only the first of many necessary steps, in the end we may fail. It may already be too late; the momentum in humanity's carbon-based economy may be too great to be reined in; at least, not in time to do any good in reducing climate-change risk.

There is no way to estimate those probabilities at present. Given what is at stake, however, we maintain that no serious case can be made for being unwilling even to try to succeed.

WHY NOT A MADE-IN-CANADA APPROACH?

Opponents of Kyoto are quick to point out that the developing world does not yet have targets for reducing their greenhouse gas emissions.

This is a serious problem. If we expect to reduce absolute global emissions, all countries must work together. The dilemma, as we have discussed, is how to do this? A made-in-Canada plan, taken to its logical conclusion, presumes that each country should simply pursue emission reductions on its volition and time frame. It's hard to imagine how such a plan could lead to the type of long-term global reductions necessary. Kyoto, on the other hand, at least begins to build a framework for global coordination, however tenuous it may be. In addition to binding targets, Kyoto has provisions for transferring technology and know-how to the developing world through the clean development mechanism. This allows countries like Canada, who might find their targets overly onerous, to take credit for lower-cost emission reductions in developing countries.

A made-in-Canada plan, if it follows the premise of the Alberta climate change plan or its U.S. counterpart, would establish *emissions intensity* targets, that is, reductions in emissions per unit of GDP. Alberta plans to reduce its emissions intensity by 50 per cent by 2020, which on the surface seems impressive. Yet there is no guarantee that absolute emissions will be reduced, particularly if we have robust economic growth.[71] The Pembina Institute has calculated that if Alberta's economy continues to grow as it has over the past ten years, then absolute emissions will actually grow under an intensity target.[72] Again, if we take these intensity targets to their logical conclusion and assume that all nations will set similar targets in the coming years, are we likely to see any reductions in absolute emissions? We suggest not.

A made-in-Canada climate strategy would also likely preclude the purchase of international credits, perhaps to the delight of some environmentalists and business leaders, who would rather we spend our money and effort at home. Unfortunately, access to valid international credits might turn out to be the cheapest way to meet our reduction targets. If we "go it alone," as the Alberta plan proposes, we cannot gain such credits. This doesn't seem to make a lot of sense. And yet, a number of industry voices call into question the propriety of emissions trading, in particular, saying that it is a "disguised transfer of wealth" to poorer countries and, more seriously, that trading doesn't benefit the environment, because we are avoiding our responsibility to make our own reductions by obtaining so-called "hot air" from allegedly unscrupulous nations.

This is a serious charge, but also a dishonest one. It has no business in this debate at all. Here's why: those who were part of the intense negotiations at Kyoto will tell you (we have talked to them) that Canadian industry pressured the government negotiators strongly and persistently on one point – if you are going to sign an international agreement on greenhouse gas emissions reductions (particularly one where we have an ambitious target), don't come home with a deal that does not allow emissions trading. At that point many in Canadian industry had been trying to get the Canadian federal government to set up an emissions trading system for a decade or more, following the lead of the United States, which pioneered this approach for sulphur dioxide and other air pollutants and now uses it extensively. So the federal negotiators made sure they got such a deal. Now a few misguided souls in industry are trying to turn the tables on them and say that it is an immoral thing to do.[73]

Why is emissions trading a valid part of good environmental policy? First, it is only a policy instrument, that is, a means to an end (some other instruments are taxes, regulations, and voluntary covenants). But it is a particular kind of instrument, namely, a market-based one, which business people – excluding those whose opposition to Kyoto apparently has caused them to forget what good business principles are – normally like and support. It is sometimes also called a "flexible mechanism," because it allows an almost unlimited range of specific strategies. Finally, but most important, it tends to be the lowest-cost type of instrument, because it encourages entrepreneurial ingenuity and technological innovation.

But the primary purpose of any such instrument is to achieve environmental protection goals. Any emissions trading regime does so by definition, because it is authorized by governments for exactly that purpose. It is called a "cap and trade" scheme and this is how it works: first, an environmental protection target is set; if the culprit is excessive emissions, then the target is set initially at some point below current emissions levels – in other words, emissions are "capped" at that level. (For Kyoto as a whole, the level is 5.2 per cent below 1990 levels.)

This means that all emitters subject to the restrictions collectively have this target. The key objective is reducing total emissions for a defined set of polluters (companies, sectors, or nations), over a specified period of time, until they are at or below the cap, which is where they are permitted to be. The permitted amount of total emissions is allocated among the players in that set. There is no trading regime without a cap, and the cap is the environmental protection guarantee. Usually the cap is lowered some time later, to increase the level of environmental protection, and this process can go on indefinitely.

When the first allocation occurs, some players will already be below their assigned targets; among firms, these are typically the most efficient or proactive ones. (They may also be planning to shut down their most inefficient plants.) These players, in effect, will have credits that they will be allowed to sell. The buyers will be other firms or sectors or countries whose current emissions exceed their permit allocations, for whom it is cheaper to buy credits than to achieve their targets in other ways, such as buying pollution control equipment. Individual firms have the flexibility to make their own choices and the market sets the prices for the permits through supply and demand.

Back to Kyoto. At the insistence of major industrial sectors, an international "cap and trade" mechanism was included in the Protocol. But only those nations that have signed and ratified the Protocol can participate in the trading. All nations that ratify the Protocol have the flexibility to choose how much they want to reduce emissions domestically and how much they want to trade on the international emissions market. Some countries, Russia in particular, will have credits to sell, because their total emissions are well below their negotiated target as of 1990.

Exactly how Canada's proposed domestic trading system will be integrated with an international system is not yet clear, although one thing is certain: without Kyoto, Canadian industry would have no access to international credits. This access, coupled with the federal guarantee that the price will not rise above C$15 per tonne of carbon dioxide equivalent, provides more than enough economic security for Canadian businesses.

For these simple reasons Kyoto is a more rational plan for mitigating climate risk than a made-in-Canada approach. The anti-Kyoto chorus has failed to provide a better plan, or indeed any plan, for engaging nations such as China, India, and Brazil in mitigating climate change.

BUT THE U.S. ISN'T IN THE AGREEMENT!

We must take up one other objection that for many Canadians may appear to trump, all by itself, all the difficulties with Kyoto – namely, our American cousins are not going to do this, and, therefore, we cannot, since our economies are so closely linked. To reduce our emissions when the Americans aren't reducing theirs will make our industries uncompetitive, it is alleged.

The Bush administration removed the u.s. from the Kyoto Protocol in March 2001. The u.s. withdrawal from Kyoto appears grounded in two arguments: the Kyoto targets for the Protocol cannot be achieved without significant economic cost; and the Protocol is ineffective because it exempts developing countries such as China and India. On the former, Bush has said "I will not accept anything that will harm our economy or hurt our American workers. I'm worried about the economy and the lack of an energy policy and the rolling blackouts in California."[74] On the latter, Bush wrote in a 13 March 2001 letter, "I oppose the Kyoto Protocol because it exempts 80 per cent of the world, including major population centers such as China and India, from compliance, and would cause serious harm to the u.s. economy. The Senate's vote, 95-0, shows that there is a clear consensus that the Kyoto Protocol is an unfair and ineffective means of addressing global climate change concerns."[75]

The anti-Kyoto campaigners may have been surprised to read the 19 March 2002, statement by Paul Cellucci, the u.s. ambassador to Canada, in which he proclaims that the u.s. intends to take strong action "over time" to "slow and, as the science justifies, stop and ultimately reverse emissions growth."[76] According to Cellucci, the u.s. government will spend $4.5 billion on emissions reductions strategies next year alone, largely on the development of energy-efficient technologies. In a May 2002 comparison of u.s. and Canadian government action on climate change, the Pembina Institute concludes that "governments in the u.s. have taken far more significant action to reduce GHG emissions than have governments in Canada."[77]

So quite likely u.s. industry, prodded by state-level initiatives and pulled by u.s. government-sponsored research funding, will become more energy-efficient, while some sectors in Canadian industry will be doing little except complaining that for us to do likewise offers no benefit. This will guarantee that some Canadian industries will indeed become uncompetitive with the u.s., not because of Kyoto ratification, but because some in our nation will have helped to prevent it from happening. Obviously the Canadian economy is not the economic powerhouse that the u.s. economy is, and Canadian governments cannot provide by themselves the huge research budgets to support technological innovations that are common there. u.s. government research subsidies are so large that it can afford to go it alone in its response to global climate change risk in the short term. Canada and most other nations cannot follow suit. But thought of another way, the u.s. decision represents an advantage for Canada, in that emissions trading credits will be cheaper in the world market, because the u.s will not be competing for them (only those that ratify Kyoto can use these credits). The only thing we will not be able to do, if we ratify while the u.s. does not, is generate any credits by transactions with u.s. entities.

The simple message to those among our captains of industry who have been propagating visions of economic doom resulting from Kyoto ratification is this: ease up on the doomsday rhetoric and get on with the job of making Canadian industry more energy-efficient. If this seems too daunting a task, a quick look at British Petroleum may help.[78] In March 2002 this large petroleum producer announced that not only had it achieved company targets for emission reductions

– 10 per cent below its 1990 levels (which includes all its growth since then) – but also it had done so at no net cost to the company as a result of energy cost savings.

CLIMATE POLICY IN CANADA: SOME MODEST SUGGESTIONS FOR A PATH FORWARD

Canada's ratification of the Kyoto Protocol, while the correct choice, was not impressive from a policy or risk management standpoint. Our major decision-making institutions – the two senior levels of government and the business community – were at each other's throats for the better part of 2002. An intensive public relations and lobbying campaign was carried out by leading industry associations under the guise of the hilariously misnamed and now inactive Canadian Coalition for Responsible Environmental Solutions. Federal and provincial politicians became openly hostile,[79] a public official in Alberta was fired for support of Kyoto,[80] and despite all the hyperbole and talk, the Canadian public seems no better informed about the serious challenges that lie ahead with climate change. We hope this is not the "business-as-usual" scenario for Canada.

The case against Kyoto ratification made to Canadians failed in part because it does not attempt to evaluate fairly the accumulated results of reputable climate science, and in part because its own rhetorical structure is a patchwork of half-articulated premises and evasive arguments.

The case to be made for Canada's ratification and ongoing support of the Kyoto Protocol rests on a straightforward application of the same principles of risk management that we use in this country every day to make decisions, where the potential adverse impacts are serious and the processes giving rise to them may have irreversible consequences.

Once these obstructions are cleared away, a fresh look at the balance of probabilities and uncertainties encourages us to believe that it is reasonable for Canadians to suppose the risks associated with accelerating growth of greenhouse gas emissions are far more serious than are the contrasting risks, namely, the chance that beginning Kyoto compliance now will cause Canada to suffer major blows to its economy for no offsetting benefits.

The downside risk in the climate forecasts is defined by the fact that we are already riding the tiger of increasing global greenhouse gas concentrations. Not only that, but the tiger's momentum is accelerating, so that the longer we stay on, the wilder the ride gets. It may not be too late to jump off now. But the longer we hang on, the scarier it will be when we eventually take the leap – as we must, sooner or later.

The Kyoto debate will be back. But before it returns, there is a small window of opportunity in which we could, if we want, design a better structure for public discourse about climate risk.

The Kyoto debate will be back because it is only the first small step towards solving the problem. The nations who assembled in Kyoto had been persuaded by the consensus judgment of the world's climate scientists that there was a problem to fix – namely, "climate forcing" by human-caused greenhouse gas emissions. That consensus, summed up in the 1990 and 1995 IPCC reports and strengthened in the 2001 IPCC report, said that we should reduce human GHG emissions to "stabilize" concentrations of GHGs in the atmosphere at some yet undefined acceptable level of risk.

All the world's nations must act to make the emissions line "go flat" and then start to decline, but even in the most optimistic scenario this is unlikely to happen before 2100 or so. The Kyoto reductions are too small to accomplish this, as everyone knows. The world will likely need a number of Kyoto or Kyoto-like agreements to adequately address climate change – if the world is capable of doing so. But no doubt a Round II at least will occur, sometime in the next few years, when those countries who want global action on climate change will try to cajole and persuade others – especially China and India – to start to control their emissions growth.

Canada will be at the table again, regardless of the fate of Kyoto. Let's imagine two plausible scenarios for the coming years:

- Russia ratifies Kyoto in late 2004 or early 2005. The parties meet in 2005 and, under Article 3, must show "demonstrable progress." One imagines that Canada will likely have little to show in the way of actual reductions. Rather, our progress will rest largely with the prospect of a domestic trading scheme, an investment in climate-related technology and innovation from the proceeds of the federal government's final shares of Petro-Canada[81] and the piecemeal benefits of all the so-called targeted measures. It is likely that a number of E.U. countries will be in a similar situation, although the E.U.-wide emissions trading program will be up and running in 2005.
- Russia chooses not to ratify Kyoto or, more likely, says nothing about its intention and simply lets the agreement dissolve. At this point, the E.U. will struggle with its commitment to unilaterally meet its Kyoto targets. Likewise Canada will surely not meet its Kyoto target without having access to valid international credits. This scenario brings our climate policy dilemma into much sharper focus, perhaps sooner than we will want.

The wildcard in these scenarios is, of course, the U.S. While the Bush administration appears unlikely to enter into a Kyoto or Kyoto-like agreement, one should not assume that a Democratic White House, led by John Kerry, would have any more leeway. While Kerry has stated his intention to support some alternative to Kyoto (it is undoubtedly too late for the U.S. to meet the Kyoto targets negotiated in 1997 without, like Canada, making significant purchase of international credits), a two-thirds majority is required to approve any international treaty. In years past the U.S. Senate has, first, unanimously rejected (the mid 1997 Byrd-Hagel Resolution) any treaty that requires the U.S. to reduce emissions without "commitments to limit or reduce greenhouse gas emissions for Developing Country Parties within the same compliance period;" and second, rejected by a majority vote the 2003 McCain-Lieberman bill on climate change (it established a domestic emissions trading scheme, albeit one that was much more timid than Kyoto's targets). Therefore it seems likely that even a Kerry administration will have difficulty bringing the U.S. into any international climate treaty. So the duality of our desire for multilateral action on climate change and our desire to maintain a close economic relationship with the U.S. is likely to remain with us for some time.

The most implausible scenario is that the climate change problem goes away, regardless of how deeply we bury our heads in the sand. That's why we wish to make the following plea: Canada must start now to find a way to conduct our public debate more sensibly and productively before the next round starts. Here are our modest recommendations to help us get ready:

1 Canadian policy makers and citizens can only benefit from robust, regular, and well-communicated national assessments of climate science and the economic costs of GHG reductions. First, we must start with a process that brings to the citizen a clear and credible account of the climate science consensus. Certainly as time passes there will be more evidence on which to base the consensus judgment, whatever that might be. However, the so-called "skeptic" viewpoints will still be around. None of us who aren't climate scientists can possibly decide for ourselves who is right when "duelling science" is presented. So we need a credible process to sort things out. Fortunately, a robust and highly credible process already exists, in the form of the IPCC.

But national context and interpretation is important for a highly complex risk like climate change. Governments frequently refer questions about how to interpret the science consensus to their national academies.[82] This is done all the time for many different types of issues for which there is a body of scientific evidence. No country uses this process more actively than the United States: the National Academy of Sciences (NAS) issues one report of this nature almost every working day of the year. The world's oldest national academy, the Royal Society (U.K.), is also very active, and our own Royal Society of Canada has performed this service numerous times.

Let's ask our governments to adopt the following process:

- On a five-year cycle, starting now, commission a series of reports on the current climate science consensus (including the range of expert opinion) from our national academies.
- On the same cycle, commission a series of economic scenario reports from our national academies on the impacts of various emissions reduction targets on our country and its regions.
- Do likewise with a series of reports on risk/cost/benefit trade-offs, where the two previous sets of reports are put together in a policy-relevant framework.

2 But don't stop there. These are highly technical issues, hard for most of us to understand. Governments should use trusted institutions, such as a network of university researchers, to ensure that these results are regularly and understandably communicated to the public. These researchers could operate a web-based public information resource that would "translate" the scientific complexities into understandable terms, without distortion, for the citizen; and also operate a variety of mechanisms for answering questions and conducting debates. These resources should include high-quality animated graphics, for ease of understanding of the very difficult concepts scientists have to use to describe and model something as complex as the global climate.

If we had such a basis for informed and intensive debate, we might also hope to have, next time around, less extreme rhetoric and scare-mongering. Climate change risk involves some extremely tricky issues and they are not going to go away. On the contrary, with each successive round the questions will become more complicated and the stakes – in terms of both risks and costs – will be higher. One way or another, our lives and prosperity, and that of our descendants, may depend on getting it right. We owe it to them and to ourselves to devise a more effective way of deciding on what is the right thing to do.

3 Consistent political direction and coordination is needed to help reduce the domestic policy uncertainty surrounding climate change. By establishing long-term (say 2030) national and provincial targets for reducing our net greenhouse gas emissions by half (interim

targets could also be established), political leaders could back-cast from the long-term target to develop an adaptive policy framework.

4 Any domestic policy framework should make comprehensive use of economic instruments to reduce greenhouse gas emissions. The creation of a domestic trading market is the first step in this direction; and the imposition of taxes on greenhouse gas emissions must be considered seriously.

5 Canada is especially vulnerable to the impacts from climate change. We need to considerably expand our ability to predict and be prepared for the eventual impacts, particularly in the Arctic.

We have argued throughout this chapter that the risks of climate change call for Canada to provide consistent leadership in establishing a globally coordinated, long-term framework for action. For now, this leadership takes the form of the Kyoto Protocol, although we must be prepared to adapt to changing international circumstances. We recognize that many of our arguments rely on our professional judgment of the risks and costs and we welcome further discussion and debate on our position.

12 Life in the Fast Lane: An Introduction to Genomics Risks

MICHAEL TYSHENKO AND
WILLIAM LEISS

PROLOGUE

Newspapers around the world picked up a story from the American Association for the Advancement of Science's annual meeting in Seattle, February 2004. The story reported on the results of a scientific study in which a virus carrying the gene for a growth hormone called IGF-1 was injected into the hind-leg muscles of rats, who were then put through an aggressive physical-training program. The targeted muscles grew between 15–30 per cent in both size and strength, in comparison with those of a control group of untreated animals. The higher levels of IGF-1 occurred in the muscle tissue, but not in the bloodstream. This raised the hope that someday a gene therapy program might be developed for humans suffering from muscle-wasting diseases such as muscular dystrophy.

Why the heavy media coverage of a rat study? The answer is contained in a remark made at the time by Lee Sweeney, the study's lead researcher: "Half of the e-mails I get are from patients, and the other half are from athletes." The prospect of gaining a quick advantage over others in competitive sports through gene therapy is irresistible to some – especially because current anti-doping tests on athletes could not detect this kind of modification. That this particular therapy has undergone no human safety testing is apparently a trivial point. The dark stories about health damage in later life to the athletes of the former East German communist regime, who were treated by their own government as experimental laboratory animals, appear to hold no terrors for them. The great irony is, of course, that every incremental step in the technological enhancement of performance acts as a spur for the next one. The cycle recurs with increasing rapidity as the rate of innovation grows, as the benefits of newer techniques leapfrog those of their predecessors.

Before too long a great flood of experimental gene therapies will be pouring out of the world's research laboratories. In the not-too-distant future the results of athletic competitions may reflect nothing so much as the differential risk tolerance among individuals for trying out the latest innovations in mixing various therapies. The trophies will recognize those with the courage to live life in the fast lane – for that day. What comes after is anybody's guess.

THE MANIPULATION OF LIFE

Almost two centuries ago a young woman engaged in a parlour game with her travelling companions, including two rather famous English gentlemen by the names of Byron and Shelley. She bore the name of her mother, the famous feminist Mary Wollstonecraft, who died shortly after giving birth to her; but the world knows her by her married name: Mary Shelley. The game – played while the three of them were vacationing in Switzerland – was to write a gothic novel, and of the three she was the only one to carry it out. The result was *Frankenstein*, first published anonymously in 1818; she was all of nineteen years old when she wrote it.[1]

Most people know her achievement only through the equally famous movie, starring Boris Karloff. This is a shame, because although it is a remarkable work of art in its own right, James Whale's 1931 film does not do justice to Mary Shelley's genius. Even her subtitle is important: *Frankenstein; or, the Modern Prometheus*. Prometheus, in Greek mythology, was the god who stole fire from Heaven and gave it to mankind; he was punished by Zeus by being chained to a rock, where an eagle fed on his liver, which regenerated daily so that his torment was endless. Even her novel's epigraph – three lines on the title page from Milton's *Paradise Lost*, where Adam is addressing God – is important: *Did I request thee, Maker, from my clay / To mould me Man, did I solicit thee / From darkness to promote me?*

Mary Shelley's novel is more "relevant" today than it was when she wrote it – a testament to her far-seeing genius. Her main theme is the responsibility of scientists for their creations. Her narrative tells how Dr Victor Frankenstein abandoned his creation – the world's first recombinant entity – at the moment the creature became alive. The scientist fled in horror from his laboratory, forcing his creation to go into the world alone. There is immense pathos in Shelley's rendition of the creature's fate, for he thinks of himself as human, and yet every encounter with humans is disastrous, for like Victor they flee from him in fear and disgust. (It is significant that he has no name, of course.)

So he hides out, in proximity to the humans who have spurned him, reading Milton and eavesdropping on the players of classical music. His encounters with humans lead to what are accidental tragedies, but humans regard him as a murderer and hunt him. Victor flees to Scotland, where his creation tracks him down and confronts him with a simple request: You made me, therefore take responsibility for my fate. Humans will not accept me as one of their own. I am dying of loneliness; you must create for me a female mate of my own kind. Victor first agrees, embarks on this task and then reneges, expressing horror at the very thought, whereupon his bitterly frustrated creation proceeds to wreak terrible revenge upon him.

About two hundred years later the modern science of genetics has turned what was a juvenile literary exercise into a stark reality of the near-term future. Research using genetics focuses on improving human health, the quality of life, and life spans – a predicted panacea of treatments for many human diseases, coming very soon. Every day in the media we read or hear about the next astonishing health or scientific breakthrough, derived from the study of our genetic material, that promises to provide revolutionary cures for various diseases. This rapid pace of new breakthroughs and promised cures in the near future provides a meaningful context that allows us, as a society, to feel that we have chosen the correct path in exploiting what we know about science, innovation, and biotechnology for the greater societal good. However, at the same time, what remains in the shadows, hidden and not discussed, is a fear that we are gaining too much power through the rapid acquisition of knowledge combined with a reduced choice over random destiny and an imposed alteration of our humanity. While this claim of enslaving ourselves with our own technology may seem fantastical at first it doesn't take long to realize that we have already altered the genetics of other species (hybrid plant varieties) on the planet so profoundly that they have become unable to reproduce successfully without our help.[2]

The limits of genetic technologies are being overcome with great speed, surpassing even the preconceived expectations of scientists themselves. This was most notable with the achievement of successful mammalian cloning in the late 1990s, since many eminent scientists had been sure that such a breakthrough was still far off in the future.[3] Cloning of animals was first proposed in 1938, by German embryologist Hans Spemann, as a "fantastical experiment" where the nucleus of an egg would be removed and replaced with a nucleus from another cell. The result of such an experiment would be to create an exact replica of the original organism, creating life without sexual procreation. Because of technical limitations, it wasn't until 1952 that American scientists Robert Briggs and Thomas King attempted the experiment using frog's eggs (they are large and easy to manipulate), transferring an adult cell nucleus to replace the egg's nucleus. This initial experiment failed but other scientists continued to refine the technique of somatic cell nuclear transfer.

Partial success was achieved in 1970 when a developmental biologist, John Gurdon, inserted the nuclei from an advanced frog embryo back into the eggs, rather than the previously tried adult cells. The frog eggs developed into tadpoles, but then all died before becoming adults. With the continued improvement of technology, in 1984 Steen Willadsen, a Danish embryologist, succeeded in cloning a sheep using a nucleus from a cell of another early sheep embryo. This result was repeated by researchers using several other animals but seemed limited, working only when other early embryo cells were used as donor nuclei. The nuclei from differentiated animal cells could not be used to clone, as they did not seem to be able to "reprogram" themselves to act like an early embryonic cell.

The mystery surrounding reproductive cloning was unveiled from knowledge of the way cells divide: it became apparent that cells don't divide until conditions are appropriate. The reason that all previous attempts at cloning failed was that the egg and the donated nucleus needed to be at the same stage in the cell cycle. In 1995 reproductive biologist Ian Wilmut succeeded in cloning a farm animal from advanced embryos by resynchronizing the host cell and donor nucleus; he cloned an adult mammal for the first time, producing a lamb named Dolly from a six-year-old ewe, using tissue taken from the ewe's udder. Out of 277 nuclear transfer attempts, Dolly was the only successful clone.[4] Within two years, the same group from Scotland created Polly, the first transgenic sheep with a human gene in every cell of its body. Since then scientists have successfully cloned a host of animals, including cats, cattle, goats, rabbits, mice, and pigs.[5]

With the cloning of a higher mammal (Dolly the sheep), public concern immediately jumped to the ability to clone humans.[6] An ominous refrain was "if we can clone a higher mammal then we can clone a human and we inevitably will," which appeared in several media articles echoing public concern.[7] A few laboratories have already shown their proficiency and ability to clone humans, but elected to stop the "experiment" at an early stage.[8] Several countries have adopted the moral position that cloning a human by nuclear transfer (reproductive

cloning) is illegal. Such emerging science, when driven by the technological imperative and proprietary business values, makes people
uneasy because something that can be done in the realm of science is
seemingly inevitable and only a question of research time and effort.
The example of the history of cloning illustrates that the barriers confronting researchers are usually technical ones and with time these
problems are usually overcome; from its inception as a fantastical
experiment to actualization took a mere fifty years. This ability to
reduce the unknown to the known scientifically because it is technically
possible leaves us with an overwhelming sense of a predestined outcome – one of inescapability: a sense that science is largely unyielding
to our concerns and therefore unstoppable. Researchers, for the most
part, are unconcerned with the gap between things that "can be done"
and things that "will be done," placing scientific innovation as a technical exercise set apart from any ethical concerns. As a result, the ethics
of science takes a quiet back seat or, even worse, it becomes completely
irrelevant to the fast pace of innovative research.

The story of Dolly provides an excellent example that ethical concerns
do have a place alongside the juggernaut of science as it applies to
human gene therapeutics. After the birth of Dolly it was determined
that a number of things were wrong with the "successful" clone. At
three years of age the DNA (Deoxyribonucleic acid or heritable material) in her cells was typical of a much older animal. All chromosomes
are capped with telomeres, tiny repeating strands of the DNA that can
be related to chronological age. Telomeres shorten each time a cell
divides, and continuously erode as an animal ages. The researchers
found that Dolly's telomeres were shorter than other three-year-old
sheep, suggesting that she was genetically much older than her birth
date.[9] By five years old, she had developed severe arthritis, but it was
unclear whether the condition was a result of the cloning process.
Dolly died at age six, euthanized after being diagnosed with progres-
sive lung disease. Sheep usually live to twice this age or longer; arthritis
and lung infections are commonly found in older sheep.[10] Human
clones, even if they don't display monstrous abnormalities in the
womb, may age prematurely at a severely accelerated rate or show
other cloning-related diseases; perhaps such technologies should
never be applied to humans at all.

We must realize that, in time, all of the mysteries of life involving
biological processes will be deconstructed by scientific research and
become known, however appealing or overwhelming their potential
application to the human condition may be. If many of the innovations
derived from science are to be realized and actualized as therapeutic
treatments we must understand the various kinds of risks that may be

associated and ask the question: should there be limits on what we do, even in the name of human health?

THE CONCEPT OF RISK AND ITS RELEVANCE TO GENOMICS

The concept of risk provides a suitable canvas on which to array and systematically describe the social, ethical, and legal issues raised by the engineering of our heritable genetic material through direct manipulation using either genetics or genomics. The concept of risk has certain intrinsic attributes that make it especially useful for this purpose. First, risk poses the two questions of greatest interest to everyone, in terms of outcomes – of either natural or technological processes – the questions that cause concern or dread to individuals and societies: how likely is it to happen? and if it does happen, what are the expected consequences? Second, risk lends itself to both qualitative and quantitative description. In both types, but especially the latter, risks can be compared with each other, across very broad domains, thus facilitating certain critical choices open to us as individuals – in particular, whether certain risks rise above the threshold of acceptability or tolerability, whereas others do not. Third, the concept of risk asks us to estimate the dimensions of the uncertainties attached to particular risky ventures, so that we know whether the risk can be controlled with the strategies currently available to us.

Risk is a powerful concept that defines the trajectory of industrial society, intent on the domination of nature for enlarged human benefit, a project envisioned by Francis Bacon in the seventeenth century. Today we seek to carry out this project in two interconnected ways: by maximizing the spread between benefit and loss; and by minimizing the "downside risk," i.e., protecting ourselves from the possible worst-case consequences. To achieve these two interconnected goals we require good risk management, which requires us to recognize the pertinent risk factors in a particular endeavour in advance; failure in this regard can be catastrophic. Recent research into improving human health and the quality of life has led us inexorably to the capacity to engineer our own genomes and to alter the randomness of passing desirable and undesirable traits to future generations. Such knowledge is perhaps the most fateful of all human powers, in that the risks to be managed go beyond specific interventions and reach into the very foundations of human civilization. Society can manage genomics and genetics risks only if the scientific community becomes actively engaged in this process, assuming its share of responsibility for their potential scope, well in advance of successfully achieving our practical objectives.

We find ourselves standing on a precarious slope, with the promise of emerging biotechnology seemingly offering all of society therapeutic benefits to cure diseases beyond anything we could have imagined a little over a decade ago. The technologies can be divided into two broad categories: "genomics," which is primarily concerned with using genetic information to create tools for human therapeutics that will involve traditional drug treatments and pre-symptomatic disease management; and "genetics," which will use the tools and information derived from genomics and apply them to other emerging technologies, again for therapeutic cures.

GENOMICS: TOOLS FOR FUTURE THERAPEUTICS

Genomics is the intersection of bioinformatics (knowledge derived from computer analysis of biological data) and genetics, and is defined as the study of genes and genomes.[11] Genomics now encompasses a broad range of molecular biology technologies, from traditional genetics to genetic databases from which new therapeutic areas of study are emerging. Computer databases of genetic information are the culmination of decades of worldwide research.

In 1865 an Augustinian monk named Gregor Mendel mated green pea plants and observed how different traits (colour, appearance) were transmitted to the succeeding generations. He described a gene as a discrete unit of heredity; much later these genes were determined to be made of DNA. The structure of DNA was worked out in 1953 by James Watson and Francis Crick, its basic unit being a nucleotide base that consists of a sugar and phosphate group to which one of four nitrogen bases are attached. The nucleotide bases are joined together to form a long, linear strand of DNA; for stability DNA exists as a double stranded helix or twisted ladder. Physically characterized, a gene is a string of nucleotide bases located somewhere along the DNA strand, and the average size of a human gene is 3,000 nucleotide bases. A single gene encodes for the trait or directions to make a single protein that is needed inside the cell.

The genome consists of all DNA inside our cells that encodes all our genes for making and expressing all the proteins. The technique of DNA sequencing was discovered independently in two different labs at around the same time. Walter Gilbert (with graduate student Allan Maxam) in the United States and Frederick Sanger in England each developed new techniques for rapid DNA sequencing. Within a decade, the technique for sequencing had been automated, along with other innovations allowing for high throughput data collection. The first genome from a bacterium was completed in 1995 and the complete genetic sequence of other model organisms (fruit fly, mouse) quickly followed. The human genome project began in 1990 as a collaborative, public domain effort; the completed draft of the entire human genome was published in April 2001. The human genome sequence revealed that our genome has 3 billion nucleotide base pairs that encode 30,000 different genes; all of the genes that we consider the important parts comprise less than 2 per cent of the entire DNA molecule.

Currently, the amount of information contained in the largest DNA database, "Genbank," is truly astounding: some ~30 billion base pairs. In addition to the complete human genome data, it contains genes and DNA sequences from other species' genomes. Collectively, the amount of sequence data is doubling every 12–14 months.[12] However, large repositories of DNA sequences by themselves, while impressive for sheer volume, have little impact on improving human health; they are a fundamental tool for genomic medicine, acting as a road map to locate disease gene loci.

A number of important areas of genomics are emerging from static databases of genetic information, including *pharmacogenomics*, which focuses on analysing single nucleotide polymorphism databases; and *transcriptomics* and *proteomics*, which will help in pre-symptomatic medical treatment, individualized disease detection, and individualized therapeutic treatments.

Pharmacogenomics: Personalized Therapeutics

The idea of "biochemical individuality" was first proposed by Roger Williams in 1956 to explain variability in disease susceptibility, nutrient needs, and drug responsiveness among otherwise seemingly healthy people. It is only now, with the ongoing genomic revolution, that the number of gene targets identified has increased and, with genetic testing, will allow medical doctors to assess true biochemical individuality.[13] The combination of pharmacology with diagnostic genomics is called "pharmacogenomics," and this emerging research branch holds the promise that drugs might one day be tailor-made for individuals and adapted to each person's own genetic makeup. Environment, diet, age, lifestyle, and state of health can all influence a person's response to medicines, but understanding an individual's genetic makeup is thought to be the key to creating personalized drugs with greater efficacy and safety. Pharmacogenomics combines traditional pharmaceutical sciences such as biochemistry with annotated knowledge of genes, proteins, and single nucleotide polymorphisms that have been derived from catalogued database sources.[14]

Single nucleotide polymorphisms (SNPs, pronounced "snips") are sites in the human genome where individual DNA sequence differs, usually by a single base. Single base-pair variations are the most common and can determine whether or not we develop a certain disease. The magnitude of deleterious effects from infectious microbes, toxins, and drug treatments is also moderated by SNPs. Analysis using SNPs is an important diagnostic tool, since they are widespread and easy to detect. One database has catalogued over 1.4 million human SNPs.[15] Some well-characterized examples of genetic polymorphisms include a mutation that causes sickle cell anemia with reduced susceptibility to malaria; polymorphism in the cytochrome P450 CYP2D6 gene that affects adverse drug responses; and alcohol intolerance influenced by aldehyde dehydrogenase gene polymorphisms.[16]

Medical research is just now beginning to correlate DNA polymorphisms with individual responses to medical treatments. Patients determined by their DNA variation will have drug treatments customized for their subgroup. During medical treatments 0.1 million people die from unexpected adverse side effects while another 2.2 million experience serious reactions, and still others fail to respond at all. Enzymes involved in drug metabolism, like cytochrome P450, are responsible for metabolizing most drugs used today, including many for treating psychiatric, neurological, and cardiovascular diseases.[17] Characterization of DNA variants in such genes will virtually eliminate adverse reactions. Tens of thousands of people are hospitalized each year as a result of toxic responses to medications that are beneficial to others. Some cancers respond dramatically to current therapeutic regimens while the same treatment has no effect on disease progression in others. Scientists in major pharmaceutical companies are trying to sort out the specific regions of DNA associated with drug responses, to identify particular subgroups of patients, and to develop drugs customized for those populations. These capabilities are expected to make drug development faster, cheaper, and more effective, while drastically reducing the number of adverse reactions.[18]

Transcriptomics

The central dogma of molecular biology states that heredity information flows from DNA to RNA (ribonucleic acid) to protein. This concept explains how the genes in our genome, made of DNA, encode the amino acids of the proteins; RNA acts as an intermediary between DNA and the proteins it encodes. Such a set-up allows the DNA to stay protected in its own separate compartment, called the nucleus, away from the caustic chemistry of the cytoplasm; and it provides an easy way to regulate the amount of a certain protein needed in the cell by making more or less of the intermediate message.

RNA has the same structure as DNA, consisting of a sugar phosphate polymer backbone; but because of slightly different chemistry RNA is too bulky to form a stable double helix like DNA, so it exists as a single-stranded molecule. There are several kinds of RNA inside the cell, but only one type, called messenger RNA (mRNA), acts as the cellular photocopier for genes. It carries the information from the DNA in the nucleus out to the cellular machinery in the cytoplasm, where it is used to make the protein.[19]

Not all genes are turned on in all cells. The subset of DNA genes that are turned on, represented by these intermediate mRNA forms in a given cell, is called the transcriptosome. Transcriptomics describes the levels or amounts of the mRNAs present in the cell under a given set of conditions and reflects the link between the genome, the proteins being expressed, and the cell's physical state and appearance. If a cell is healthy and functioning normally it will express a number of mRNAs as it should, but if sick or malfunctioning the amounts of the mRNA expressed could be significantly altered for a number of genes; for example, a cell that becomes cancerous and is dividing rapidly has many genes for cell growth turned on, and this is easily detected when tested for. The regulation of highly variable gene expression of mRNA within the cell can be tested and monitored using a technique called DNA microarray analysis.[20]

A microarray slide consists of a set of known DNA genes, derived from the human genome sequencing project, stuck onto the surface in individual, discrete spots, usually laid out in a grid-like pattern. The technology of spotting the DNA onto the slide to create the microarray has been miniaturized; genes representing the entire human genome (all 33,000 genes) are now available on two microarray slides each no bigger than a few centimetres.[21] To see what genes are turned on or off the mRNAs are isolated from the cell or tissue and a reverse copy linked to a fluorescent dye is made. In this way the amount that binds to its corresponding gene on the microarray slide can be detected; computer-enhanced laser detection quantifies the signal. Microarray technology uses the sequence data from genome projects to determine which genes are differentially expressed in a particular cell type of an organism, at a particular time, under particular treatment conditions.[22] Although only recently created, the microarray databases already contain significant amounts of experimentally generated data. Transcript profiling has already been used to identify possible drug targets and biological markers that allow for the prediction of a patient's response to chemotherapy drugs.[23]

Proteomics

The largest sequence repositories (NCBI, PIR, Swiss-Prot, TrEMBL and Uniprot) contain all known protein sequences, mostly derived from conceptual translation of DNA gene coding regions. Most entries do not contain any information about individual protein function or activity.[24] A subset of protein databases deals with distinct protein families and these are well annotated, usually maintained by interested researchers wishing to share research results. A more functional subset of databases for pharmacogenomics covers proteomic databases that use analytical techniques (2D gel analysis) to separate and catalogue all the proteins of a cell under particular growth conditions.[25] Much like transcriptomics and microarrays, the proteome information can determine which genes are expressed in a particular cell type of an organism, at a particular time, under particular treatment conditions.

Current Genetic Diagnostic Testing (Adults)

DNA-based tests are among the first commercial applications arising from genomics. Genetic testing for known disease loci can be used to diagnose disease, confirm the existence of a disease in asymptomatic individuals, and help predict the risk of disease in healthy individuals or their progeny. Individuals who are asymptomatic can take preventive treatments to delay the onset or reduce the severity of symptoms. The diagnostic tests reveal a disease condition or estimate the likelihood for developing one. Gene tests involve looking at the DNA sequence obtained from any tissue, scanning it for specific mutations or changes that have been linked to a known disorder. Although several hundred DNA-based tests exist for different disease conditions, most are still offered as informative research tools only. Fewer than 100 gene tests are available commercially, and most are for mutations associated with rare diseases in which just a single gene is involved. Common diseases that involve the interaction of several genes do not have, at this time, accurate predictive tests.[26]

INTRINSIC AND EXTRINSIC RISKS OF GENOMICS

Databases and profiling of diseases by pharmacogenomics, transcriptomics, and proteomics will allow for individualized drug treatment plans and pre-symptomatic disease treatments. The therapeutic treatments will consist of drug regimes, prescribed by medical doctors, that will use approved pharmaceuticals well regulated under Canadian law.

However, the use of genetic sequences derived from databases and the classification of an individual's SNPs, transcriptosome, and proteome data for personalized therapeutics faces complex social, moral, and legal issues.

Several areas of intrinsic risk relate to the protection of individuals, the privacy of genetic information, and the possibility of using data in a discriminatory manner.[27] The results of genetic testing may lead to social stratification, with expensive pre-symptomatic drug treatments being available only to those who can afford them. Employers, insurance companies, and even potential mates could also discriminate against individuals who are tested and found to carry certain disease loci. The emotional trauma of knowing that you carry and will get a number of serious diseases predetermined by your genetics is a burden that some individuals may not want to carry, which raises the question of the personal right "not to know" if close relatives are tested. Moreover, because many diseases that can be currently tested for have no known cure or treatment and are rare, many pharmaceutical companies will not see any profit in spending research and development money to deliver orphan drugs. Finally, issues arise over the confidentiality and privacy concerns of who should have access to personal information derived from personal genetic profiling.[28]

Extrinsic risks also exist with genomics technologies. The large-scale database collection of information on entire populations could have transformative social effects. Like individuals, entire ethnic communities could face widespread stigmatization and be considered pariahs if it is found that they are carriers for a high number of deleterious gene polymorphisms. A bigger problem is expansion and linkage to other databases that could transform the data for individuals, cohorts, or communities far beyond their original intention. Police and police states would find the collective and personal polymorphism databases an easy way to perform racial profiling, when linked to other personal information. Companies could exploit personal pharmacogenomic data to market and target specific segment groups and communities for a variety of consumer products based on their level of risk for specific future diseases.

GENETICS — BEYOND "OMICS" RESEARCH

The biology of genetically engineering ourselves falls into three major categories: first, making chimeras by creating quasi-human animal hybrids through mixing genetic materials between species; second, eugenics/gene therapy, which alters the existing genetic material to fix or replace undesired diseases and improve desirable qualities of beauty, health, intelligence, or longevity; and third, xenotransplants, which mix human and animal genetic material to harvest animal organs for human use without fear of immunologic rejection.[29,30,31]

The most promising of these three is gene therapy, for a number of reasons. Genomics is already providing the working gene targets for gene enhancement and gene therapy. Gene-therapy techniques are being refined in laboratories with the promise of a virtuous benefit – to repair gene defects and cure diseases in adults and in unborn children. It is a far less contentious prospect, morally, than creating new chimeric life forms or human-animal entities. Moreover, gene therapy using therapeutic cloning and stem cell techniques will avoid the problems of any immune rejection that complicates work on xenotransplants. Researchers who are commercializing this work have chosen, out of practicality, the least perilous system to champion first.

All of these new genetic techniques rely on genetic engineering, which can be defined as the process of manipulating the pattern of proteins in an organism by altering its existing genes. Either new genes are added or existing genes are changed so that they are made by the body's DNA at different times or in different amounts. Because the genetic code is similar in all species, genes taken from one person or animal can function in another human. In addition, the promoters or "on-off switches" from one coding sequence can be removed and placed in front of another coding sequence to change when or where the protein is made. The various types of "omics" research will provide the tools and broaden the array of identified gene targets available to be manipulated.

Research has been perfecting the ability to manipulate genes in lower life forms, and favourable characteristics from a wide range of organisms have been introduced into recipient plant species, creating genetically modified crops. These new characteristics can be introduced using a number of techniques, including: injection into the nucleus of the cell with a tiny needle; an electrical shock to the cells, which briefly depolarizes the membrane allowing for DNA uptake; attachment of the DNA to small metal particles and use of a "gene gun" to shoot the particles into the cells; and use of viruses and bacteria engineered to infect cells with the foreign DNA. The newly introduced DNA must find its way into the nucleus and then become incorporated into the recipient's own genetic material. Once incorporated into the host at the DNA level, the introduced gene functions like all other genes of the host. This process of transplanting desired traits from one organism to another is called "transformation," or more commonly "gene splicing." The resulting products from recombinant manipulations are termed "transgenics" or "genetically modified organisms" (GMOS). Repair and replacement of defective human genes requires slightly more sophisticated technologies; current developments use delivery systems (viral, liposome mediated, naked DNA) similar to those already worked out in plant systems. Humans receiving gene-therapy treatments will be rightly considered to be GMOS or, in the case of therapeutic cloning that uses stem cells maintained on a layer of mouse feeder cells during growth, they will be considered to be xenotransplants.

Gene Enhancement

Genetic enhancement refers to technologies that transfer genetic material to modify non-pathological human traits. Unlike gene therapy, which treats disease conditions, gene enhancements are used to treat non-disease characteristics, mainly to provide cosmetic alterations. Enhancements will be used to make someone who is already in good health even better by optimizing what society deems to be "desirable" attributes. Physical traits that could be altered include appearance, such as hair or eye colour, height, physical build, increased muscle mass, decreased body fat, improved strength, and increased endurance; behavioral traits could be changed as well to improve intelligence or temperament, and to alter basic personality traits to make individuals outgoing.[32]

Athletes have been well aware of the importance of single nucleotide gene polymorphisms and how they influence sports performance for many years. At the 1964 Winter Olympics in Innsbruck, Austria, a cross-country skier from Finland who won two gold medals was later found to have a genetic mutation that increased the number of red blood cells in his body because he could not switch off erythropoetin (Epo) production; this mutation increased his capacity for aerobic exercise. Synthetic Epo is currently used to treat anemia, but it has also been abused by athletes as a way to improve their stamina. During the 1998 Tour de France professional bicycle race, an entire team was disqualified and two top cyclists admitted taking the drug. Recent efforts to deliver the Epo gene into patients' cells would eliminate the need for regular injections, but this could also be abused by athletes.[33]

As mentioned in the prologue, experiments at the University of Pennsylvania have revealed that when rats or mice are injected with a modified virus that adds an essential growth gene (insulin-like growth factor, IGF-1) to their cells, they develop into heavily muscled, superstrong animals (nicknamed mighty mice by the scientists who created them). The effects were doubled when the gene therapy was coupled with an exercise-training regime that forced them to climb ladders.

The added IGF-1 gene also stopped the ageing process in older mice: none suffered from typical old age muscle wasting.[34] Now being developed to treat patients with muscular dystrophy and other muscle-wasting diseases, this gene therapy could be used as a gene enhancement given to athletes to deliver vast improvements in speed, power, and strength. Gene enhancements have the potential to boost sport performance more radically than any combination of existing drugs, such as anabolic steroids and Epo.

Dr Lee Sweeney, the lead scientist, has already been approached by coaches and athletes, mainly bodybuilders, seeking to try this gene therapy, even though the technique is barely ready for patient trials. He lamented: "This is but one example of a number of potential gene therapies that are being developed with disease treatment as the goal, but if given to a healthy individual would provide genetic enhancement of some trait." It is highly likely that gene enhancements will be used by professional and amateur athletes alike for performance enhancement, just as many drugs are used and abused today. The chairman of the World Anti-Doping Agency said he was concerned that gene doping would become a major problem for Olympic sport, with gene-enhanced athletes "certainly realistic" by the 2012 games and beyond.[35]

The genes for enhancement are already being well characterized from genomics research and will be used to supplement the functioning of normal genes or perhaps engineered to produce a desired enhancement. Gene insertion into adults for enhancement purposes will be intended to affect only the single individual through somatic cell modification.[36] Trying to differentiate between therapeutic modifications and enhancements can lead to confusion. For example, enhancements for anticipatory resistance to disease in already healthy individuals, or for resistance to environmental or workplace toxins, or for improving "normal" eyesight are all enhancements that do not correct an actual disease state but do have some potential individual benefit. The real prize of gene enhancement will be treatments to increase intelligence, memory, logical thought, and critical reasoning. At present agreement is widespread that germline engineering (see following section) should be banned for both therapeutic and enhancement applications, but how effective this will be in practice remains anyone's guess.

Gene Therapy

Human gene therapy is the introduction of DNA into humans or human cells with the purpose of treating or curing diseases. To perform gene therapy the defective gene must be identified; genetic engineering techniques can then create copies of the normal, functioning gene and transfer this correct copy into the target cells. Gene therapy can correct a gene defect in several ways: a normal gene may be inserted into a nonspecific location within the genome to replace a nonfunctional gene(this is the most common approach); the abnormal gene could be swapped for the normal gene using site specific homologous recombination; the abnormal gene could be repaired inside the cell nucleus by selective reverse mutation changing the single base pair; or, finally, the regulation (how much gene product is made) could be altered.[37]

There are two kinds of gene therapy: "somatic gene therapy," in which DNA is introduced into cells or tissues other than germ cells (sperm and egg); and "germline gene therapy," in which DNA is introduced only into male or female germ cells. The germline (or sex) cells are responsible for making our gametes (sperm or egg) for reproduction, so changes to genes in these cells would affect all subsequent generations. The transformative ability of germline gene therapy is already a known ethical issue; in 1983 the U.S. President's Commission endorsed somatic, but not germline, gene-therapy treatments. Many other countries, including Canada, have adopted this distinction as part of the legislation surrounding gene therapy. Gene therapy has much potential for treating and curing genetic and acquired diseases, including various cancers, by using normal genes to supplement or replace defective genes. In the future gene therapy will cure various classes of diseases: inherited single-gene diseases (cystic fibrosis, Parkinson's disease, familial hypercholesterolemia, Fanconi anemia, to name a few); infectious chronic diseases (HIV); acquired disorders (peripheral artery disease and rheumatoid arthritis); and multi-gene diseases (cancers).

One of the earlier, tragic attempts at gene therapy that failed involved the death of 18-year-old Jesse Gelsinger, who suffered from a genetic disease called ornithine transcarboxylase deficiency (OTCD), a rare liver disease that causes failure to properly control ammonia metabolism. His death was triggered by a severe immune response to the modified adenovirus vector that was being used to carry the healthy copy of the transcarboxylase gene. Adenovirus is a class of viruses with double-stranded DNA genomes that cause respiratory, intestinal, and eye infections in humans – it is the same virus that causes the common cold. The goal of the gene-therapy treatment was to deliver and express the transcarboxylase gene, but the transfer efficiency in this procedure is low (only 1 per cent of all injected adenovirus with the good gene gets delivered to the cells and recombined into the human genome). The doctors sought to overcome this limitation by using an extremely high infection dose of 38 million viral particles, which was calculated from animal testing and was believed to be accurate. But less than twenty-four hours after they injected Jesse with this amount of virus, his entire body began reacting adversely. He went into a coma and died two days later from multiple organ failures, just four days after starting the treatment, his death a direct result of the gene-therapy experiment.

In January 2003 the u.s. Food and Drug Administration, which oversees gene therapy, placed a temporary halt on all gene-therapy trials using retroviral vectors in blood stem cells, after learning that a second child, treated in a French gene-therapy trial, had developed similar leukemia-like conditions after being treated for x-linked severe combined immunodeficiency disease (x-scid), also known as "bubble baby syndrome."[38]

Despite the tragedies, over 600 clinical gene-therapy trials occurred worldwide in 2002, with most trials focusing on various cancer types, infectious diseases, and vascular diseases.[39] Worldwide, the majority (~75 per cent) of all gene-therapy protocols, trials, and patient treatments occur in the United States. Canada has relatively few gene-therapy trials and gene-therapy patients (~3 per cent worldwide).[40] Current protocols in the formative stages are focused on establishing the safety of gene-delivery procedures rather than effectiveness. The technology itself still faces many obstacles before it can become a practical approach for treating disease. In Canada, gene therapy is regulated by Health Canada (the Biologics and Genetic Therapies Directorate, bgtd) with responsibility for biologics and biotechnology products used for gene therapy. Prior to gene-therapy product approval, bgtd requires data for safety and efficacy with provisions to monitor products after approval. Because of the ethical considerations that surround gene therapy, granting agencies for research in Canada, including the Natural Sciences and Engineering Research Council (nserc), the Social Sciences and Humanities Research Council (sshrc), and the Canadian Institutes of Health Research (cihr) have ethical conduct and policy requirements for research involving human subjects.[41]

Often overlooked in discussions of snps for use in gene therapy or enhancements is the acknowledgement of the complexity of human gene expression, involving both epistatic[42] interactions and pleiotropic[43] expression. These terms refer to the fact that many traits such as height, body type, weight, and metabolic rate are governed by the cumulative effects of many genes. Polygenic traits, or those traits involving multiple genes, are not expressed as absolute or discrete characters but are expressed as a continuous variation or gradation of small differences. Gene expression is not only temporal (some genes are turned off or on at various stages of development) but it is also tissue specific: inappropriate expression of a particular gene product or a knockout of another unrelated gene product, when the new gene from gene therapy is recombined into the genome at random in non-target tissues, could have serious detrimental effects.

Therapeutic Cloning and Stem Cell Research

One of the major problems with current disease treatments is the body's immune response system. When foreign cells from donated organs, tissues, or blood are transplanted, transfused, or xenografted, the recipient mounts a rejection response, attacking and destroying these cells. People using donated organs and tissues that are a close match must endure a lifetime of immuno-suppressive drugs. Using a patient's own cells as a source for the treatment would circumvent the problems of rejection and scarcity of compatible donor organs. Special undifferentiated cells, called stem cells, if somehow harvested and used from the patient, would avoid the immunological rejection, as the cells and tissues would genetically be a match. Therapeutic cloning is a way to obtain these needed stem cells by using somatic cell nuclear transplantation.[44]

"Adult DNA cloning," such as the method used to clone Dolly, on the one hand, and "therapeutic cloning," to produce cells and tissues for transplant, on the other, are quite different procedures, but they both begin by transplanting a nucleus into a donor egg and both terms contain the word "cloning." This causes a great deal of confusion among those who wish to understand exactly what therapeutic cloning is.[45] Cloning, as in the production of Dolly, means making an identical genetic copy of an individual by nuclear transfer from a somatic donor cell to an enucleated host egg; this is called "somatic cell nuclear transplantation" or "adult DNA cloning." The multi-cell embryo at the blastocyst stage is implanted back into the uterus of a surrogate host and pregnancy is allowed to proceed normally.

With therapeutic cloning the somatic cell nuclear transplant also creates a blastocyst, but there is never any intention of implanting to create a living being. At day 5–6 the blastocyst is a ball of cells organized into an outer layer that will become the placenta and an inner layer called the inner cell mass containing the stem cells which are harvested for use. The inner cell mass will form the tissues of the developing body and can differentiate into any other cell types; this ability of the stem cells is called "pluripotency."[46]

The great potential of pluripotent stem cells for therapeutic purposes is that they can create any required cell type needed. This plasticity of cell fate has resulted in an exponential growth in stem cell research; however, because of the demand compared to the small numbers of starter cells, very slow growth, and problems of bacterial contamination of tissue culture, the supplies of stem cells for research are very limited. Embryonic stem cells can be derived from several sources, but a central, contentious ethical issue remains regarding the use of a human embryo as the initial source of stem cells. Stem cell research has potential for use in regenerative medicine to supply replacement cells for degenerative diseases and traumatic injuries. Stem cells can be used as a supply of nerve cells for the treatment of Parkinson's disease and spinal cord injuries; pancreatic islet cells to treat diabetes; blood cells to treat anemia; and muscle cells to treat muscular-wasting diseases. Transplantation can be done with unmodified or genetically modified stem cells or subsequently differentiated cells.[47] The potential individual medical benefits of using stem cells in therapeutics are enormous.

DISCUSSION: MANAGING MODERN RISKS

An orientation to the world where systematic risk-taking is the norm rests on a more fundamental notion, namely, that the world of nature is essentially a field in which human ingenuity can be exercised without restriction. The phrase "without restriction" is crucial: it means that no other interests subsist there, no other entities possessing a will and consciousness – no gods or spirits or demons – that can oppose us with an alternative plan as we proceed to manipulate nature to our benefit. This world is simply full of latent "power" (what we now call matter – energy) that can be appropriated and turned to human benefit. The traditional competitions among people within society are zero-sum games, where gains are won only at the expense of others. But the contest with nature is different, because there are no competing interests.[48]

Yet all powers are two-edged swords. As the scope of the good they can do for us expands, so does that of the harm they might do, either inadvertently or by someone's deliberate choice. Two examples must suffice. Unlocking the power of the atom yields a new energy source and a fearsome new weapon of mass destruction at the same time. The technique of "DNA shuffling" and the creation of "daughter genes" makes possible the creation of new biological traits – as well as the possibility of so-called "synthetic pathogens" and the prospect of confronting novel infectious diseases against which no immunity exists.[49]

A simple lesson flows from this perspective. The challenge of effectively managing the risks we create – to ourselves, other creatures, and ecosystems – in the search for human benefits grows in proportion to our

technological prowess. Managing risks means adopting a precautionary mode of behaviour, trying to identify and limit potential trouble
before it hits us in the face. We have a collective responsibility – an
ethical duty, if you will – to act in this way. Yet, quite obviously,
discharging this responsibility is easier said than done and gets harder
with each passing day. This is so because the global reach of innovation
demands effective international collaboration in managing risks, a
capacity that presently exists at a primitive stage of development.[50]

The purpose of risk management, as first developed in the financial
sector and later extended into the health and environmental zones,
is to bring a systematic perspective to bear on the propositions already
enunciated. Another way of saying this is to recognize that through
risk management we seek to introduce a foundation of precaution
beneath our risk-taking activities. This occurred first in the domains
of public health and occupational health and safety. The introduction
of sanitary measures to control the spread of infectious disease is an
attempt to head off the adverse consequences, or at least a certain
proportion of them, before they arise. Establishing allowable limits of
exposure to hazardous substances in the workplace is an alternative
to ignoring the casualties and just replacing sick workers with others
not yet sick, without bothering to ask whether it was the workplace
that sickened them.

The management of health and environmental risks, considered as
a precautionary exercise, developed as a step-wise procedure for controlling risk:

- Hazard identification and characterization, specifying all relevant
  possible adverse outcomes (population average and subpopulations,
  e.g., gender and age-specific), including a dose-response curve;
- Exposure estimation, often using surrogate data;
- Risk assessment, as probabilities of occurrence for each adverse
  outcome and relevant subpopulation, identifying uncertainties;
- Risk reduction strategies, where probabilities are above the level of
  "tolerable" or "acceptable" risk;
- Risk management options: risk-risk, risk-benefit, risk-cost-benefit
  tradeoffs;
- Monitoring and evaluation of new data.

Advances in methodologies for toxicology, epidemiology, and statistical analysis have been one of the primary drivers of progress in this
area. In this respect risk assessment resembles detective work, where
the "culprit" sought is the significant association between risk factor
and adverse outcome, which can be deeply hidden, especially in

epidemiological data. To be sure, these "technical" aspects of the risk management approach are only one side of the whole story, for important social interests can be affected.

Risk is unequally distributed in many ways – in occupations, socio-economic levels, neighbourhoods, race, and so on – bringing matters of justice, equity, and equality to the fore. Risk is also unequally distributed as a result of idiosyncratic variations in personal proclivity (degree of risk aversion) and preferences or choices. This means that very important dimensions of health risk can be, at least in principle, under substantial personal control – affected by personal choices in patterns of diet, exercise, intake of alcohol and other drugs, recreation, driving behaviour, tobacco smoking, and many other domains. In addition, people can perceive the nature and significance of many hazards, especially those that they believe are being imposed on them without their consent, in terms radically opposed to those who are using formal methodologies to perform quantitative risk assessments.

So bitter battles over risks can erupt and have done so regularly. These battles began a century ago with respect to occupational risks. Firms routinely denied that there was sufficient cause-and-effect proof (using a legal standard of proof) to justify lowering allowable exposures, since expenses were incurred in doing so. Evidence was often hard to come by, and in many cases was concealed when it surfaced. Few cases are as notorious and long-lasting, or as fraught with catastrophic health consequences, as that of occupational exposure to asbestos, which goes on to this day. The history of occupational risk is important for showing us that social and economic interests come into play whenever changes are sought to the prevailing community standards for acceptable levels of risk.

In public health no battle has been as bitter as that with the tobacco industry, which fronted the longest-running battle against epidemiological science that has ever been waged. At its height in the 1980s and 1990s, before the industry finally capitulated, specialists were recruited with secret payments to cast doubt on epidemiological studies.[51] More recently, the perceived economic costs of complying with greenhouse-gas emissions reduction targets, to control the risks associated with climate change, resulted in attacks on the credibility of the scientists who support the reports of the Intergovernmental Panel on Climate Change. Science itself, as represented by toxicology and epidemiology, is drawn into the fray when controversies erupt among social interests about risk assessment and management.[52] Risks associated with the engineering of genomes, especially the human genome, will without a doubt be intensely controversial, and the scientists working in those areas will be drawn into those controversies, along with the rest of us.

RISK FACTORS ASSOCIATED WITH GENETIC ENGINEERING

Considered simply as areas of scientific investigation with practical applications for human benefit, molecular biology and genetics are immensely important fields of inquiry. In particular, the sequencing of complete genomes and (ultimately) what will follow – full knowledge of individual gene functions, gene-expression mechanisms, and the pleiotropic effects of gene alteration – will have nothing less than revolutionary consequences for us as the data will be applied to gene therapy. And these steps will introduce us to a range of risks that we have never before confronted. At present, we do not know even where to start in confronting them. Some types of downside consequences associated with genomics, if they come to pass, will have the following results: either they will produce catastrophic harms or they will so frighten the population that there will be a demand for an end to research and development in this area; or both.

The term "risk factor" connotes a probable cause of an adverse effect, taking into account not only varying degrees of uncertainty but also the fact that risk is by definition probabilistic. When one says, for example, that tobacco smoking is a risk factor for cancer (lung, mouth, pharynx, larynx, esophagus, pancreas, uterus, cervix, kidney, and bladder) and dozens of other diseases, it means that (a) the existence of an association between the two is highly plausible; (b) a scale of harmful dose is known; and (c) a certain percentage of smokers will fall victim to these diseases. About 10 per cent of regular smokers will get lung cancer, on average, but the distribution of the risk is also very important: women have double men's risk of lung cancer, and are at risk for more serious type of this disease, at an equivalent dose.[53] This terminology is very widely used and is relatively easy to communicate, although some difficulties in understanding remain.[54]

A risk factor, then, has to do with adverse consequences only and thus begs the question as to what benefits accrue as a result of the risk-taking behaviour. As a general rule we can assume that risks in this sense are encountered as a result of the search for benefits, even with something like smoking. A fair description of a risk domain, therefore, requires a sketch of both benefits and costs (where costs are the probabilities of harm, or risk factors), and both sides of these equations may be phrased in either monetary or non-monetary terms.

Risk factors for technologies can be sorted into two categories; for want of better terms they are divided into "intrinsic" and "extrinsic." In the former are those hazards inherent in either the nature of the technology itself or in its normal applications. To give an example from the world of chemicals: trihalomethanes and their cancer risk are created as byproducts of using chlorine to disinfect water. The occupational hazards associated with producing chlorine, or the risk of accidental releases to those who live in proximity to the plant boundary, are other examples of intrinsic risk factors. "Extrinsic" refers to the impacts that specific technologies can have on a wide range of institutional subsystems in society – law, ethics, religion, and politics. As a society, we need to have as accurate an idea as possible about the nature and scope of the hazards we face in this domain. Equipped with this idea as well as with the precautionary approach, we would then be in a position to engage a wider public in a discussion on how to manage the associated risks, proactively, and not wait to be confronted with the actually existing harms.

A general description of the two distinct classes of risk factors associated with genomics and genetics might be as follows: Intrinsic risks arise inevitably out of achieving the ability to undertake genetic alterations in existing genomes, or to construct entirely new genomes, with predictable and reliable results in achieving the expression of desired traits. Intrinsic risks of genetics include many of the same problems of intrinsic risks associated with genomics: concerns of privacy, safety, and efficacy, for example, apply to all branches of genetics, as medical information is compiled into large databases. Unintended effects due to gene therapy include altered metabolism, altered brain functions, or unforeseen gene actions, insertions, and recombination events that would occur to individuals as a result of the technology. Some technologies, such as stem cell research and therapeutic cloning, have special intrinsic concerns, with the ethical uncertainty of creating life solely for the purpose of therapeutics and the underlying valuation of one life over another. Likewise, xenotransplantation could have psychological ramifications with individuals who have become part animal and are treated differently, or unforeseen problems of zoonotic diseases from retroviral sequences that will infect the tissue recipient with a life-long non-transmissable infection.

Extrinsic risks are the impacts that this almost certainly will have on a wide range of institutional subsystems outside the bounds of scientific discovery itself – law, ethics, religion, and politics, including such things as the concept of the person and the family. A provisional list of extrinsic risks associated with gene therapy and its convergence with other technologies is outlined below.

Genetically Engineering the Works of Creation
(Including Ourselves)

First, we must be clear about the scope of the "power over nature" that genetics science seeks. Altering smaller or larger sections of the genomes of existing entities (plants, animals, humans), to achieve otherwise unattainable human benefits, is what most people would think of right away. But a much larger prize is lurking in the background: creating *de novo* the biological "platform of life" onto which any desired set of traits whatsoever could be grafted. This is known as the "minimally necessary genome" and it is now a prize being sought by – among others – the irrepressible Dr Craig Ventner of the Human Genome Project fame:

Scientists in the United States plan to build a tiny new germ from scratch, promising it will be harmless to people and could someday be used to produce new forms of energy. The scientists ... want to keep portions of their work secret to prevent terrorists or hostile nations from using the new organism to make biological weapons. If the experiment works, the synthetic germ would begin to reproduce on its own.

A Stanford University bioethicist was quoted as saying that she wasn't too worried by this project "partly because I have a sense that the scientists are aware of the possible risks of what they're doing."[55] We would certainly hope so, but a second example shows that researchers are already delving into using humans as a "platform of life" to introduce desired traits. The absolute transformative nature of genetics and gene therapy has the ability to change what we are as a species, quite possibly including the creation of various isolated (non-breeding) sub-species of humans. Ongoing research into gene therapy is currently struggling to overcome the technical barrier to introducing good genes, but one avenue of research is trying to leapfrog this problem by introducing a new, artificial chromosome:

Researchers also are experimenting with introducing a 47th (artificial human) chromosome into target cells. This chromosome would exist autonomously alongside the standard 46 – not affecting their workings or causing any mutations. It would be a large vector capable of carrying substantial amounts of genetic code, and scientists anticipate that, because of its construction and autonomy, the body's immune systems would not attack it. A problem with this potential method is the difficulty in delivering such a large molecule to the nucleus of a target cell.[56]

The words "not affecting their workings or causing mutations" presumes that those researchers already have some understanding of the long-term implications of their proposed molecular tinkering. Considering that evolution is a slow process occurring over tens of millions of years, introducing an entirely new chromosome, engineered by humans, moves us into the zone of unfathomable risks; for example, the potential of giving rise to post-zygotic isolating mechanisms that could create a number of reproductive problems in the human species. Those with extra chromosomes could experience one of the following conditions:

- Hybrid inviability, where the embryo development proceeds abnormally and the hybrid is aborted (the hybrid egg formed from the mating of a sheep and a goat will die early in development);
- Hybrid sterility, where the hybrid is healthy but sterile (the mule is the hybrid offspring of a donkey and a mare but is sterile, unable to produce viable gametes because the chromosomes inherited from its parents do not pair and cross over correctly during gamete formation);
- Hybrids that are healthy and fertile, but less fit, or where infertility appears in later generations (this occurs in laboratory crosses of fruit flies, where the offspring of second-generation hybrids are weak and usually cannot produce viable offspring).[57]

Exchanging health for procreation in the name of therapeutics, or worse, the potential creation of a sub-species of humans, are hardly risk-benefit choices we should even be considering. At the very least, scientists – when presenting the miraculous upside benefits of gene therapy's future – should make note of potential risks and problems.

The amount of money spent each year on weight-reduction products and services, including diet foods, products, and programs in North America is close to $33 billion; to combat baldness more than $1 billion is spent each year; and consumers spend roughly $800 million on herbal remedy products to boost their immune systems and to treat illnesses.[58] Without a doubt, gene enhancement technology to correct non-disease conditions will be readily accepted and likely widely used by consumers seeking a "quick fix." W. Gardener argues that the technology of gene enhancement used for cosmetic reasons in the future may be so dispersed and so easy to apply as "junk medicine" that it will be virtually impossible to contain it from widespread use:

There are some controls over the proliferation of nuclear weapons, but only because H-bombs require distinctive tools and materials that can be tracked.

The knowledge required to build a bomb is everywhere. Generations from now, the human biology required for enhancement may be everywhere. But whereas bombs require esoteric tools and materials, genetic enhancement is likely to require the tools and materials of gene therapy, which may be distributed throughout medicine.[59]

The ultimate biological result of widespread, indiscriminate use of gene enhancements will be a skewing of gene allele frequencies[60] for certain traits within a large population and a reduction in genetic biodiversity. There are single gene alterations for enhancing weight loss or improving stamina that would affect a number of other inter-related metabolic pathway genes; many enzyme pathways are intercon-nected, both up- and down-regulating other genes by feedback loops. Treatments for one cosmetic condition may create an entire popula-tion of enhanced individuals that may be at higher risk for other diseases as a result. It is already known that allele frequencies in a population can both fortuitously protect them from or selectively predispose them to different disease states.[61]

Convergence of Genomics and Commerce: Sterile Seed Technology

This is the neutron bomb of agriculture.[62]
Camila Montecinos, agronomist,
Chilean-based Center for Education and Technology

Not all of the examples for extrinsic risk involve human therapeutics derived from genetics and genomics by the manipulation of human genetic material. One ongoing example of a technology that has extrinsic risk and the power to subvert entire societies and cultures, not only in affluent countries but also in developing countries, is "terminator gene" plant technology that results in genetically modified (GM) food crops that produce sterile seeds.

In 1997 the Canadian-based Rural Advancement Foundation Inter-national (RAFI, now called ETC group) called upon the U.S. Govern-ment to deny the patent pending on the terminator gene, submitted by the Monsanto corporation (now owned by Pharmacia), on the grounds that it is contrary to public and social morality. ETC group contacted government officials and civil society organizations in the eighty-seven countries where the terminator patent was pending to ask them to reject the patent by invoking the legal mechanism of "*ordre public.*" When patent offices invoke this mechanism, they not only reject the specific claim; they also reject the whole technology and its use by anyone within their borders. ETC group also wanted international regulatory agencies to rule that the terminator can't be sold as "seed," since it is the opposite of what a seed is – something that can reproduce itself from generation to generation.[63] The ETC group failed in their attempt to stop commercialization of the first terminator gene plant technology. The Delta and Pine Land Company, a seed company owned by Monsanto Inc., in collaboration with the United States Department of Agriculture, was awarded U.S. Patent Number 5,723,765, entitled "Control of Plant Gene Expression," in March 1998. The patent covers several applications, but the main invention is to engineer crops that produce seeds that are reproductively sterile in the second generation. This would make it impossible for farmers to save and replant seeds, leaving them dependent on the seed suppliers.

Modern agriculture relies on hybrid varieties to produce genetically uniform food crops; that is, all plants look identical in size and height and possess desirable traits not present in either parent alone. When these hybrids make seeds, however, the second generation is quite variable because of the natural shuffling of genes that occurs during sexual reproduction. Large-scale industrial agriculture requires uniformity, because the plants must mesh with harvesting combines. Farmers in North America who grow hybrid corn varieties usually buy over 80 per cent new seed every year to avoid harvesting losses and loss of the characteristics found in the hybrid strain.

Non-hybrid variety food crops include several major food crops: wheat, rice, soybeans, and cotton. Farmers in some of the most populated parts of the world (India, Asia) often save the seeds from these crops, and may not go back to the seed company for up to a decade or more before purchasing more seeds or a new crop variety. The genetic engineering mechanism of sterile seeds is a complicated process involving the expression of three genes (repressor gene, recombinase gene, and a toxin gene) and a reshuffling of the plant DNA after treatment with an inducer chemical.[64] Sterility in the second generation is ensured if the seeds are treated with the inducer, usually an antibiotic like tetracycline, before they are planted.

Since 1997 the first terminator strategy has been refined by researchers and now two different kinds of technologies have been developed as a way for large corporations to maintain control over their GM technologies. Both are "Genetic Use Restriction Technologies" or GURTs. The terminator gene technology is an example of a V-GURT and results in genetically engineered crops that produce sterile seeds when grown.

The second type is called T-GURTs, dubbed "traitor technology" by opponents. These engineered plants require chemical triggers to switch on or off important traits during growth. The crop's basic functions – germination, flowering, ripening, and immune deficiency – rely on hormone chemicals and the plants have been genetically engineered to respond only to a specific corporation's agrochemical applied externally; failure to treat the seeds results in the seeds not growing at all.[65]

Serious ecological and health questions need to be addressed regarding sterile seed technologies. v-GURTs are activated by soaking large quantities of seeds in kilogram quantities of tetracycline, an antibiotic still used widely in medicine; this will rapidly increase tetracycline resistance in bacteria. That the large life science companies would knowingly do this given the medical warnings against increasing antibiotic resistance worldwide seems unscrupulous.[66] T-GURTs require using large-scale amounts of an inducer chemical (chemical hormone mimic) that will definitely affect other plants in the environment in unforeseen ways. Moreover, the presence of high amounts of toxin products (expressed ribosomal inhibitor protein) in seeds left accidentally in the fields year after year will have unknown long-term effects on the ecosystem.

It is doubtful that farmers or consumers will still have a choice between sterile or non-sterile (hybridized or open-pollinated varieties) in the near future, since a handful of other big Life-Pharma companies have been aggressively purchasing all seed-producing companies since 1997 in an attempt to monopolize the market. By the end of the year 2000 the biotech-seed market was already dominated by a very few large corporations. By 2001, the main six corporations (Syngenta, Bayer Aventis, Monsanto, DuPont, BASF, and Dow) based in the u.s. and Europe controlled 98 per cent of the market for GM crops and over 70 per cent of the world's pesticide market.[67]

The proposed use of terminator sterile seeds has infuriated critics, who believe the technology will force farmers in developing countries to buy seed each year. The large companies producing sterile seed argue that the genetic manipulation is designed solely to protect their unique varieties, not to subvert entire societies' "way of life." The u.s., Canada, Argentina, and China grew 99 per cent of the world's GM crops in 2002, with South Africa and Australia accounting for most of the remaining 1 per cent. Another twelve countries grew under 50,000 hectares.[68] Genetically engineered plant technology and associated agrochemicals are definitely aimed at the biggest and richest food producers and are not being created intentionally to subvert third world countries.

But unintentionally this technology gives one reasons to worry. Crop geneticists who have studied the terminator seed genetic modifications believe it is almost certain that pollen from crops with the terminator trait will infect neighbouring fields of farmers who either refuse or can't afford the technology. Their crop won't be affected initially but when the farmers sow seed the following season they could find that a portion of their seed stock is sterile, the result of sterile pollen being blown onto their crops from nearby terminator fields. The resulting seed loss, crop yield loss, food security loss, and potential increased human suffering may be quite astounding, all affecting the poorest farm communities. It has been estimated that 50 per cent of the world's farmers are too poor to purchase commercial seed every year. Half the world's farmers feed 20 per cent of the world's population, or 1.4 billion people in Africa, Asia, and Latin America. The potential risk, human cost, and dire effects to entire societies make the terminator gene technology questionable.[69]

The public backlash associated with GURT technologies has been nothing less than incredible. Intense hostility and attempts to block the patents have occurred in several countries, and even farmers from North America, who are the most accepting of GM plants, condemn this developing technology. The GM plant offers no advantageous characteristics to the consumer and farmer while threatening the survival of non-hybridized crops. It appears that the GURT technologies are being pursued for purely economic control in the face of huge opposition.

Syngenta was formed from the agrochemical merger of AstraZeneca (formerly Zeneca) and Novartis on 13 November 2000. The next day the company won a terminator patent approval, U.S. Patent 6,147,282, "Method of controlling the fertility of a plant." With 1999 sales of $7 billion U.S., Syngenta is the world's largest agrochemical multinational, the third largest seed corporation. In a letter from the Zeneca Research and Development director, dated 24 February 1999, the company stated: "Zeneca is not developing any system that would stop farmers growing second-generation seed, nor do we have any intention of doing so."[70] Moreover, corporate competitors like Monsanto also bowed to public pressure in late 1999 vowing "never to commercialize sterile seed technology."[71] Syngenta now controls at least six terminator plant type patents and a host of new patents on genetically modified plants with defective immune systems. It seems that Syngenta is intent on creating plants that will not survive to a second generation, or even grow successfully during a first generation without the application of the company's own chemicals.

Other companies also have GURT technologies under development that could easily be turned into sterile seed terminators. Given that the global market value for GM seeds alone in 2002 was estimated to be $4.25 billion, it is not surprising that each of the large biotechnology companies is racing at breakneck speed to develop its own version of suicide seed. Seed sterility is a profitable goal for the multinationals with large investments in seed companies, because close to 75 per cent of the world's farmers routinely save seed from their harvest for re-planting.

The issue of terminator genes must be put into the larger context of genetically engineered food crops. Large-scale use of genetically engineered food crops such as Bt corn to resist insects places severe selection pressure on insect and pest populations, making them super-resistant within a relatively short time. The result is an increased risk that reduced yield and potential food shortages will occur more frequently. However, Bt corn with terminator technology could be used exclusively until resistance appears; then it could be removed entirely from the world marketplace and replaced with a different resistant GM corn species until insect and weed resistance becomes widespread again, and so on. As long as the seed companies can develop transgenic plants with safe, novel resistance mechanisms quickly enough, they will maximize food yields. The use of the terminator technology ensures that outbreeding to wild relatives will not occur and that insect and pest resistance will never arise. Hypothetically, all farmers (globally or by continent) could switch over synchronously to the new pest-resistant GM food crop in the same year. While many may be uncomfortable with a large food biotech company oligopoly, this would be one of the best ways to implement a global insect/weed resistance control strategy.

Convergence of Genomics and Bioweapons

The best example of extrinsic risks in genetics (driven in this case by international politics) is the bioengineering of virulent bacteria and viruses for warfare. Research on chemical weapons and viral pathogens for biowarfare has continued since the end of World War II – although it is useful to remember that biological weapons have been in existence since medieval times, when invading soldiers catapulted plague-ridden corpses over city walls to infect and destroy the besieged population.[72]

However, so far biological terrorism has been rare and the use of biological weapons during warfare has been limited. Japan first used biological weapons during the 1930s against China, and from 1980 to 1988 biological weapons were used during the Iran-Iraq war by both countries. In 1942 British officials allowed the military to conduct anthrax tests on sheep just off the Scottish coast on Gruinard Island; today the island is still uninhabited and still infected with deadly anthrax spores. During the 1950s and 1960s the United States expanded its offensive biological warfare program initiated during World War II. In 1992 Dr Kanatjan Alibekov, former first deputy director of Biopreparat (the civilian arm of the Soviet Union's biological warfare program), defected to the United States. He revealed what some had already suspected, that Russia had an extensive offensive biological program, including its use of smallpox stock to make new deadlier bioweapons.[73] This was the first indication that genetic engineering was being used to make deadlier "designer" viruses.

Twenty years ago only two countries – the former Soviet Union and the United States – were actively developing biological weapons programs. Now at least seventeen countries are reportedly known or suspected to be developing biological weapons. Countries with active bioweapons programs include Iran, Syria, Libya, North Korea, Taiwan, Israel, Egypt, Vietnam, Laos, Cuba, Bulgaria, India, South Korea, South Africa, China, Russia, and the United States.[74] In an increasingly global world connected by transcontinental travel it is likely that biological weapons engineered for virulence would easily spread beyond the target country. That the indiscriminate use of biological weapons has not yet occurred is largely because of the inability to target bio-engineered weapons accurately.

The extrinsic risk involved here is that genomics will reveal the sequence of human and many viral pathogens, thus providing any group with sufficient knowledge of genetics to begin designing bioweapon agents (bacteria or viruses) that target specific gene alleles in a given ethnic population. Populations are known to have skewed gene allele frequencies for many cell proteins. The cell surface proteins to which viruses bind could be singled out as targets, cross-referenced to human populations, and engineered to a specific gene polymorphism, with the ultimate goal of targeting virulence to specific populations.

The 1925 Geneva Protocol, appealing to "the conscience and the practice of nations," forbade the use of chemical and bacterial agents as offensive weapons, stating that they were "justly condemned by the general opinion of the civilized world." The 1972 biological weapons international convention describes biological germ warfare agents as "repugnant to the conscience of mankind." Dr Joshua Lederberg, who received the Nobel Prize in 1946 for the discovery of gene swapping in bacteria, is a member of a working group of scientists who advise the American government on biological weapons and are actively trying to maintain an open dialogue with Russian biologists. He has stated: "There is no technical solution to the problem of biological weapons. It needs an ethical, human, and moral solution if it's going to happen at all." It would be naïve to think that the horror and the ability to infect many countries along with the intended target would prevent the use of genetically modified biological weapons.[75]

Extrinsic risks can also occur from genetic engineering of organisms during routine government-funded research. Australian researchers recently demonstrated extrinsic risk: when designing a contraceptive for mice for use in pest control they accidentally created a genetically engineered mousepox virus with 100 per cent lethality.[76] Mousepox virus does not affect humans, but it was speculated that a similar genetically engineered virus with human genes would likely be extremely virulent.[77]

Convergence of Preimplantation Genetic Diagnostics and Gene Therapy

Preimplantation genetic diagnostics (PGD) are tests that screen for genetic flaws among embryos created by *in vitro* (in-glass) fertilization (IVF). Embryos from IVF can be tested for a variety of abnormalities (abnormal number of chromosomes, Down's Syndrome), sex determination, and gene defects (cystic fibrosis, Duchenne muscular dystrophy, fragile X syndrome, hemophilia, retinitis pigmentosa, Tay-Sachs disease, and others). The technique involves extracting one cell from the eight-cell embryo, then testing and freezing the embryo until the results of genetic testing are known. Fertility specialists can use the results of this analysis to select only mutation-free embryos for implantation into the mother's uterus; the technique is designed to avoid termination of affected gestations later in a pregnancy.[78]

Before PGD was available, couples at higher risk of conceiving a child with a particular disorder would have to initiate the pregnancy and then undergo chorionic villus sampling in the first trimester, or amniocentesis in the second trimester, to test the fetus for the presence of disease. If the fetus tested positive for the disorder, the couple would be faced with the dilemma of whether or not to terminate the pregnancy. With PGD, couples are much more likely to have healthy babies. Although PGD has been practised for years, only a few specialized centres worldwide offer this procedure.[79,80]

In the future PGD could be coupled with gene therapy to correct the early embryo's defective genes. Treatment by gene therapy at this stage is enticing, since repair of four to eight cells is much easier to deal with than is gene therapy on adults, who have on average about 100 trillion cells. Given that this is currently only a technical problem, it is likely that once gene therapy delivery systems are perfected, correcting diseases of IVF embryos, as well as of early embryos *in utero*, will be feasible. Individual couples wanting "the best" for their children may be seduced by the prospect of correcting both disease and non-disease traits (enhancement of intelligence, height, and body symmetry) in their offspring. The extrinsic risk is two-fold: first, the impact on society will be profound, with a skewing of social ideas of what exactly "normal" intelligence, height, physical strength, and beauty are; second, a stratification will occur between those who are enhanced and those who are not.

Convergence of Nanotechnology and Gene Therapy

Nanotechnology is an emerging field using technologies and processes, materials, devices, and structures that occur on the scale of nanometres (a nanometre is one billionth of a metre). The use of DNA-derived tools in the fields of molecular and medical nanotechnology promises a plethora of medical benefits with potential applications to gene therapy.

Even in nanotechnology's infancy, early-stage products for medical treatment are being constructed. A "nanodevice" composed of titanium oxide nanocrystals attached to short DNA fragments is being developed to target defective genes. After binding the nanodevice with DNA to its defective, homologous gene in the cell, the nanodevice is exposed to light; titanium oxide is photocatalytic and therefore can cut out the defective gene. Researchers developing this technology state that the titanium oxide DNA scaffolding is also amenable to attaching other molecules for repair (enzymes that would rearrange, copy, or join DNA pieces) as a way to introduce a good gene copy.[81]

This type of DNA-repair device does create a form of "active nanotechnology" with the potential to perform unwanted DNA manipulations if it were to enter an organism. Because of their extremely small size (under 70 nanometres in diameter), such devices would not trigger an immune response from the body, and the particles could disperse eventually from the tissues being treated and enter all cells, including germline cells. Since there is no way to turn off the repair enzymes, they could continue to rearrange and join DNA segments causing other serious genetic damage to sex cells (sperm or eggs).

Convergence of Gene Therapy and Unforeseen Recombination Events

The DNA used in gene therapy will likely consist of either short fragments or segments carried on viruses or other carriers (liposomes, synthetic polymers) that will be rapidly degraded inside our cells to short fragments. Research has shown that DNA injected intravenously into pregnant mice was detected in fetuses, suggesting that if used to deliver gene-therapy treatments the DNA fragments would dissipate and persist internally, affecting somatic and germline cells (sex cells).[82] It is also known that short double-stranded DNA oligonucleotides are internalized into cells by endocytosis (pinching in of the outer cellular membrane) and easily cross membranes before the majority are degraded. A small fraction does escape degradation.[83] Gene modification by homologous recombination is one of the techniques that may eventually be used for gene-replacement therapy. Evidence shows that small, synthetic, single-stranded DNA fragments are capable of participating in homologous recombination in human cells and are incorporated into the genome.[84] Gene therapy for treatments using millions of injected fragments undoubtedly has the potential to induce unwanted recombination events in germline cells.

Subversive Uses of Gene Therapy and Gene-enhancement Technologies

Some extrinsic risks of these technologies may not be obvious at first, but their use, development, and widespread availability could easily lead to exploitation, with the application used in ways that are morally corrupt to the point of abhorrence.

Use by criminals.   One of the advantages of genetics is the improvement in forensic methods to match criminals to violent crimes, rapes, and murders, or to exonerate innocent individuals by DNA testing of crime scene evidence. Those committing crimes and wishing to avoid being found guilty would simply have to undergo gene therapy to alter a number of polymorphic sites known to be used in diagnostic DNA testing. The change of specific DNA markers would alter their diagnostic DNA profile when tested, introducing a level of doubt as a defence. Gene therapy could also be used to change the physical ridge pattern found on our fingers and thumbs, or the blood type cell antigens, making crime scene fingerprint and blood matching useless. This presumes that "underground" gene-therapy treatments would be available.

Creating cheap designer drugs.   Humans have used opiate drugs such as morphine and heroin for thousands of years to lessen pain and produce euphoria. The discovery of proteins called opiate receptors in the brain showed how drugs like morphine and heroin affect the brain and led to characterization of opiate-like chemicals produced in the body to control pain, immune responses, and other body functions. Research on opiate drugs has given rise to many discoveries that could revolutionize not only pain relief but also the understanding of addiction, reproduction, and the immune system. The opiate receptor is a protein located on the surface of nerve cells or neurons, which communicate with each other by releasing signalling chemicals called neurotransmitters. These chemicals attach to receptors on nearby neurons in the same way a key fits a lock.[85]

With gene therapy it would be possible to alter the protein receptor genes expressed in specific regions of the brain for several different kinds of hallucinogenic drugs, changing them so that they would bind to simpler molecules, for example sugars or other small, inert, organic molecules that are cheap and abundant. Such gene therapy would result in substances that would cause neurotransmitter release in the same way that psychoactive drugs do. The ability to become euphoric on an ever-changing number of readily available, cheap, innocuous substances would make drug enforcement impossible. Other brain receptors could also be altered in this way.

Modulating existing brain chemistry.   Cannabinoid receptors in the brain respond to marijuana and do not require mind-altering substances or any other chemicals to activate. The cannabinoid receptor (CB1) is one of the brain's most plentiful, with multiple activities of controlling mood, learning, perception of pain, memory, and the immune system; stimulating the appetite; and controlling nausea, all at the same time. Unlike opiate receptors that are turned on by specific chemicals, cannabinoid receptors are already stimulated, signalling about 30–40 per cent of the time. Cannabinoid receptors often dominate other receptors in the cell by holding onto important activating proteins (G proteins) that regulate calcium ion channels. The CB1 receptor binds to the G protein and shuts down the calcium channel, keeping neurotransmitters inactive. In certain parts of the brain, gene therapy could be used to alter the CB1 receptors to prevent its binding or to introduce a protein agonist to bind the CB1, thus leaving the calcium channel open, with the effects of reducing pain, decreasing memory, and inducing a permanent marijuana-like high.[86]

A second example is research into severe obesity, where brain scans have revealed that, like drug addicts, severely obese people have fewer receptors for dopamine, a neurotransmitter that helps produce feelings of satisfaction and pleasure. Scientists speculate that people overeat to stimulate the dopamine "pleasure" circuits in the brain, just as addicts do by taking drugs. "This is the first scientific contribution that the addictive pathways are deficient in the obese and it may explain their cravings," said Dr George Blackburn, an associate professor of nutrition at Harvard Medical School. In animal studies, exercise has been found to increase dopamine levels and to raise the number of dopamine receptors. Gene therapy could be used to increase the number of dopamine receptors by adding multiple gene copies. The treatment could be exploited by those who are only slightly overweight seeking a quick diet fix for their poor eating habits or as a way to avoid exercising. A number of brain functions for mood and personality could be significantly altered in specific segments of society. Young adults may "experiment" with cannabinoid receptor alteration and young women worried about body image may find alterations to dopamine receptors an easily acceptable alternative. Widespread usage would have transformative social impacts on ideas of normalcy.[87]

Creating human GURT technology.   Currently 6 billion people inhabit the earth, with population predictions of over 9 billion by the year 2050.[88] Control of population growth is a serious sustainability concern for some over-populated countries. Governments may consider using mass gene therapy to alter reproduction by linking it to a specific drug or inducing chemical. Much like the sterile seed T-GURT technology developed in plants, similar gene therapy could be used to prevent functional gametes from developing; for example, by altering key genes for egg maturation or sperm motility. Given as a mass public inoculation to adults or newborns, gene therapy targeting sex cells would ensure sterility and zero population growth. Couples wishing to procreate would apply to the government for permission to conceive a child and be given the inducer chemical, or would otherwise remain reproductively sterile. This technology, given the correct gene delivery vehicle (virus delivery in genetically modified plants or nanoparticles in water), could be turned into a clandestine weapon for genocide or ethnic cleansing.

Given the magnitude of the extrinsic risks it is clear that genomics and genetics can intersect with a number of other technologies with potentially destructive outcomes. The use of genetics applied to other areas creates a synergy and resulting applications that can have far-reaching consequences when used in ways we may not be able to control. A full list of risk factors within these two categories should be compiled, to make it as accurate and complete – from a scientific standpoint – as possible. We must also make an effort to describe the risk factors in terms that are understandable to the public. Once this is done, undertaking three important tasks will become feasible: first, engaging the public in an informed and sustained dialogue about risk management options; second, identifying the areas where proactive, precautionary risk control measures should be instituted by researchers and research sponsors, such as funding agencies; third, identifying the areas where changes in laws and regulations are needed.

A simple and familiar example of this typology is provided by the case of genetic screening. Here the benefits include taking precautionary health measures, adjusting one's lifestyle with the knowledge of special risk factors, and making informed choices about mating and reproduction. The intrinsic risk is the psychological damage that could be done to an individual by gaining the knowledge that he or she is carrying certain types of defects, which carry the "sentence" of premature death, or debilitating disease, or social stigma. The extrinsic risk is the possibility that adverse effects will follow from others gaining access to this knowledge: effects on private health or life insurance coverage, employment prospects, and judgments made by others about one's suitability as a mate.

Typology of Intrinsic Risk Factors in Genomics and Genetics

The types of intrinsic risks inherent in any technological intervention – using products of industrial chemistry, say, or DNA manipulations – are, by definition, closely tied to the benefits we seek in making that intervention in the first place. For example:

- Gene therapy
  Benefits: control of inherited disease in individuals
- Germline gene therapy
  Benefits: elimination of inherited disease in populations, such as the so-called "French-Canadian variant" of Leigh's Syndrome[89]
- Gene enhancement (physical traits)
  Benefits: enhancement of athletic performance, endurance, skills, etc., in individuals
- Genetic modifications of behavioural traits
  Benefits: control or elimination of anti-social behaviour (e.g., criminality, aggression) in individuals[90]

From this we can derive an illustrative list of intrinsic risk factors associated with the above set of manipulations:

- Minor unintended adverse genetic and health consequences, resulting from pleiotropic effects
- Major unintended adverse genetic and health consequences, resulting from pleiotropic effects

- Unintended germline effects in individuals
- Unintended behavioural consequences

Typology of Extrinsic Risk Factors in Genomics and Genetics

Extrinsic risks are the impacts that this ability almost certainly will have on a wide range of institutional sub-systems outside the science itself – law, ethics, religion, and politics. An illustrative list of extrinsic risk factors associated with the above set of manipulations is:

- Discriminatory or perverse distributional effects in society of gene therapy and gene enhancement resulting from social differentiation (impacts on differences in income, wealth, race, employment, health, etc.)
- Possibility of creating isolated genetic sub-populations designed to restrict genetic advantages within certain socio-economic groups and nations
- Unintended or intended germline changes through private choices that spread into the wider population
- Manipulations of behavioural traits imposed on individuals or groups by governments

A further provisional accounting of intrinsic and extrinsic risks associated with genomics and genetics using the framework outlined above is given in tables 12.1 and 12.2.

DIFFICULT CHOICES: AN ILLUSTRATION

Using the concept of risk helps us greatly to systematically array the risk factors involved in genomics and genetics. But it does not, and cannot, yield a simple decision rule to resolve difficult matters of judgment in this area. Each of these genomics techniques has known competing risks and benefits; determining the level of the likely risks to benefits outcome is not an easy task – it is open to a great deal of interpretation and speculation.

A good illustration of these difficulties is supplied by the matter of therapeutic cloning. Two opposing interpretations of the risk and benefit trade-offs here have been given by members of the academic community in Canada. Tim Caulfield made the case for permitting this form of cloning in the context of Bill C-13, arguing in effect that the future health benefits are substantial and that the downside risk could be controlled by effective regulation.[91] Françoise Baylis and Jocelyn Downie have argued the opposite case, saying that the

Table 12.1
Genomics technologies with benefits and risks

Genomics Technology	Anticipated Benefits	Intrinsic Risks	Extrinsic Risks
SNP detection	• Identification of single and multiple gene associated diseases • Identification of SNPs that confer greater risk or protection from diseases • Clarification/confirmation of medical diagnosis • Identification of responders/non-responders to certain drugs, improving treatment	• Knowledge of untreatable multigene diseases with no cure • Resulting treatments only for those who can afford it • Discrimination against individuals or groups • Fairness and access to databases • Individual privacy concerns • Personal right "not to know" • Burden on those identified as carriers (psychological impacts) • Errors of testing	• Widespread social stigmatizing of carriers • Deliberate misuse of polymorphism data to target bioweapons to specific ethnic groups • Partitioning of public database and accumulated testing data into private databases • Racial, ethnic profiling • Expansion of database use/linkage far beyond original intention
Pharmacogenomics	• Identification of safer drugs • Improved disease screening • Better vaccine designs • Decreased costs to health care • Targeted health care for individuals • Tool for increased public education for health risks • Evidence for making informed health policy decisions	• Use of gene testing to validate harmful lifestyle choices (it is okay to smoke because of lack of lung-cancer related polymorphisms)	
Pre-symptomatic therapeutics	• Identification of predisease genes for treatment		
Transcriptomics	• Identification of gene expression for disease and treatment efficacy		
Proteomics	• Identification of gene expression for disease and treatment efficacy		
Identifying medical responders	• Effective drug treatment based on DNA profile		
Genetic screening (karyotype, PND, microarray chips)	• Identification of micro-organisms contaminating soil, air, water, and food • Pinpointing of disease sources • Improved forensics, genealogy, and military dog-tags		
Assisted reproduction/ Prenatal diagnostics	• Identification of gross abnormalities and diseases in embryos		

Table 12.2
Genetics technologies with benefits and risks

Genetics Technology	Anticipated Benefits	Intrinsic Risks	Extrinsic Risks
DNA medical nanotechnology (active nanotech)	• Targeted drug delivery using nanodevices or nanocages	• Increased toxicity • Health hazards of increased particulates, e.g., asthma and allergies	• Creation of viral-like active nanotechnology devices (infective nanotechnology) • Unintended germline changes by somatic nanotech gene therapy
Gene therapy	• Treatment and correction of diseases in adults and children	• Privacy of genetic information • Safety and efficacy of tests/treatments • Social stratification and eugenics • Unintended gene insertions • Unintended alteration of metabolism • Unintended alterations to other emotions and higher brain functions • Manipulation of embryos by ART or *in utero* treatments deleterious	• Recombination (scrambling) of inserted viral vector genes creating new contagions • Synergism of inserted viral vector genes potentiates other viruses (manifestation of more severe, transmissible disease symptoms) • Method of population birth-control/extreme skewing of sex ratios • Use by criminals for anonymity/innocence
Gene enhancement	• Correction of a wide array of non-disease traits largely for cosmetic purposes (intelligence, strength, height, youthful skin, baldness, metabolism, stamina, strength)		• Unintended germline effects of widely used cosmetic treatments • Skewing societal perceptions of "normal"
Gene modification of behaviour	• Treatment of violent criminals, pedophiles, and sociopaths		• Creation of an easily controlled docile citizenry • Modification of individuals deemed dangerous by the state (outspoken academics, political leaders) • Creation of altered neuron receptors for modified designer drugs • Altered social values of normal behaviour and attitudes towards health

Table 12.2 (continued)

Genetics Technology	Anticipated Benefits	Intrinsic Risks	Extrinsic Risks
Stem cell research	• Unlimited reprogramming of cells to make skin, nervous tissue, muscle for transplants	• Ethical uncertainty of creating life for therapeutic treatments	• Use of stem cells to create chimeras (hybrid human and non-human entities)
Therapeutic cloning	• Compatible replacement tissues, cells, organs		• Unexpected zoonosis from feeder cell contact
Xenotransplantation	• Alleviation of organ shortages for those most in need	• Psychological trauma of being part animal • Individual non-transmissible zoonotic diseases (retrovirus from donor animal tissue)	• Unforeseen recombination events creating new virulent transmissible zoonosis • Transmissible zoonotic diseases from donor animal • Societal backlash against individuals with animal organs
Pronuclear/Nuclear transplantation (cloning)	• Use of cloned transgenic animals as bioreactors, biofactories (producing drugs in milk) • Assisting infertile couples	• Medical problems of clones and endangerment of surrogate	• Cloning of infamous leaders, religious figureheads to perpetuate social control • Cloning to obtain "spare parts"
Convergence of technologies	• Synergistic benefits to overcome technical barriers	• Creation of new unforeseen problems (see this chapter)	• Creation of new unforeseen problems (see this chapter)
Genetic engineering (non-human)	• Improved crop yield • Crop or animal resistance to disease, drought • Plants as biofactories, improved nutrient content, produce/contain drugs and vaccines	• Health and environmental issues from genetically modified (GM) foods, animals and microbes	• Oligopolization and control of world food supply • Subversion of third world by GURT technologies • Undetected detrimental health effects from GM foods on a subpopulation of susceptible "responders"
Other (catch-all)	No intended benefit	• Any form of accidental event (catch-all) • All unforeseen pleiotropic, epistatic, polygenic, position effect, or other genetic interactions	• Any form of accidental genetic event (catch-all) as a result of genetic technology e.g., accidental creation of virulent pathogens during research

health benefits may be achievable in other ways and that the downside risk is too great.[92] The difference between the two views lies largely in the conception of the nature and the scope of the downside risk.

For Baylis and Downie, permitting therapeutic cloning will make human cloning more likely, because it will generate technological advances in the art of mammalian – and thus human – cloning generally. This is an excellent beginning for an informed debate, but it must be pushed further. Baylis and Downie, it seems to us, have the more persuasive argument, largely because the regulation proposed by Caulfield would hold sway only in Canada, whereas the techniques perfected by Canadian researchers would become the property of the global community, where no regulation is even imaginable at this time.

The risks posed by the internationalization of science are illustrated in the following report:

A respected Chinese scientist ... Lu Guangxiu, 61, who heads a team of 60 scientists at a high-tech laboratory in Changsha, south central China, said last week she had created more than 80 embryos containing the genetic blueprint of an existing adult ... Lu also disclosed that she had created cultures of human cells capable of proving 'spare parts' for a variety of fatal human diseases ... In four cases, the embryos have been kept alive to the stage where they are clusters of hundreds of cells and would normally be transferred to the wombs of mothers if they were being used to create babies.[93]

Unless and until effective international regulation of molecular biology applications is a reality, the precautionary approach suggests that therapeutic cloning should be prohibited by law in Canada, and that Canada should press the international community to establish appropriate and enforceable safeguards against human cloning.

CONCLUSIONS

We know that emerging branches of genomics and genetics hold significant promise for generating therapeutic treatments, presymptomatic disease treatment, replacement or regenerative tissue treatments, and cures for a number of diseases. Emerging technologies, such as human cloning, force us to examine the very essence of what it means to be human. Stem cell research, coupled with nuclear transplantation, with the ability to reprogram cells into gametes to create new embryos from somatic cells, confronts us with the morality of the value of life and the question of the legal rights of human somatic cells.

Convergence of emerging technologies may give rise to extrinsic risks far beyond the capacity of our social and regulatory institutions to control or manage. The far reach of these issues demands that we enter into some form of informed dialogue to understand the implications and impact of these emerging technologies. With each new emerging technology the ability to ultimately exert control over every aspect of our humanity comes closer. While the intrinsic and extrinsic risks discussed here deal mainly with individual choices, the role and responsibility of society in seeking to minimize harm should be considered. Thus we have two competing value sets: reducing suffering and harm to individuals by adopting new emerging genomics technologies versus ensuring societal safety by a stringent precautionary approach that would delay or ultimately deny the benefits to those who require them the most.

The emergence of new technologies like pharmacogenomics, cloning, or stem cell research should not automatically translate into availability, absence of regulation, and commercialization of the technology without regard for public safety and well-being. Genomics technologies have outpaced and are continuing to outpace the development of appropriate forward-thinking policies in many of the areas outlined (the lack of regulation for genetic testing, medical privacy, and genetic discrimination, for example). The recent cloning of humans, creating a number of embryos, and the ensuing media frenzy reveal our current societal sensitivity to technologies that have the power to create, control, alter, and manipulate life.[94] Given the current status of mammalian cloning, we already know the tremendous potential risks for both mother and child. Mammalian cloning has revealed medical risks, severe problems of developmental delays, heart defects, lung problems, malfunctioning immune systems, and accelerated aging. In one example that seems like science fiction come true, some cloned mice that were normal as young adults suddenly grew grotesquely fat.[95] Current cloning techniques are not adequate to abolish the downside risks and provide a minimum level of safety and efficacy.

A precautionary approach is needed for emerging genetics technologies. Some technologies, such as pharmacogenomics, DNA testing, and PGD may require only slight caution, while other areas of research, such as gene therapy, therapeutic cloning, and convergent genetic technologies, should have a more rigorous precautionary approach applied to minimize the downside risks, as well as the extrinsic risks that we may not yet be aware of. An open, informed debate is essential, to guide public policy about rapidly advancing genomics and genetics technologies.

Genomics gives rise to types of intrinsic and extrinsic risks that are not only unique but also exceptionally "potent" for individuals and societies, for the following reasons. Both the potential benefits and the risks touch on aspects of life that are intensely personal and private and, at the same time, crucial to social interactions. These include most of the factors thought to be important for individual happiness and social acceptance: appearance, pleasing personality, health, sociability, intelligence, attractiveness to mates, fecundity, livelihood, and on and on. As individuals, we each should have the choice of deciding whether or not we will pursue purely cosmetic alterations based on our notions and values.

However, the risks associated with genomics touch on aspects of life that are fundamental to social organization: the concept of personal responsibility in law and religion, an individual's autonomy with respect to their parentage (the "accidental" character of genetic mixing in animal reproduction), the character of political freedom (the development of the "free" individual unconstrained by genetic heritage), and the great values of democracy: justice, equity, and equality. The level of genetics and genomic science does not give rise to any of these extrinsic risk factors today but there is a fear that, generations from now, the human biology required for enhancement may be everywhere, with the capability to transform society.[96]

What is important – given the sensitivity of these types of risks – is that we look ahead to the capabilities that are undoubtedly sought after now, and almost certain to be achieved in the future. For the types of possible impacts in this domain remediation after the fact would not be appropriate. On the contrary, the potential consequences are such that we must resolve to deliberate and act in a precautionary way, so as to prevent certain types of consequences from ever arising. Such deliberation must start within the academic community, where issues are clarified and posed in an appropriate way. Then, of course, it must move out to the public domain, where credible information resources should be provided to the public well in advance of engaging citizens in prolonged dialogue.

Society can manage genomics risks appropriately only if the scientific community becomes actively engaged in this process, by assuming its share of responsibility for their potential scope, well in advance of successfully achieving the practical objectives stemming from research. Under a system of innovation and research that separates the communities of experts in the usual way – where media reports about scientific discovery elicit passing comments from a few "ethicists" – the results are utterly unsatisfactory, because the two rarely or never engage each other in public dialogue.

In a moving scene at the end of Mary Shelley's novel the creature delivers a eulogy while standing over his creator's lifeless body:

Fear not that I shall be the instrument of future mischief. My work is nearly complete. Neither yours nor any man's death is needed to consummate the series of my being, and accomplish that which must be done; but it requires my own.[97]

Perhaps this may serve as an appropriate forewarning, at the beginning of our journey into genomics and genetics research, which will move us inexorably towards the fateful endgame of widespread genetic manipulation. Our capacity to engineer genomes is perhaps the most fateful of all human powers, in that the risks to be managed go beyond specific interventions, and reach into the very foundations of human civilization. Therefore we must be proactive in managing these risks, acting in a precautionary mode rather than waiting for unthinkable consequences to emerge.

Appendix

THE USE OF MEDIA ANALYSIS IN
RISK COMMUNICATION RESEARCH

Media analysis, like public opinion surveys, is a tool to understand the formation of public opinion – to look at what people are saying and what they are being told. Previous research has demonstrated that consumers receive much of their science information from the media.[1] When asked about sources of information for health risks in Canada, people identified news media as the primary source. This helps explain the high perceived risks relating to ozone depletion and breast implants, ranked number two and three respectively in a 1992 survey, when those issues were prominently covered in general news media.[2]

Reliance on the media helps to define the public's sense of reality and its perceptions of risks or benefits.[3] Media messages have several origins, including journalism, public education, and public relations; and on any particular risk issue there is not one but many publics, including the passive public, the attentive public, and the active public.[4] The media both reflect public perceptions of an issue (journalists do not "make up" newsworthy stories but rely on sources and interviews) and also shape public perceptions by telling society what to think about: Kone and Mullet (1994) found a "practically totally determinant effect of the media in risk perception." As such, the way in which the media portray issues about biotechnology and food safety, for example, will have a profound effect on consumer perception and behaviour.[5] Just how profound, though, remains a controversial point.

Media messages can be evaluated both quantitatively and qualitatively. The first studies of newspaper content analysis can be traced back to Mathews, who attempted to illustrate the overwhelming space devoted to "demoralizing, unwholesome, and trivial" matters as opposed to worthwhile news items through the measure of story column inches.[6] As recounted by Gamson (1987), World War I marked the first systematic effort at nationwide manipulation of public opinion, and it was widely successful. This experience gave rise to the so-called hypodermic model of information transmission, using the metaphor of a hypodermic needle injecting ideas into the bloodstream of a trusting public.[7] Shortly after the conclusion of the war, the public relations industry was created, and its mission was summed up in the 1923 book by Edward Bernays, *Crystallizing Public Opinion*. In 1955 Bernays wrote that public relations "is the attempt, by information, persuasion and adjustment, to engineer public support for an activity, cause, movement or institution."

During World War II the American Library of Congress housed a propaganda analysis group devoted to basic issues of sampling, measurement problems, reliability, and validity of content categories in decoding public messages. Another group at the U.S. Federal Communications Commission relied on domestic German broadcasts to understand and predict events within Nazi Germany. A British group accurately predicted the date of deployment of the German V-weapon against Great Britain, based on analysis and interpretation of speeches by German government ministers.[8]

Despite these successes, many researchers began to question the simple counting of variables in public messages. Quantitative indicators can be insensitive and shallow in providing political insights. Even if large amounts of data are available, as required for statistical analyses, they do not lead to the "most obvious" conclusions that political experts are easily able to draw and to agree upon by observing qualitative changes.[9] In 1974 McLeod and Becker announced that the hypodermic needle metaphor of mass communication effects was finally dead. Yet as noted by Coleman (1993),[10] it is not unusual to find communication practitioners and scientists who still cling to the belief that messages relayed through mass media channels will result in well-informed and rational publics.[11]

Other models have been advanced to explain the impact of media messages on risk perception and consumer behaviour. The notion of media framing suggests that perception of a specific issue is organized – within discrete boundaries – for citizens and journalists alike to create a range of positions, allowing for a degree of controversy among those who share a common frame.[12] The agenda-setting model of the

1970s posits that media do not directly influence what the public thinks but are successful in making issues salient or significant.[13] Twenty years later Shaw and Martin (1992) suggested that, in addition to setting the agenda, the press may unconsciously provide a limited and rotating set of public issues around which the political and social system can engage in dialogue: "The press does not tell us what to believe, but does suggest what we collectively may agree to discuss, and perhaps act on."[14] In an experiment to predict public opinion from a content analysis of German television news regarding the importance of various political issues, Fan *et al.* (1994) found not only that media set the agenda but also that media content typically leads public opinion.[15]

Mazur (1981) argued that a rise in the opposition to a specific technology coincides with a parallel rise in the amount of media coverage on a specific technology, regardless of whether such coverage is positive or negative. Further, the more technical information the media provide, the more concerned the audience becomes, even if the information is thought by scientists to be reassuring.[16] Austin and Dong (1994), in an experiment to determine the effects of message type and source reputation on judgments of believability, discovered that experimental subjects based judgments of news believability more on the apparent reality of the message content than on source reputation.[17] In other words, a newspaper is simply a newspaper, and a story stands or falls largely on its own merits, regardless of who is quoted in the story. However, this study, like many others, used students from an introductory communication course at a university as research subjects, which may say more about the perceptions of college students than about the general public.

An additional theory – the so-called "magic seven" – suggests that issues such as microbial food safety will rise to a place of social prominence only when accompanied by elements of drama, and must displace a current social problem from one or more public arenas because only seven (plus or minus two) issues attract public attention at any one time.[18] While explaining how and why issues cycle in media attention, Hertog *et al.* (1994) commented that the public agenda can accommodate additional issues without displacing others.[19] With media narrow-casting – the targeting of niche markets – and the growth of electronic communications, there seems to be more room for additional public discourse on the issues of the day.

Applying a concept of drama, both Gibson and Zillmann (1994) and Brosius and Bathelt (1994) found that readers attribute more significance to stories that begin with exemplars (i.e., personal examples).[20] Zillmann *et al.* (1992) used different versions of a news magazine

report on the "yo-yo" diet phenomena, where people regain weight
after participating in a weight control program.[21] Those stories that
began with exemplars caused respondents in recall interviews to estimate that 75 per cent of dieters were unsuccessful in maintaining their
weight loss, even though base rate information stated that on average
one-third of dieters regain their weight. Following an outbreak of
cryptosporidium in Milwaukee's water supply, Griffin *et al.* (1994)
noted that it was worry that motivated audience members to seek
cryptosporidium information actively, both by enhancing their reliance
on mass, interpersonal, and – in particular – specialized media (such
as information brochures and government information), and by mag-
nifying their attention to the cryptosporidium information they
encountered through routine use of mass media.[22] Worry was found
to be intensified by past personal experience with cryptosporidiosis,
and directly or indirectly by risk perception. In other words, those who
were personally impelled gathered the most information. Still other
researchers such as Zelizer (1993) argue that communication research
has failed to explain journalism. Today it is generally agreed that the
effect press messages will have depends on the social context in which
they are received.[23]

MEDIA AND SCIENCE

In 1919 the *New York Times* published a series of editorials on the
public's inability to understand new developments in physics, and what
the newspaper regarded as the disturbing implications for democracy
when important intellectual achievements are understood by only a
handful of people. Not much has changed in the intervening period.
Nelkin (1987) has noted that public understanding of science and
technology is critical in a society increasingly affected by the impact
of technological change, one in which policy decisions are determined
in large part by technical expertise.[24] Yet in her analysis of science
journalism in the print media, she concluded that imagery often
replaces content, with little discussion of the scientific questions being
posed, that issues are covered as a series of dramatic events, that
different message providers are intensely competitive with one
another, and that scientists themselves are increasingly seeking favourable press coverage as a means of enhancing their research support.
Science has become politics, and politics has become a series of media
events and photo-ops.

Today's style of science writing can be traced back to the formation
of the u.s. Science Service in 1921, which was set up to translate the
arcane language of science into something that could be understood

by a wider audience. However, because the syndicate was controlled by trustees from the most prominent science associations, the editorial policies were dominated by the values of the scientific community.[25] Whereas most journalists seek to analyse and criticize, science writers and much of science writing seek to elucidate and explain, resulting in many accounts that rely on only one (scientific) source or press releases from promoters of science.

In 1919 the American Chemical Society (ACS) became the first scientific association to organize a news service hiring a professional science writer to translate technical reports for the public and to write descriptions of scientific research for the press. In the 1930s, in conjunction with the rise of the public relations profession, a number of other associations followed ACS's lead, seeking to generate public interest and support. DiBella *et al.* (1991) observed that most scientists who were interviewed reported a willingness to *allow* – emphasis added – media interviews in order to educate the public and to engender interest in the scientists' own specialty.[26] Dunwoody and Ryan (1985) found that 86 per cent of scientists felt publicity about scientists' work could sometimes help them get research funds.[27] In a public controversy over risks related to electromagnetic frequencies (EMF), Newman (1991) quoted EMF researchers who said the most positive effect of increased media coverage from 1989–91 was a rise in funding provided by the U.S. Congress.[28]

In 1961 the U.S. federal government had 1,164 people working as writers-editors and public affairs specialists. By 1990 the number in public information jobs was nearly five thousand, making the federal government the nation's largest single employer of public information officers.[29] Today journalists often obtain material for their stories from press releases, conferences, interviews, and selected journals, especially *Science, Nature,* the *New England Journal of Medicine* (*NEJM*) and *JAMA,* the *Journal of the American Medical Association.*[30] The AMA makes available weekly video and radio news releases by satellite to eight hundred television and five thousand radio stations nationwide.[31] Under the terms of the *NEJM* embargo arrangement, 250 advance copies of the journal are delivered to the media at least three days prior to formal publication date. In turn, the media agree not to disclose details until the publication date, ensuring that journalists have equal access and sufficient time for analysing and interpreting a study.[32] Such embargo agreements are now routine with most of the major journals and many of the specialized ones. Those sources that are best organized to provide technical information to journalists in an efficiently packaged form have a great deal of control over what ultimately appears as news.

Yet despite this level of control over science news, much of what is actually reported is rife with errors. In comparing media accounts (newspaper, television, and magazine) with the original scientific reports, Singer (1990) found it was common to introduce errors of omission, emphasis, or fact in an attempt to make the reports more lively.[33] Two-fifths of a sample of forty-two stories had one or more statements that were substantially different from statements in the original research report. Science in the popular press, states Singer, is livelier and easier to read than science in the scholarly journals; it is also simpler, sharper, and less ambiguous than science in those journals; and science in the scholarly journals is already simpler, sharper, and much less ambiguous than the science that takes place in the laboratory or in the field. The result is that in the popular press, science and scientists come across as more authoritative than they really are, and that scientific findings are regarded with more confidence than may be warranted.

Scientists and journalists both use explanatory devices to convey the meaning of their work: science is about models, explanation, and representation, while journalists often resort to metaphors. According to Layoff and Johnson (1980), a metaphor is not just a rhetorical flourish but a basic property of language used to define experience and to evoke shared meanings.[34] Nelkin (1987) argues that the use of metaphors in science writing is particularly important in the explanation of technical detail, to define experience, to evoke shared meanings and to allow individuals to construct elaborate concepts about public issues and events.[35] Nelkin (1987) has also shown that the metaphors used by science writers in general have cycled over the past five decades, with the notion of progress resurrected as innovation, and the celebration of technology present once again as high technology promotion.[36]

In 1985 Nobel Prize winner Kenneth Wilson helped convince the U.S. National Science Foundation to spend $200 million to help establish four university-based supercomputing centres.[37] The most crucial factor, said Wilson, was a single newspaper article quoting a scientist who said that such a program was necessary for the United States to retain its lead in supercomputing technology: "The substance of it all (supercomputing research) is too complicated to get across – it's the image that is important. The image of this computer program as the key to our technological leadership is what drives this interplay between people like ourselves and the media and forces a reaction from Congressmen."[38]

This is a powerful statement, one that opens the way for serious abuse and manipulation of the decision-making process. Journalists also convey values through the way stories are selected, the choice of headlines and leads, and the selection of details; in short, journalists equip readers to think about science and technology in specific ways. Journalistic sources themselves also convey values in the statements they provide. Priest and Talbert (1994), in an analysis of newspaper coverage of biotechnology in the United States, showed that different social actors – government, scientists, consumer groups, and others – are quoted in such stories in differing frequencies and use different types of arguments to support their positions.[39]

A random sample of 1,250 American adults, commissioned by the u.s. based Scientists' Institute for Public Information (1993), concluded that the number of American adults who want serious scientific news is substantial, and that science news provides basic, functional information necessary for living in the modern world, especially in the areas of personal health and the environment.[40] A majority of respondents (56 per cent) said they are regular viewers of TV programs on science, technology, and nature, and roughly 40 per cent of the public were solid followers of science news. For example, 38 per cent were weekly readers of science news in the newspaper; 43 per cent read books or magazines on science every month; and 40 per cent said they discussed issues related to science with someone else approximately once a week. An interest in health issues was leading the way for interest in other kinds of science news, a view echoed by Chew *et al.* (1995), who found that health-related topics enjoy relatively stable media coverage and represent at least a quarter of all daily newspaper articles.[41]

Media Analysis and Risk Communication

Public communication about issues of technological risk often involves messages from diverse individuals or communities that are translated and synthesized by media outlets and other members of the public. At each step message providers, journalists, and audience members are framing a specific event using their own value systems, constraints, and the filters of experience and expectation in a way that makes the most sense to the particular individual. Different people use different sources to collect information related to issues of scientific and technological risk. It is therefore incumbent on the provider of risk messages to determine how a specific target audience receives and perceives risk information.

Schanne and Meier (1992), in a meta-analysis of fifty-two studies of media coverage of environmental risk, concluded that journalism constructs a universe of its own, a "media reality" that does not mirror

actual reality.[42] Specifically, the journalistic construction of environmental issues and environmental risk mirrors only partially, or not at
all, the scientific construction of environmental issues and risk. While
the professional isolation of both scientists and journalists presents an
ongoing impediment to communication, it is mistaken to view journalists and the media always as significant, independent causes of
problems in risk communication.[43] Further, many media analysts, who
may never actually write for public media, often fail to recognize the
chaos of everyday life (especially that of a newsroom), fail to acknowledge the constraints imposed by a media industry which is geared for
profit, and fail to acknowledge the critical faculties of any particular
reader. Rather, the assumption seems to be that an uncritical public
is waiting to be filled with educational material from a variety of media
– residual effects of the hypodermic needle model – and that media
is more influential than common sense and practical experience may
suggest. Many problems in scientist-journalist interactions and pronouncements can be traced to the myth of objectivity resident in both
disciplines. Scientists and journalists who acknowledge that a degree
of bias is normal are likely to be better prepared to distinguish facts
from value judgments in both expert statements and media accounts
of food safety debates.[44]

The role of the media in shaping public perceptions in technological controversies has been well documented.[45] Yet the actual impact
of media coverage on citizen decision with respect to a particular risk
remains unclear. Protess *et al.* (1987) found when examining the
impact of reporting on toxic waste controversies that media disclosures
had limited effects on the general public but were influential in changing the attitudes of policy makers.[46] Dunwoody (1993) argues that
while mass media tells people something about the risk present in a
society, interpersonal channels are used to determine the level of risk
to individuals.[47] How much information these secondary sources originally receive from media stories has not yet been determined. Further
research is on-going in this area.[48]

Communicating uncertainty is also the focus of more recent
research. While it is often argued that a more thorough explanation
of uncertainty surrounding a technological risk may enhance trust and
citizen decision-making,[49] Johnson and Slovic (1994) found that
media accounts containing details relating to health effects and exposure pathways to a dangerous chemical had no apparent effect on risk
perceptions.[50] Similar findings have been reported elsewhere. Burns
et al. (1993) concluded that media and public response appears to be
determined by perceptions that a reported event was caused by man-
agerial incompetence and is a signal of future risk.[51] Presentations of

technical detail and uncertainty have little effect on risk perception.[52] Research in health-related risk communication has shown that the presentation of risk statistics has little meaning to a public audience, and that attitudes about how science and technology are controlled are better predictors of risk levels than are the cost-benefit considerations, judgments about effects, or concerns about how science and technology are used.[53]

For the media analysis used in several of the chapters in *Mad Cows and Mother's Milk*, the Science and Medicine section of the u.s. based *Associated Press* wire service was searched daily and the appropriate stories retrieved (*AP* is available as part of the basic service of the electronic information provider, CompuServe). The daily North American edition of the *New York Times* was also chosen because, as noted by Nelkin (1991), the *Times* is critically important for setting agendas in the media world. The *Globe and Mail*, which is the agenda-setting outlet in Canadian media, was also scanned daily, as was the *Kitchener-Waterloo Record*, a local paper based in Kitchener, Ontario, one hundred km west of Toronto.[54] Notably, the *Record* is one of the few newspapers in Canada that has a reporter devoted to the agriculture beat (albeit a half-time beat since 1994). With recent layoffs in Saskatoon, the *Record* may now be the only one.

These four media outlets can be deemed representative of the newspaper coverage of medical, food, and health issues because of the agenda-setting effect of the outlets chosen, and because of the increasing homogeneity amongst news outlets.[55] Manual searches were conducted for two reasons. First, they provided timely information, which is crucial in an evolving risk scenario. Second, relying on searches of electronic or paper indexes – which have been found to be inconsistent and unreliable – can lead to erroneous results.[56] Although full-text electronic databases of specific newspapers are increasingly available, they are relatively expensive to access and tardy.

Nevertheless, while useful for determining broad trends, quantitative data analysis has many limitations. Smythe (1954) called the simplistic reliance of content analysis on counting quantitative data an "immaturity of science" in which objectivity is confused with quantification.[57] Krippendorf (1980) notes that simply analysing a representative sample of the *New York Times* may be specific about the data "but vacuous regarding target and context. In fact, the analysis may have completely ignored the symbolic qualities of this medium."[58] Newspapers like the *Times* and the *Globe* are targeted to an elite audience that may not be representative of the wider public.[59] Yet these newspapers and the stories they cover – while perhaps not setting the public agenda – do tend to set the news agenda, the issues that get reported, the stories that get told. This in turn shapes the public discussion of an issue.

The measures presented here are only intended to provide a quantitative estimation of what the public is exposed to. This does not account for varying perceptions of risk on a particular issue or quantify sometimes dramatic changes in the coverage of a specific topic.

A Note on the Media Search Method for E. Coli O157:H7

For the period 1993 to 1995, all articles dealing with *E. coli* O157:H7 were obtained by manually scanning the daily editions of the *New York Times*, the *Globe and Mail*, the *Kitchener-Waterloo Record* and the *Associated Press* wire service (via the electronic information provider Compu-Serve). Articles from other media outlets were obtained through database searches, although these were not used in the quantitative assessments of media coverage.

Published research regarding *E. coli* O157:H7 was obtained by searches in three widely used databases: *Agricola, Food Science & Technology Abstracts,* and *Medline.* Key words used were "coli O157" or "enterohaem" or "enterohem."

As well, two periodicals covering the three years preceding the 1993 outbreak were manually searched to attempt to determine information that might have been more widely read by quality-control or production people, especially in the meat industry. To further ensure that material intended for a broader food scientist audience was reviewed, the journals *Food Technology, Dairy Food,* and *Environmental Sanitation* were searched manually from 1982–93.

Those articles recognized by more than one database were not separated. However, there were differences in the types of journals searched by each database: *Agricola* was more extension and agriculture based, including studies of colonization and control of O157:H7 on the farm; *Medline* more clinically focused; and *Food Science and Technology* more inclined to food-processing related articles.

Notes

CHAPTER ONE

1 Madelaine Drohan, "Britain Struggles with Aftermath of Mad Cow Scare," *Globe and Mail,* 11 October 1996, B7.
2 Stephen Dorrell, statement in Parliament, 20 March 1996.
3 "How BSE Crisis Forced Europe out of Its Complacency," *Nature* (2 January 1997).
4 Rowan Dore, "BSE Crisis Bill," *Press Associated News* [hereafter PA *News*], 3 Feb 1997.
5 Bradley and Wilesmith, "Epidemiology and Control of Bovine Spongiform Encephalopathy."
6 U.K. Institute of Food Science & Technology, *Bovine Spongiform Encephalopathy (BSE) Position Statement.*
7 For review, see Prusiner, "The Prion Diseases."
8 Brandner *et al.,* "Normal Host Prion Protein Necessary for Scrapie-Induced Neurotoxicity," *Nature* (January 25, 1996): 339–43; Patino *et al.,*"Support for the Prion Hypothesis for Inheritance of a Phenotypic Trait in Yeast"; Glenn *et al.,* "Evidence for the Conformation of the Pathologic Isoform of the Prion Protein Enciphering and Propagating Prion Diversity," 2079–82.
9 Marianne McGowan, "Disease Killing British Cattle," *New York Times,* 24 January 1990, C13.
10 Sheila Rule, "Fatal Cow Illness Stirs British Fear," *New York Times,* 20 May 1990.

11 Steven Greenhouse, "Anger in Britain Growing over France's Ban on Beef," *New York Times*, 2 June 1990, I9.

12 *The Economist*, 19 May 1990.

13 John von Radowitz, "Government Blocks Inquiry into 'Mad Cow' Death Link," PA *News*, 15 August 1995.

14 Ibid.

15 Mark Thomas, "Two More Human 'Mad Cow Disease' Cases Reported," PA *News*, 24 October 1995.

16 John von Radowitz, "Health CJD Substitute," PA *News*, 27 October 1995.

17 Gavin Cordon, "BSE Warning to Slaughterman," PA *News*, 10 November 1995.

18 Alan Harman, "Television Report Sparks Fears of BSE-Infected Meat," *Western Producer*, 30 November 1995.

19 Ibid.

20 "School Bans Beef over BSE Fears," PA *News*, 17 November 1995.

21 Ibid.

22 Andrew Evans, "Government Forecasts End of Mad Cow Disease," PA *News*, 23 November 1995.

23 See Barry Wilson, "Canada Challenges EU Beef Ban," *Western Producer*, 26 September 1996.

24 "Doctors Demand More Research into Mad Cow Disease," *Reuters*, 24 November 1995.

25 "Government Claims Challenged," *Manchester Guardian Weekly*, 26 November 1995.

26 Brian Farmer, "Action Call after New 'Mad Cow' Alert," PA *News*, 1 December 1995.

27 Gavin Cordon, "Dorrell Bids to Allay 'Mad Cow' Beef Fears," PA *News*, 4 December 1995.

28 Rowan Dore, "Minister Warns against 'Overreaction' on Mad Cow Disease," PA *News*, 6 December 1995.

29 Brian Farmer, "Major Seeks to Ease Beef Fears," PA *News*, 7 December 1995.

30 Brian Farmer, "Pressure Grows for 'Mad Cow Disease,'" PA *News*, 7 December 1995.

31 Brian Farmer, "BSE Scare Causes 'Worrying' Drop in Beef Sales," PA *News*, 18 December 1996.

32 John von Radowitz, "BSE Beef 'Probably Safe' Say Scientists," PA *News*, 20 December 1995.

33 Brian Unwin, "Suspected CJD Victim Worked in Abbatoir," PA *News*, 22 December 1995.

34 Sue Leeman, "Britain – Mad Cow Disease," *Associated Press*, 9 January 1996.

35 Nick Robinson, "Supermarkets in Bid to Boost Beef," PA *News*, 17 January 1996.

36 The scientific paper appeared as Will *et al.*, "A New Variant of Creutzfeldt-Jakob Disease in the U.K.," 921–5.

37 See end of chapter for full text.

38 Jo Butler, "We Always Followed Medical Advice – Dorrell, " *PA News*, 20 March 1996.

39 John von Radowitz, "Fatal Disease Which Leaves Brain Riddled with Holes," *PA News*, 21 March 1996.

40 Sarah Womack, "Half-Compensation Blamed for BSE Cattle Risk," *PA News*, 20 March 1996.

41 Maxine Frith, "Intensive Farming to Blame for Mad Cow Disease," *PA News*, 21 March 1996.

42 Geoff Meade, "Mad Cow Crisis 'an Act of God'," *PA News*, 8 October 1996.

43 Kate Chattaway, "Government Handling of Beef Crisis under Fire," *PA News*, 17 April 1996.

44 Hamish Macdonell, "Slaughterhouses Failing to Comply with New BSE Controls," *PA News*, 30 April 1996.

45 John von Radowitz, "Uncovering Links between BSE and CJD," *PA News*, 24 April 1996.

46 Ehsan Masood, "BSE Transmission Data Pose Dilemma for UK scientists," *Nature* (8 August 1996).

47 Ibid.

48 "Transmission Dynamics and Epidemiology of BSE in British Cattle," *Nature* (29 August 1996): 779–88.

49 Amanda Brown, "Government Halts Beef Cull," *PA News*, 19 September 1996.

50 B.E.C. Schreuder *et al.*, "Preclinical Test for Prion," 563.

51 Hsich *et al.*, "The 14–3–3 Brain Protein in Cerebrospinal Fluid As a Marker for Transmissible Spongiform Encephalopathies."

52 "Britain Too Slow on Mad Cow Tests, Journal Says," *Reuters*, 27 September 1996.

53 "BSE Researchers Bemoan 'Ministry Secrecy,'" *Nature* (10 October 1996).

54 Declan Butler, "Panel Urges Precautionary Approach," *Nature* (17 October 1996).

55 Collinge *et al.*, "Molecular Analysis of Prion Strain Variation and the Aetiology of 'New Variant' CJD," 685–90.

56 Sian Clare, "Europe Gets Even Tougher over Beef," *PA News*, 24 October 1996.

57 "U.K. to Slaughter 100,000 Cattle: E.U. to Study Plan," *Dow Jones News*, 16 December 1996.

58 Sarah Hall and John Von Radowitz, "Hundreds to Die Each Year from Eating BSE Beef," *PA News*, 27 November 1996.

59 Peter Beal, "Girl, 19, Is 13th to Die from New CJD Strain," *PA News*, 16 December 1996.

60 Nelkin, *Selling Science: How the Press Covers Science and Technology,* 224.

61 Collinge *et al.,* "Molecular Analysis of Prion Strain Variation and the Aetiology of 'New Variant' CJD."

62 Bill Schiller, "Crusading Scientist Locks Horns with Beef Barons," *Toronto Star,* 28 January 1996, C6.

63 "Hsus Expert Available to Discuss Mad-Cow Disease," *Humane Society of the United States,* 21 March 1996.

64 Casey Mahood, "'Destruction Justified,' Canadians Say," *Globe and Mail,* 22 March 1996, A10.

65 "USDA to Increase Inspections of Beef Imported from U.K.," *Dow Jones News,* 21 March 1996.

66 Powell, D., personal communication, 3 July 1996.

67 Powell, D., personal communication, 23 October 1996.

68 "U.S. Group Calls for Animal Meal Ban for Cattle," *Reuters,* 28 March 1996.

69 Ibid.

70 Heather Jones, "BSE Debate May Provide Avenue for Moving U.S. Beef to the EU," *Feedstuffs,* 29 April 1996.

71 "USDA, U.S. Public Health Service Announce Additional Steps, Support for Industry Efforts to Keep U.S. Free of BSE," *PR Newswire,* 29 March 1996.

72 "A Joint Statement by National Livestock and Professional Animal Health Organizations Regarding a Voluntary Ban on Ruminant Derived Protein in Ruminant Feed Recommended," *PR Newswire,* 29 March 1996.

73 Mike Cooper, "U.S. Orders More Checks on 'Mad Cow' in Humans," *Reuters,* 8 August 1996.

74 Eddie Evans, "Oprah Winfrey Challenges U.S. Beef Industry," *Reuters,* 16 April 1996.

75 Brian Laghi, "Cattle Ranchers Get the Word out about Beef Safety," *Globe and Mail,* 28 March 1996, A4.

76 Courtney Tower, "Canadian Officials Attempt to Squelch Consumer BSE Fears," *Western Producer,* 4 April 1996.

77 "FDA Sees Animal Protein Ban for Cattle Feed in 6–12 Months," *Dow Jones News,* 14 May 1996.

78 Sarah Muirhead, "CGMP, HACCP-Based Plans for BSE Prevention Offered," *Feedstuffs,* 17 June 1996.

79 Charles House, "Renderers Say BSE Proposal Based on Fear, Not Science," *Feedstuffs,* 4 November 1996.

80 "FDA Proposes Precautionary Ban against Ruminant-to-Ruminant Feeding," *FDA Press Release,* 2 January 1997.

81 "Statement by the National Cattlemen's Beef Association Regarding FDA's Precautionary Ban against Feeding of Ruminant Protein to Ruminants," *National Cattlemen's Beef Association Press Release,* 2 January 1997.

82 Lawrence Altman, "FDA Proposal Would Help Prevent Mad Cow Disease," *New York Times,* 3 January 1997, A1.

83 Laura Rance, "High Stakes Surround Proposed Meat Meal Ban," *Manitoba Co-operator,* 2 May 1996.

84 Stephen Strauss, "AIDS Triumphs, Martian Fossils, Mad Cows and the Internet," *Globe and Mail,* 28 December 1996, D6; "School Bans Beef over BSE Fears," *Globe and Mail,* 17 November 1995.

85 Mike Strathdee, "Fears about Mad Cow Disease Take Toll in Ontario Sheep Industry," *Kitchener-Waterloo Record,* 6 July 1996, B8.

86 Kathy Kaufield, "Canada 'Unjustified' in Mad Cow Actions," *Charlottetown Guardian,* 8 July 1996, 3.

87 Don Stoneman, "U.S. Rethinks Offal Ban," *Farm & Country,* 16 July 1996.

88 Patrick Gallagher, "CCA Supports Ban on Animal Based Protein," *Ontario Farmer,* 27 August 1996.

89 Don Stoneman, "Meat Meal Ban for North America?" *Farm & Country,* 27 August 1996.

A list of references relevant to chapter 1, particularly on-line material and U.K. legislation related to BSE, is found at the end of the bibliography.

CHAPTER TWO

1 We borrow the concept of "risk amplification" from the pathbreaking article by Kasperson *et al.,* "The Social Amplification of Risk."

2 An excellent introduction is Rodricks, *Calculated Risks.*

3 This is the year of the earliest uses of the phrase risk communication, according to the references listed in Rohrmann *et al.,* ed., *Risk Communication: An Interdisciplinary Bibliography,* 26, 56, 111.

4 Leiss, "New Applications of Communications Theory."

5 The wide purview now enjoyed by the risk approach stems from a few sources, including Lowrance, *Of Acceptable Risk,* and Rowe, *An Anatomy of Risk.*

6 The seminal work is Covello *et al., Risk Communication.*

7 For example, see Siddall and Bennett, "A People-Centred Concept of Society-Wide Risk Management," 272.

8 A good summary of the errors in judgment to which experts are prone is the U.S. National Research Council, *Improving Risk Communication,* 44–7.

9 Another way of putting this point is to say that "risk is a construct," that is, an understanding of a risk-type situation that is related to the situation of each participant. See Bayerische Rück, ed., *Risk Is a Construct.* This transition represents a complete change of emphasis within the components of the phrase "risk communication": in phase one, the emphasis is on the adjective; in phase two, on the noun.

10 Slovic and MacGregor, "Social Context of Risk Communication," 17.

11 In this period institutional risk managers in government and industry were often told that up to 75 per cent of "message content" – as received by audiences – was based on the non-verbal dimensions of the message delivery format itself (body posture, hand gestures, style of dress, facial expression, etc.).

12 See Leiss, "'Down and Dirty.'"

13 The best guide is Slovic and MacGregor, "Social Context of Risk Communication," 17.

14 See appendix, "Use of Media Analysis," for an overview of the methodological issues involved in this use of media content.

15 The dotted line indicates that a readily comprehensible version of the scientific results is not reaching public audiences. The double-headed arrow indicates, among other things, that, in the absence of the good information exchange prevented by the formation of a risk information vacuum, the fears and misunderstandings that fester in poorly informed public opinion undergo a process of self-amplification.

CHAPTER THREE

1 David Burnham, "Scientist Urges Congress to Bar Any Use of the Pesticide 2,4,5-T," *New York Times*, 10 August 1974; Clyde Hertzman, personal communication; Sheila Copps, *Kitchener-Waterloo Record*, 14 September 1994; and Environment Canada, "News Conference Notes for the Honourable Sergio Marchi, PC, MP, on the Occasion of the Tabling of the New Canadian Environmental Protection Act," National Press Theatre, 10 December 1996.

2 Usage varies between the singular and the plural form, with the latter preferred because dioxins are a "family" of seventy-five related chemical compounds, which differ markedly in their toxicity profiles. Collectively these seventy-five are referred to as polychlorinated dibenzodioxins (PCDDs). They are closely related to another family of 135 compounds, the polychlorinated dibenzofurans (PCDFs), and so one will often see the phrase "dioxins and furans," or the collective abbreviation PCDD/Fs. The singular form "dioxin" usually refers to the most toxic member of the PCDD/F family, 2,3,7,8-TCDD [tetrachlorodibenzo-*p*-dioxin], sometimes just TCDD. See part 1 for further discussion.

3 In September 1994 representatives of a number of Canadian environmental groups asked the federal minister of the Environment, Sheila Copps, to "declare a dioxin emergency in Canada" (*Kitchener-Waterloo Record*, 14 September 1994). It is impossible to say what such a declaration might have meant in terms of public policy or environmental regulation. There has been no further mention of this request since that time.

4 Cf. Gregory et al., "Technological Stigma."

5 Jon R. Luoma, "Scientists Are Unlocking Secrets of Dioxin's Devastating Power," New York Times, 15 May 1990 (discusses Ah receptor binding).

6 The first two selections are from an article by Ralph Blumenthal, "Files Show Dioxin Makers Knew of Hazards," New York Times, 4 July 1983. The memo and letter were part of a large file of company documents which had been supplied to a court in connection with the Agent Orange class-action lawsuit filed against the manufacturers by Vietnam war veterans, and which were not otherwise publicly available. The memo was written in connection with a meeting convened by Dow of chemical companies making 2,4,5-T. The documents make clear that Dow was concerned that *other* manufacturers were allowing excessive amounts of dioxin impurities to develop in the herbicide during the production process; apparently Dow had learned from the German firm Boehringer how to control the process so as to keep the dioxin relatively low, and it wanted others to adopt this process. (See M. Gough, *Dioxin, Agent Orange*, 188–90.) Most of the contents of the memo reproduced above are also in the Greenpeace document "Dow Brand Dioxin," 16. The third selection is drawn from: Anon., "Another Herbicide on the Blacklist," *Nature* 226 (25 April 1970): 309–10. For the fourth: Tschirley, "Dioxin," 34–5.

7 Portier et al., "Ligand/Receptor Binding for 2,3,7,8-TCDD."

8 Gough, *Dioxin, Agent Orange*.

9 Adapted from Rawls, "Dioxin's Human Toxicity."

10 Expanded from Webster and Commoner, "Overview: The Dioxin Debate."

11 Masuda, "The Yusho Rice Oil Poisoning Incident"; and Hsu et al., "The Yu-cheng Rice Oil Poisoning Incident."

12 P.H. Schuck, *Agent Orange on Trial*, 19; and D. Ecobichon, "Toxic Effects of Pesticides," 673.

13 Long and Hanson, "Dioxin Issue Focuses on Three Major Controversies in u.s."

14 Schuck, *Agent Orange on Trial*, 5.

15 Carter et al., "Accidental Poisoning," 738–40.

16 Gough, *Dioxin, Agent Orange*, 121–56.

17 Pocchiari et al., "Accidental Release."

18 Gough, *Dioxin, Agent Orange*, 151–53.

19 See generally Harrison and Hoberg, *Risk, Science and Politics*, ch. 3. The u.s. number is derived by taking the animal test result in the most sensitive species (guinea pigs, in this case) and adding a hundred-fold safety factor. The setting and revising of such numbers is a highly "political" process, especially in the United States; for the dioxin case see Finkel, "Dioxin: Are We Safer Now Than Before?" 161–5; and Roberts, "Dioxin Risks Revisited," 624.

20 Extensive discussions will be found in the following sources: DeVito and Birnbaum, "Toxicology of Dioxins," 139–62; U.S. Environmental Protection Agency, *Health Assessment Document*; Gough, *Dioxin, Agent Orange*, ch. 14; Moore *et al.*, "The Dioxin TCDD"; Tschirley, "Dioxin"; and Greenpeace, *No Margin of Safety*, an excellent and comprehensive overview.

21 Cited in Luoma, "Scientists Are Unlocking Secrets," *New York Times*, 15 May 1990.

22 DeVito and Birnbaum, "Toxicology of Dioxins," 147.

23 The phrase is from Roberts, "Dioxin Risks Revisited," 624; and the number from *Casarett and Doull's Toxicology* (table 2–1), 14.

24 Gough, *Dioxin, Agent Orange*, 185–8.

25 Fingerhut *et al.*, "Cancer mortality in workers," 212–18.

26 Bertazzi *et al.*, "Cancer Incidence."

27 Gough, "Human Health Effects," 149.

28 Holloway, "A Great Poison," 16, 20. Endocrine disruptors, also called endocrine disrupting chemicals or endocrine modulating substances, are compounds that are known to have, or are suspected of being capable of having, specific effects on the functioning of endocrine systems in humans and other mammals. See Kavlock and Ankley, "Endocrine-Disruptive Effects," 731–9.

29 Portier *et al.*, "Ligand/Receptor Binding for 2,3,7,8-TCDD."

30 U.S. Environmental Protection Agency (1) *Interim Report on Data and Methods for Assessment of 2,3,7,8-Tetrachlorodibenzo -p-dioxin Risks to Aquatic Life and Associated Wildlife*, March 1993; (2) *Health Assessment Document for 2,3,7,8-Tetrachlorodibenzo -p-dioxin (TCDD) and Related Compounds*, 3 vols (June 1994) 1,100 pages; (3) *Estimating Exposure to Dioxin-like Compounds*, 3 vols. (June 1994) 1,300 pages. Greenpeace had its interpretation of the whole reassessment out on the street within a month (Thornton's *Achieving Zero Dioxin*) and followed this up with an extensive commentary on EPA's exposure study in January 1995.

31 *Health Assessment Document for 2,3,7,8-Tetrachlorodibenzo -p-dioxin (TCDD) and Related Compounds*, vol. 3, 9–81. "Background human exposures" are the average exposure levels found in human body tissue resulting from all sources of a particular substance. Cf. Hrudey and Krewski, "Is There a Safe Level of Exposure to a Carcinogen?"

32 First epigraph: see notes 42, 43; second: Michael Keating, "Dioxin Discovered in Human Tissue Test," *Globe and Mail*, 25 June 1982; third: Kimberly Noble, "Pulp, Paper Mills Linked to Dioxin Contamination," *Globe and Mail*, 14 October 1987.

33 "Vietnam: A Medical Consequence of War," *New York Times*, 16 September 1972, article by George Perera, an American professor of medicine who had visited North Vietnam. The French spelling ("dioxine") in this article reflects the colonial tradition in Vietnam. This is the first entry

under "dioxins" in the *New York Times* index. We have located a few earlier mentions of dioxins, beginning in 1970, but they are all passing references which provide no information beyond the fact that dioxin had been discovered to be a contaminant of 2,4,5-T.

34 Boyce Rensburger, "E.P.A. Ends Drive to Ban Defoliant," *New York Times*, 27 June 1974; David Burnham, "Scientist Urges Congress to Bar Any Use of Pesticide 2,4,5-T," *New York Times*, 10 August 1974.

35 "Death of Animals Laid to Chemical," *New York Times*, 28 August 1974.

36 A rich background discussion of the Agent Orange and Times Beach episodes will be found in Wildavsky, *But Is It True?*, ch. 3.

37 *New York Times*, 19 September 1972, 28 August 1974, 29 July 1976, and 27 June 1980.

38 Quoted in Richard D. Lyons, "Contamination of Fish in Vietnamese Waters Laid to U.S. Defoliant," *New York Times*, 6 April 1973.

39 D.G. McNeil Jr. "3 Chemical Sites near Love Canal Possible Hazard," *New York Times*, 22 December 1978.

40 Richard Severo, "Two Crippled Lives Mirror Disputes on Herbicides," *New York Times*, 27 May 1979.

41 *Associated Press*, 30 May 1980; Frances Cerra, "Garbage Recycling Plant Stays Closed over Dioxin," *New York Times*, 2 August 1980; "Inmates in 60's Test of a Poison Sought," 18 January 1981; Wayne Biddle, "10 Years Later, Missourians Find Soil Tainted by Dioxin," 10 November 1982.

42 *Globe and Mail*, 29 November 1980, 3, 4, 9, 10 December 1980; and 13 August 1981.

43 *Globe and Mail*, 9 December 1980; 14 May, 17 July, 13 August, and 27 October 1981; 5 and 6 January, 2 April, and 25 June 1982.

44 See generally Eric Ouellet, "Organizational Analysis and Environmental Sociology," 321–38.

45 Greenpeace, *Achieving Zero Dioxin*, 16.

46 *Harvard Report on Cancer Prevention*, Harvard School of Public Health, Boston, November 1996.

47 Canadian Council of Resource and Environment Ministers [CCREM], *Dioxins and Furans: The Canadian Perspective*, n.p., n.d.

48 Health Canada's dioxins pamphlet is easily accessible on the department's Internet website. In February 1997 one of the research assistants for this book project, based in Vancouver, was given the assignment to seek general information on dioxins (not technical reports) by telephone from Environment Canada, representing himself as a member of the public. After two days and numerous calls to various officials (more commonly to their voice-mail message systems), our dedicated RA still had no information, and he was finally referred by an Environment Canada official to the British Columbia Ministry of Environment. After

repeating the fruitless cycle of phone calls with a series of officials there, he came up empty-handed once again. His research notes conclude as follows: "Everyone I talked to was very pleasant and tried to be helpful, but the system does not seem to be set up in a way to allow the public to easily get basic information."

49 Our dedicated RA was given a similar assignment involving EPA. With some difficulty he traversed EPA's sizeable website and, finding no general publications on dioxins, managed to locate the telephone number of the agency's Public Information Center in Washington, DC. The personnel there reported having no brochures on dioxins and referred our caller to EPA's Research and Development Office in Cincinnati, Ohio. No publications were available from that office either, but our RA was offered a third telephone number in a different state, an office from which two publications could be purchased – at a cost of $140 and $133, respectively. His note concludes: "I let her know that this was out of my price range and asked if there was anywhere I could get a three- or four-page summary of what dioxins were. She suggested that I could probably get something like that from Washington but that she didn't know whom I should contact there."

50 See, for example, Globe and Mail, 22 March 1996 (column by Cameron Smith) and 26 March (column by Terence Corcoran); Toronto Star, 4 March 1996, 2 (article by Paul Moloney).

51 Greenpeace, Polyvinyl Chloride (PVC) Plastic: Primary Contributor to the Global Dioxin Crisis, 3, is the source for the quotation. Alternatives are discussed in Alternatives to PVC Products and PVC at the Hospital: Use, Risks, and Alternatives in the Health Care Sector, both issued in 1995 by Greenpeace Austria.

52 An assortment of these materials was furnished to us by the Vinyl Council of Canada.

53 A leaflet prepared by Fisheries and Oceans Canada in March 1996 states that dioxins in B.C. coastal pulp mill effluents decreased by 94 per cent between 1989 and 1995.

54 Three points are relevant here: (a) The chemical industry – and later pulp and paper – have borne the brunt of the dioxins issue, and in response have made massive investments in new processes to reduce emissions; it is not widely known that other industrial sectors are implicated (see Rappe, "Sources and Environmental Concentrations of Dioxins and Related Compounds"), and to some extent they have been free riders so far as the public issue is concerned. (b) Currently there is a major initiative under way in Canada, known as ARET (Accelerated Reduction and Elimination of Toxics: see Environment Canada, Environmental Leaders 1) in which many companies from various sectors have agreed to substantial reductions of substances including dioxins. (c) The

point in the text to which this note refers is that the public communications from industry have been woefully inadequate for a long time, and still are so, even when there is "good news" to communicate.

55 The actual wording is as follows: Virtual elimination "means, in respect of a substance released into the environment as a result of human activity, the ultimate reduction of the quantity or concentration of the substance in the release below any measurable quantity or concentration that is at or approaching the level of quantification" (*Canadian Environmental Protection Act*, tabled in the House of Commons on 10 December 1996, section 64). Since dioxins are already classified as "toxic" under this act, the virtual elimination requirement pertains to these compounds. See generally Leiss, "Governance and the Environment." We believe that environmental organizations and others will interpret s.64 as a no-detectable-level action threshold. In January 1997 EPA's New England office announced a new "non-detectable" dioxin effluent limit for a pulp mill in Maine.

56 For the shellfish grounds see the two-pager by Fisheries and Oceans Canada, "Backgrounder: Dioxin/Furan Reductions and Coastal Fisheries Re-openings," 18 April 1996. The earliest technical document is: National Research Council of Canada, Associate Committee on Scientific Criteria for Environmental Quality, "Polychlorinated Dibenzo-*p*-dioxins." The most recent is "Priority Substances List Assessment Report No. 1" for PCDD/FS (1990), prepared by Environment Canada and Health Canada as a prelude to the making of regulations under the *Canadian Environmental Protection Act*.

57 Health Canada, *Dioxins and Furans*, 4.

58 Ever since the appearance of Dow's notorious "trace chemistries of fire" hypothesis in 1979, the chemical industry has maintained that combustion of all kinds, including natural occurrences such as forest fires, is the primary source of dioxin. See Rawls, "Dow Finds Support, Doubt for Dioxin Ideas," 23–8.

59 Zook and Rappe, "Environmental Sources, Distribution, and Fate of Polychlorinated Dibenzodioxins, Dibenzofurans, and Related Organochlorines"; cf. Brzuzy and Hites (1996); Thomas and Spiro (1996); and R. Duarte-Davidson *et al.* (1997). A recent (1996) review noted that there are natural sources but also that the "identified primary sources are mainly anthropogenic" (Rappe, "Environmental Concentrations of Dioxins," 1782).

60 Zook and Rappe, "Environmental Sources."

61 Environment Canada and Health Canada, *Priority Substances List Assessment Report No. 1*, 8. The CCREM pamphlet (above, note 47), p. 4, gives the ratio as 10,000 times less toxic.

62 Hayes, *Pesticides Studied in Man*, 484–8; the quotation is on p. 484.

CHAPTER FOUR

1 D. Waltner-Toews, *Food, Sex and Salmonella,* 175

2 R. Grover, "Boxed in at Jack-in-the-Box," 40.

3 T. Egan, "Tainted Hamburger Raises Doubts on Meat Safety," *New York Times,* 28 January 1993.

4 Griffin and Tauxe, *"Escherichia Coli."*

5 Riley *et al.* "Hemorrhagic Colitis," 681–5.

6 H. Lior, *"Escherichia Coli* O157:H7 and Verotoxigenic *Escherichia Coli* (VTEC)," 378–82.

7 P.M. Griffin, *"Escherichia Coli* O157:H7 and Other Enterohemorrhagic *Escherichia Coli";* L.K. Altman, "Studying the Puzzle of Tainted Hamburgers," *New York Times,* 9 February 1993, B5–B10.

8 E.C.D. Todd, "Costs of Foodborne Disease in Canada."

9 Council for Agricultural Science and Technology (CAST), *Foodborne Pathogens,* 87.

10 Todd, "Costs of Food-Borne Disease in United States."

11 T. Roberts, "Human Illness Costs of Food-Borne Bacteria. "

12 Todd, "Costs of Food-Borne Disease in United States."

13 Garthright *et al.,* "Intestinal Infectious Diseases."

14 T. Roberts and E. Van Ravenswaay, *The Economics of Food Safety,* 1–8.

15 I.D. Wolf, "Food Safety, 1991–2001," 64–70.

16 MacDonald *et al., "Escherichia Coli* O157:H7, an Emerging Gastrointestinal Pathogen," 3567–70; Remis *et al.,* "Sporadic Cases of Hemorrhagic Colitis Associated with *Escherichia Coli* O157:H7," 624–6.

17 L.K. Altman, "Studying the Puzzle of Tainted Hamburgers," *New York Times,* 9 February 1993, B5–B10.

18 D. Powell, "Hamburger Hell," *Globe and Mail,* 3 July 1993, D8.

19 American Meat Institute, "Fact Sheet: *E. coli* O157:H7, Microbiological Testing and Ground Beef," PR *Newswire,* 28 October 1994.

20 Riley *et al.* "Hemorrhagic Colitis Associated with a Rare *Escherichia Coli* Serotype," 681–5.

21 *New York Times* began on 8 October 1982, 13.

22 *New York Times,* 9 October 1982, 9.

23 L.W. Riley *et al.,* "Hemorrhagic Colitis," 681–5.

24 M.P. Doyle and J.L. Schoeni, "Survival and Growth Characteristics of *Escherichia Coli* Associated with Hemorrhagic Colitis," 855–6.

25 *Globe and Mail,* 4 October 1983, B9.

26 Neill has provided an overview of the major discoveries relating to *E. coli* O157:H7: Neill, *"E. Coli* O157:H7 Time Capsule: What Do We Know and When Did We Know It?" 374–7

27 M.B. Cohn and R.A. Giannella, "Hemorrhagic Colitis Associated with *Escherichia Coli."*

28 R.W. Johnson, "Microbial Food Safety," 1987; E.M. Foster, in "A Half Century of Food Microbiology," likewise identified *E. coli* O157:H7 as an emerging pathogen.

29 Genigeorgis, "Problems Associated with Perishable Processed Meats."

30 J.E. Line *et al.*, "Lethality of Heat to *Escherichia Coli* O157:H7: D-Value and Z-Value Determinations in Ground Beef," 762–6.

31 *New York Times*, 17 July 1985, III-12.

32 Waltner-Toews, *Food, Sex and Salmonella*.

33 *Globe and Mail*, 12 October 1985, A25.

34 *New York Times*, April 30, 1986, III-12; June 8, 1988, III-8.

35 *New York Times*, March 28, 1989, III-1.

36 *New York Times*, 18 September 1990, B11.

37 J.E. Foulke, "How to Outsmart Dangerous *E. Coli* Strain," 22.

38 Ibid.

39 U.S. Centers for Disease Control and Prevention, "Preliminary Report: Foodborne Outbreak of *Escherichia Coli* O157:H7 Infections from Hamburgers, Western United States," 85–7.

40 Foulke, "Dangerous *E. Coli* Strain," 22.

41 *New York Times*, 23 January 1993, A8; *Globe and Mail*, 29 January 1993, with an *Associated Press* [hereafter *AP*] wire story, A9.

42 *Globe and Mail*, 9 February 1993, A6.

43 "New Inspection Rules Planned," *New York Times*, 6 February 1993, A1.

44 "Clinton Proposes to Change the Way Meat Is Inspected," *New York Times*, 17 March 1993, A1.

45 C.O. Felix, "Outbreak Creates New Cooking Standard."

46 *AP*, 28 March 1993.

47 "Milk Blamed in Bacteria Case," *AP*, 21 April 1993; "Apple Cider Can Be Dangerous," *New York Times*, 5 May 1993; "Bacterial Outbreak," *AP*, 16 August 1993; and "Salami Recall," *AP*, 6 December 1994.

48 MacDonald and Osterholm, "Emergence of *Escherichia Coli* O157:H7," 2264.

49 Robert Greene, "Meat Safety," *AP*, 15 January 1994.

50 Ibid.

51 "Bad Bug," *AP*, 9 January 1994.

52 Ann O'Hanlon, "Changes Come Slowly in Meat Inspection; Proposal to Give USDA Recall Power Is Still on Its Way to Congress," *Washington Post*, 1 February 1994.

53 Carole Sugarman, "Espy Announces Quick Meat Bacteria Test; Industry, Consumer Groups Doubt Significant Progress Has Been Made," *Washington Post*, 26 August 1994.

54 For review, see A. Griffiths, "The Role of ATP Bioluminescence in the Food Industry."

55 "Personal Health," *New York Times*, 12 October 1994.

56 "Meat Safety," *AP*, 15 October 1994.

57 *PR Newswire*, 28 October 1994.

58 "What's for Dinner? Could Be Disease and Death," *PR Newswire*, 1 November 1994.

59 Marian Burros, "Food Industry Groups Sue to Stop Federal Testing of Ground Beef," *New York Times*, 3 November 1994, A14; "Testing Meat," *AP*, 29 October 1994.

60 "The Meat Industry's Bad Beef," *New York Times*, 20 November 1994, E-14.

61 "Salami Recall," *AP*, 6 December 1994.

62 Alexander *et al.*, "Commercially Distributed Dry-Cured Salami." "Deadly Bacteria Found in Salami," *New York Times*, 10 March 1995, A11.

63 "The Virulent *E. Coli* Bacteria Is Found in Salami," *New York Times*, 25 June 1995; see also K.A. Glass *et al.*, "Fate of *Escherichia Coli* 0157:H7."

64 "Meat Safety," *AP*, 14 January 1995; "U.S. Plans to Tighten Meat Testing," *New York Times*, 15 January 1995, Y12.

65 "*E. Coli* Infections More Common," *AP*, 8 June 1995.

66 "Let Them Eat Poison," *New York Times*, 3 July 1995, Y19; "Bad Meat and Politics," *New York Times*, 7 July 1995, A13; "Health and Safety Wars," *New York Times*, 10 July 1995, A11.

67 U.S. Centers for Disease Control and Prevention, 1995; "Illness Blamed on Rare *E. Coli*," *AP*, 13 July 1995.

68 "Clinton Mixes Microbiology, Politics," *UPI*, 15 July 1995.

69 "Meat Safety," *AP*, 18 July 1995.

70 "Earns – Foodmaker," *AP*, 2 August 1995.

71 Daniel Puzo, "On the Hamburger Trail: A Simple Burger? In the World of Fast Food, There's No Such Thing...," *Los Angeles Times*, 22 September 1994.

72 Ingersoll, B. "Meat, Poultry Regulations Issued by U.S.," *Wall Street Journal*, 8 July 1996.

73 Knutson, L. "Clinton – Meat Safety," *AP*, 7 July 1996.

74 "Upgrading the Safety of Meat," *New York Times* editorial, 9 July 1996.

75 "Poorly Fed Cattle May Harbor Bacteria," *Kitchener-Waterloo Record*, 1 June 1995, B7; "Study Identifies Deadly Bacteria on Dairy Farms," *Kitchener-Waterloo Record*, 3 March 1995, B7.

76 Freidman, 1996; Leiss and Chociolko, 1994, ch. 6.

77 J.E. Foulke, "How to Outsmart Dangerous *E. Coli* Strain," *FDA Consumer*, January/February 1994.

78 MacDonald and Osterholm, "Emergence of *Escherichia Coli* O157:H7," 2264.

79 See Covello, "The Perception of Technological Risks," 285–97, for a review of the psychological factors affecting public risk perception.

80 Personal communication, D. Powell.

81 Ibid.

82 "Growing Concerns and Recent Outbreaks Involving Non-O157:H7 Serotypes of Verotoxigenic *E. Coli.*" J. Johnson *et al.*, 1996, Food Protection 5910: 1112–22.

83 Wilson *et al.*, "Vero Cytogenic *Escherichia Coli* Infection in Dairy Farm Families," 1021–7.

CHAPTER FIVE

1 *Stern v. Dow Corning*, 1984. This unreported case is referred to by Rebecca Weisman in "Reforms in Medical Device Regulation: An Examination of the Silicone Gel Breast Implant Debacle," *Golden Gate University Law Review* 973, n. 66, 981. For an extensive discussion of Dow Corning's response to this award, see John A. Byrne, *Informed Consent*, chapter 6. Dow Corning appealed the decision, and while the appeal was pending, reached an out-of-court settlement with Maria Stern for an undisclosed sum, and an agreement that the internal Dow Corning memos used by the plaintiff to allege Dow Corning suppression and misrepresentation of risk information on the implants would remain secret. This agreement is considered by many commentators to be one of the most significant reasons why the *Stern* case was not followed by a flood of similar litigation against Dow Corning until nearly ten years later. Actually, the successful first lawsuit against Dow Corning came in 1977, when a Ohio woman, who claimed that her ruptured implants and subsequent operations had caused pain and suffering, received a $170,000 settlement from the company.

2 *Hopkins v. Dow Corning Corp.*, No. C-91–2132, 1991 U.S. Dist. LEXIS 8580 (N.D. Cal. May 27, 1992). Appellate court judgment (33 F. 3d 1116, 9th Cir. 1994).

3 Bryne, *Informed Consent*, 174.

4 It is estimated that over two million women in the United States, and over 100,000 in Canada, had silicone breast implants. Eighty per cent of these implants were for cosmetic reasons only – the other 20 per cent for breast reconstruction after surgery for cancer. The $4.5 billion (U.S.) global settlement later fell apart after Dow Corning's bankruptcy announcement and the realization that the number of potential claimants would far outstrip the funds remaining from the other manufacturers. A revised settlement by Judge Pointer applied only to Dow Corning's competitors and allowed lower settlement amounts for claimants, unless they were able to meet more stringent criteria for illness. It also allowed women to opt out of the settlement and sue the manufacturers directly.

5 "Supreme Court Upholds Award over Breast Implants," *Kitchener-Waterloo Record*, 22 December 1995, A6. The Supreme Court of Canada paved the way for liability claims against Dow Corning by upholding an award of $95,000 by a British Columbia court to Susan Hollis in *Hollis v. Dow Corning Corporation* (4 S.C.R. 634, 1995). The Canadian court ruled that Dow Corning had a "duty to warn" the medical community of the risks posed by the implants, risks of which it had been aware. See "Implant Makers Had 'Duty' to Warn," *Globe and Mail*, 22 December 1995, A1.

6 The first case won against Dow Chemical was *Mahlum v. Dow Chemical*, in Reno, NV, in 1995. An estimated 13,000 cases have been reported to be filed against Dow Chemical, many by women who were unable to share in the $4.5 billion global settlement due to Dow Corning's bankruptcy declaration.

7 Gabriel *et al.*, "Risk of Connective-Tissue Diseases and Other Disorders after Breast Implantation."

8 Angell, "Do Breast Implants Cause Systemic Disease?" 1748–9.

9 Angell, *Science on Trial.*

10 A second study at Brigham and Women's Hospital: Jorge Sanchez-Guerrero *et al.*, "Silicone Breast Implants and the Risk of Connective-Tissue Diseases and Symptoms," *New England Journal of Medicine* (June 22, 1995): 1666–70, examined the incidence of rheumatic disease among 121,700 American registered nurses from 1976–90. The use of breast implants among those with confirmed rheumatic disease was compared to use in a randomly selected age-matched control group. The authors "found no association between silicone breast implants and connective-tissue disease." Studies at the University of Michigan (1994) and John Hopkins Medical Institutions (1992) also found no evidence of a connection between implants or silicone and scleroderma. Studies carried out at the University of Toronto and other research institutions around the world have reached the same conclusions. For a summary and analysis of these studies, see Angell, *Science on Trial*, 100 ff.

11 *Daubert v. Merrell Dow Pharmaceuticals, Inc.* (113 S. Ct. 2786 [1993]).

12 Robert Scheer, "Breast Implant Hoax?" 232.

13 Michael Fumento, "A Confederacy of Boobs," 36–43.

14 Joe Nocera, "Fatal Litigation," *Fortune*, 16 October 1995, 60.

15 Jane E. Brody, "Simple Tests May Soon Identify Those at Risk for a Heart Attack," *New York Times*, 13 June 1995, C3.

16 Gina Kolata, "Why to Science, the Law's an Ass," *Globe and Mail*, 17 May 1995, A-10.

17 See Kathy McNamra-Meis, "It Seemed We Had It All Wrong," *Forbes*, Winter, 1996.

18 The Dow Corning implant case has been written up as a case study of unethical conduct in many business schools across North America, including the Harvard Business School. At a recent meeting of the Society of Business Ethics in Quebec City, several panelists in a discussion of the Dow Corning case indicated that the scientific evidence brought forward in the period since the 1995 bankruptcy declaration by the company requires a revision of this widespread ethical analysis of the case.

19 Hennekens *et al.*, "Self-reported Breast Implants and Connective-Tissue Diseases in Female Health Professionals," 616–21. This study of nearly 400,000 American women in the health professions included about eleven thousand with breast implants. The study has been questioned, however, because it did not attempt to verify the reported diagnoses by examining medical records. A second phase of the study will attempt to do this. See Angell, *Science on Trial*, 100.

20 Silverman *et al.*, "Reported Complications of Silicone Gel Breast Implants," 744–56. This study was conducted by the FDA.

21 Dow Corning's explanation of these studies was that they did not indicate immunological responses but only foreign body reaction and, in the case of the rat sarcomas, the tendency of rats to develop sarcomas in response to any irritant (Angell, *Science on Trial*, 58). See also Byrne, *Informed Consent*, 176–7.

22 Dow Corning's package insert for the Silastic MSI mammary implant, p. 8 (1991). Angell comments that "The company was right about the lack of evidence that implants were dangerous. But there was also little evidence that they were safe, because the manufacturers had not fulfilled their responsibility to look for it" (*Science on Trial*, 57).

23 Ibid.

24 R. Weisman, "Reforms in Medical Device Regulation," 973, 978, n. 35.

25 Byrne, *Informed Consent*, 74–6.

26 Dow Corning did issue some warnings about certain risks to the surgeons who implanted them. These included warnings about the risks of fibrous capsule formation as well as of the possibility of implant rupture during implantation, and recommendations of certain implantation techniques for prevention of such rupture. See "Dow Corning's Disclosure of Gel-Breast Implant Complications, 1960's – 1985," *Dow Corning Corporation and the Silicone Breast Implant Issue: Case Study Source Materials*, Dow Corning Canada, Inc. (1996). We are grateful to Dow Corning Canada for furnishing us with a collection of company documents.

27 See the FDA *Consumer*, 29 November, 1995, 11; Silverman *et al.*, "Reported Complications of Silicone Gel Breast Implants," 744–56; National Breast Implant Task Force, *NBITF News* 1, no. 1 (June–August 1986): 6; and Angell, *Science on Trial*, 42.

28 Robinson *et al.*, "Analysis of Explanted Silicone Implants," 6–7. A 1994
study of women who had their implants removed due to complications
or dissatisfaction with them, conducted at Toronto's Wellesley Hospital,
found that only 7 per cent of implants in place for five years or less
had ruptured. But of the implants in place for six to ten years, 59 per
cent were ruptured and another 10 per cent were leaking. Similar rates
were observed among even older implants. See also Peters *et al.*, "Factors Affecting the Rupture of Silicone-Gel Breast Implants," 449–51;
A.J. Park, J. Walsh, P.S.V. Reddy, V. Chetty, and A.C.H. Watson, "The
Detection of Breast Implant Rupture Using Ultrasound," 299–310;
Sherine E. Gabriel *et al.*, "Complications Leading to Surgery after Breast
Implantations," 677–82.

29 *Facts You Should Know about Your New Look,* Dow Corning brochure,
1970, 1972, 1976, 1980. However, the brochures added qualifying
statements to the effect that it was not possible to give an unequivocal
answer, given the limited time to observe implants to date. A 1996
"Implant Information Booklet" published by the company for women
who have had implant surgery makes the following statement: "Based
on examination of explants, some doctors have suggested a correlation
between an implant's age and the likelihood that it is ruptured or leaking. However, it is inappropriate to draw conclusions only on the status
of explanted implants" (25). And further, "It is impossible to predict
the life expectancy of an implanted mammary prosthesis" (35).

30 The memo suggests that this warning was issued as early as 1976 (Dow
Corning, "Dow Corning's Disclosure of Gel-Breast Implant Complications, 1960's – 1985," 4). It cites a series of brochures entitled "Suggested Surgical Procedures for Silastic Mammary Prosthesis" (Dow
Corning Corporation, 1976, 1979, 1981), which warns surgeons to
advise patients that "following implantation, abnormal squeezing or
trauma to the breasts could conceivably rupture the implant." It is not
clear that this warning referred to the closed capsulotomy technique
explicitly until 1983. Angell, in *Science on Trial,* 42, claims the warning
was issued in 1980.

31 *FDA Consumer,* 29 November 1995, 11.

32 Dow Corning, "Dow Corning's Disclosure," 1.

33 Bryne, *Informed Consent,* 87.

34 Angell, *Science on Trial,* 59.

35 Bryne, *Informed Consent,* 78.

36 Bryne, *Informed Consent,* 79.

37 Robertson and Bragley, "Toxicologic Studies," 100–3.

38 Bryne, *Informed Consent,* 103–4.

39 Ibid.

40 Tim Smart, "Breast Implants," 94.

41 Bryne, *Informed Consent*, 176–7.
42 "Detailed Background on 1970 Dog Study," *Dow Corning Corporation and the Silicone Breast Implant Issue: Case Study Source Materials*, 2–5.
43 In Europe the news of the court settlements against the manufacturers of implants on the basis of local and systemic health risks was widespread, forcing the regulators to decide whether to follow the lead of the FDA in removing them from their markets. Great Britain, for example, never did remove silicone implants from its market. Its Department of Health issued its own report in 1993 stating that it found no scientific reason for banning or limiting breast implants, and it reiterated this conclusion in 1994. The French have imposed bans, lifted them, and imposed them again, seemingly unable to decide. Spain at first imposed a ban and then lifted it (Angell, *Science on Trial*, 201). So the implants have remained on the market in many countries, despite widespread controversy about the known and alleged risks elsewhere. Further, the silicone implants have now been replaced in the North American market by saline filled implants, which produce nearly the same local complications (capsular contracture, with its associated problems – pain, desensitization, and malformation, as well as rupture risk). These risks are now well known but have not significantly inhibited the acceptance of the new product in the market.
44 Byrne, in *Informed Consent*, chapter 8, recounts an attempt by senior D-C management in 1990 to suppress internal information indicating much higher levels of risk from breast implants than the company was admitting it knew about to the public, the Congress, and the FDA. Robert Rylee, vice-president and general manager of the health-care business, and the person who was representing D-C to the public on the implant safety issue, had demanded that a memo written by a D-C research scientist, reporting on an independent study indicating much higher rates of complication with the implant than D-C was admitting publicly, be destroyed (125–7). The scientist's superior objected that this was unethical conduct, and brought it to the attention of John Swanson, chair of the Business Conduct Committee.
45 Mr Justice J.C. Major, speaking notes (9 November 1996); see the article by Susan Lightstone, *Globe and Mail*, 20 December 1996, B6.
46 See W. Leiss, "On the Vitality of Our Discipline."
47 Thomas M. Burton, "Dow Corning Proposes $3-Billion Reorganization" (article reprinted from the *Wall Street Journal*), *Globe and Mail*, 3 December 1996; "Breast-Implant Cases: Let the Science Decide," *Business Week*, 16 December 1996; Burton, "Creditors Propose Getting Stake in Dow Corning" (article reprinted from the *Wall Street Journal*), *Globe and Mail*, 18 December 1996; Gina Kolata, "Judge Rules Breast Implant Evidence Invalid," *New York Times*, 19 December 1996.

CHAPTER SIX

1 Cancer Prevention Coalition, Food and Water, news conference, National Press Club, Washington, DC, 23 January 1996.
2 *International Journal of Health,* January 1996.
3 D. Nelkin, *Forms of Intrusion,* 379–90.
4 Burton *et al.,* "A Review of Bovine Growth Hormone," *Canadian Journal of Animal Science* 74 (1994): 167–201; U.S. Executive Branch of the Federal Government, *Use of Bovine Somatotropin (BST) in the United States: Its Potential Effects,* Washington, D.C., 1994.
5 D.E. Bauman, "Bovine Somatotropin: Review of an Emerging Animal Technology," *Journal of Dairy Science* 75 (1992): 3432–51.
6 Ibid.
7 Ibid.
8 Ibid.
9 J.C. Juskevich and C.G. Guyer, "Bovine Growth Hormone: Human Food Safety Evaluation," *Science* 249: 875–84.
10 W.H. Daughaday and D.M. Barbano, "Bovine Somatotropin Supplementation of Dairy Cows," *Journal of the American Medical Association,* 22 August 1990, 1003–5, 1028.
11 Editorial, *JAMA,* 22 August 1990.
12 U.S. National Institutes of Health, *Technology Assessment Conference Statement on Bovine Somatotropin,* Department of Human Health and Services, Bethesda, MD, 1990.
13 Smith and Warland, "Consumer Responses to Milk from BST-Supplemented Cows," 243–64.
14 A 1990 study for the U.S. National Dairy Board estimated that 20 per cent of 592 survey participants would reduce or completely eliminate milk and dairy product purchases after hearing anti-rBST messages.
15 Hoban *et al.,* "Consumer Attitudes," 15.
16 Harlander, Land 'O Lakes, personal communication, 1994.
17 B. Zechendorf, "What the Public Thinks about Biotechnology," 870–5.
18 Optima Consultants, *Understanding the Consumer Interest in the New Biotechnology Industry,* 35.
19 CCGD, "Trends in Canada: Survey on Consumer Shopping," 55.
20 Statistics Canada, 1994 (citation).
21 Creative Research International, *Consumer Environment Study,* 22.
22 "Heavy Meat Diet Is Costing Billions," *Victoria Times Colonist,* 18 March 1996, C3.
23 Ibid.
24 Kathleen Day, "Experimental Journey: Biotech Firms Face an Uphill Struggle for Funding, Findings and Survival," *Washington Post,* 27 March 1995.

25 *NewYork Times,* 16 March 1981, IV, 5.

26 *New York Times* 19 October 1985, I, 29.

27 *New York Times,* 28 October 1985.

28 *New York Times,* 29 April 29 1989, I, 1.

29 *New York Times,* May 5, 1989.

30 *New York Times,* 25 March 1990.

31 *New York Times,* 1 May 1990.

32 *New York Times,* 4 December 1990

33 A. Gibbons, "NIH Panel: Bovine Hormone Gets Nod," 1506.

34 *New York Times,* 11 August 1992.

35 Sarah Muirhead, "BST Use in Pastoral Systems Possible with Good Management," *Feedstuffs,* 12 December 1994; Jane Fyksen, "Feeding Skills, BGH Boost Production Averages of Top Herds," *AgriView,* 27 January 1995; Jeff DeYoung, "Management-Intensive Grazing Takes Planning," *Iowa Farmer Today,* 4 February 1995.

36 *Associated Press,* 9 November 1993.

37 "Welcome High Tech Milk," *USA Today,* 10 November 1993.

38 Philip Elmer-Dewitt, "Brave New World of Milk," *Time,* 10 February 1994.

39 "Crack for Cows," an alert issued by Rifkin's Foundation on Economic Trends.

40 Tracy Connor, "Protesters Step up Attack against 'Bionic Milk,'" *UPI,* 10 February 1994.

41 "Speaking for an Industry," *World of Ingredients,* November 1993, 26–7.

42 Robert Greene, "Milk Hormone," *AP,* 8 February 1994.

43 "The Milk Brouhaha," *New York Times,* 10 February 1994.

44 Marian Burros, "The Debate over Milk and an Artificial Hormone," *New York Times,* 18 May 1994, B1.

45 Keith Schneider, "Despite critics, farmers increase use of a growth hormone in cows," *New York Times,* 30 October 1994.

46 "FDA Finds No Unusual Problems with Milk Production Drug," *AP,* 16 March 1995.

47 *Globe and Mail,* 7 April 1981, B13.

48 "Shot Raises Milk Output up to 25%," *Globe and Mail,* 25 February 1985, B16.

49 "Hormone Use Shaking Milk Industry," *Globe and Mail,* 14 August 1986, B1.

50 "Milk of Human Genetics," *Globe and Mail,* 8 May 1989, A6.

51 Robert Kozak, "Hormone May Aid Creation of Barnyard Hulk Hogans," *Globe and Mail,* 7 October 1987, B14.

52 Burton *et al.,* "A Review of Bovine Growth Hormone," 167–201.

53 "Pfizer's Genetically Engineered Food Additive Hits Market, First in U.S.," *Globe and Mail,* 27 March 1990, B12.

54 Mary Gooderham, "Battle Lines Drawn over Bovine Hormone," *Globe and Mail,* 17 April 1993, A4.

55 Mary Gooderham, personal communication, 20 April 1993.

56 Jim Romahn, "BST Information Kit Planned," 3 May 1993, *Kitchener-Waterloo Record,* B5.

57 December 1993, *Kitchener-Waterloo Record.*

58 Jim Romahn, "Growth Hormone Decision Delayed," *Kitchener-Waterloo Record,* 15 December 1993.

59 "Farm Industry Faces Hard Sell on Hormone," *Canadian Press, Kitchener-Waterloo Record,* 28 December 1993.

60 NDC and Dairy Farmers of Canada, staff members, personal communication, 13 February 1995.

61 Keith Ashdown, the Canadian coordinator of the Pure Food Campaign, quoted in "Debate over Milk Hormone Heats Up," Mary Gooderham, *Globe and Mail,* 14 February 1994.

62 The original application had been submitted by Monsanto Canada in 1990.

63 Peter Tabuns, Toronto Board of Health chairman, personal communication, 20 March 1994.

64 Patrick Gallagher, "Ontario Farmer Dairy Council Wants Delay on BST," *Ontario Farmer,* 15 December 1993.

65 The Canadian federal agriculture committee held public hearings on rBST and subsequently passed a resolution asking Cabinet to delay the use of rBST, "to allow public fears about the hormone to be addressed" (18 March 1994).

66 Alex Boston, Council of Canadians, personal communication, 17 August 1994.

67 David Nattress, former director of the animal science division, Monsanto Canada, personal communication, 13 December 1994.

68 *Canadian Press,* 3 March 1994.

69 Mike Strathdee, "Consumer Fears of Milk Hormone Overestimated, Researcher Feels," *Kitchener-Waterloo Record,* 15 November 1994, B6.

70 Strathdee, "Customs Won't Prevent Farmers from Buying Cow Hormone in U.S.," *Kitchener-Waterloo Record,* 20 May 1995, B8.

71 "Milk Study Wary," *Globe and Mail,* 11 May 95, A2; Larry Johnsrude, "Little Benefit in Milk Hormone," *Kitchener-Waterloo Record,* 11 May 95, B12.

72 rBST Task Force, "Review of the Potential Impact of Recombinant Bovine Somatotropin (rBST) in Canada," Ottawa, 1995.

73 Larry Johnsrude, "Controversy over Supercharged Cows Still Not Settled," *Canadian Press,* 12 May 1995.

74 Laura Rance, "Consumers Don't Want BST," *Manitoba Co-operator,* 8 June 1995.

75 "Dairy-Rhetoric Mounts as rbst Decision Nears," *Farm & Country*, 20 June 1995.

76 "Milk Hormone Battle about to Heat Up," *Globe and Mail*, 22 June 1995, A10.

77 "Drug Firms Upset about Expected Ban," *Globe and Mail*, 27 June 1995, B7.

78 *Vancouver Province*, 26 June 1995.

79 For example, see D.W. Hecht, "Bovine Somatotropin Safety and Effectiveness," 120–6.

80 "Another Special View," *Manitoba Co-operator*, 13 July 1995.

81 *Globe and Mail*, 13 July 1995, A13.

82 For privacy reasons Groenewegen's phone number is excluded.

83 Paul Groenewegen, personal communication, 22 February 1996.

84 *Rachel's Environment and Health Weekly* 454, Annapolis: Environmental Research Foundation, 10 August 1995.

85 Deborah Pearce, "Suspect Stimulant May Lurk in Milk," *Victoria Times Colonist*, 12 September 1995, A1.

86 *Ecologist*, September/October 1989.

87 A. Levitt, "The Flap Over Bovine Growth Hormone," 21.

88 "Dairy Coalition Statement Regarding Samuel Epstein's News Conference," *PR Newswire*, 23 January 1996.

89 Dennis Bueckert, "Study Says Cow Hormone May Raise Cancer Risk for Humans," *Canadian Press*, 23 January 1996

90 *CJAD News*, Montreal, 23 January 1996; *CHFI-FM News*, Toronto, 24 January, 1996; *CJRN News*, Niagara Falls, 23 January 1996.

91 "Consumer Groups Urge Officials to Heed Research on bst," *Montreal Gazette*, 12 February 1996, A8; for example, "Cow Hormone Tied to Cancer," *Calgary Herald*, 12 February 1996, A4; "Growth Hormone Warning Raised," *Windsor Star*, 12 February 1996, A2.

92 Mike Strathdee, "Delay Won't End Lobbying on Milk Hormone, Activists Say," *Kitchener-Waterloo Record*, 30 September 1995, B12.

93 Jim Romahn, "Requests for Animal Health Data Will Delay bst a Year," *Ontario Farmer*, 10 October 1995.

94 *Manitoba Co-operator*, 8 February 1996.

95 *Ottawa Citizen*, 19 June 1995.

96 *Western Producer*, 22 June 1995.

97 Barry Wilson, "Both Sides Bare Teeth as bst Decision Nears," *Western Producer*, 29 June 1995.

98 Leiss and Chociolko, *Risk and Responsibility*.

99 Health Canada public affairs office, personal communication, September 1992.

100 "Milk Lobbyists Fear Hormone Will Scare off Consumers," *Kitchener-Waterloo Record*, 9 March 1994, B7.

101 Franklin Loew, dean of Tufts University's School of Veterinary Medicine, in *Boston Globe*, 10 October 1989.

102 Peter Morton, "Milk-Tariff Panel Appointed after Six Months of Haggling," *Financial Post*, 23 January 1996, 3.

103 "A Scientific Case for BGH," *Wisconsin State Journal*, 12 May 1991.

104 R.D. Yonkers, "Potential Adoption and Diffusion of BST among Diary Farmers," 177–92.

105 Susan Semenak, "Stirring up Fears of Spiked Milk; Nothing Wholesome about BST: Critics," *Montreal Gazette*, 13 May 1995, A1.

106 D. Nelkin, "Forms of Intrusion," 379–90.

107 Burton and McBride, "Is There a Limit for Biotechnology?"

108 Powell, personal communication, 18 December 1996.

109 N. Ball, "Essential Connections," 11–28.

CHAPTER SEVEN

1 W.J. Hayes, *Pesticides Studied in Man*, 172–264.

2 House of Commons, Standing Committee on Environment and Sustainable Development, *It's about Our Health!*

3 Durant, *Biotechnology in Public*.

4 90/220/EEC: Directive on the Deliberate Release into the Environment of Genetically Modified Organisms.

5 Science Council, 1980.

6 B. Davis, *Genetic Revolution*; Sheldon Krimsky, *Biotechnics and Society*.

7 Agriculture and Agri-food Canada, "Field Trial," http://aceis.agr.ca/fpi/agbiotec/fieldt96.html. Accessed 4 January 1997.

8 Greenpeace, *Environmental Risks*.

9 H. Hobbelink, *Biotechnology and the Future of World Agriculture*; M. Kenney, "University in the Information Age," 60–7.

10 Rural Advancement Fund International communique, January/February 1994.

11 "Canola Genes," *Globe and Mail*, 6 April 1995, A1.

12 Agriculture Canada, *Environmental Sustainability*; OECD, "Biotechnology, Agriculture and Food, 4–8"; UNCED, *UN Conference on Environment and Development*.

13 A. Griffiths, "Implementation of Biotechnology Research and Development Policy."

14 Leiss, "Biotechnology in Canada Today."

15 See generally Limoges *et al.* (1993). The discussion that follows may be compared with chapters 2 and 3 in Krimsky and Wrubel, *Agricultural Biotechnology and the Environment*, which we saw after we had completed the research for this chapter; the entire volume is an outstanding discussion of biotechnology issues.

16 Statistics Canada, *Cereals and Oilseeds Review.*

17 Canola Council of Canada, *The Canola Growers Manual;* Griffiths, "Biotechnology Research and Development Policy."

18 Ollsen (1955) in Scheffler *et al.*, "Frequency and Distance of Pollen Dispersal," 356–64; Eckert, "The Flight Range of the Honeybee," 257–85.

19 N.C. Ellstrand, "Pollen As a Vehicle for the Escape of Engineered Genes?"s30–2.

20 Mikkelson *et al.*, "The Risk of Crop Transgene Spread," 31; *rapa* is the name by which *campestris* is now known.

21 Science Council, *Biotechnology in Canada.*

22 Interview with M. Kenny and others, 10 September 1996.

23 AFFC, *Workshop on Food Biotechnology: An Information Session to Increase Awareness of Food Biotechnology within Agriculture Canada,* 3.

24 This quote is interesting in light of the assertion by the current head of BSCO, cited above (note 22), that its mandate does not encompass the promotion of biotechnology.

25 AAFC, *Biology of Brassica Napus L. (Canola),* Regulatory Directive 94-09 (1994).

26 C. Frankton and G.A. Mulligan, *Weeds of Canada,* 2.

27 Griffiths, "Implementation of Biotechnology Research and Development Policy"; Klein *et al.*, "Farmer Acceptance of Biotechnology," 71–88.

28 AAFC, "All about Canada's Vegetable Industry"; Boiteau and LeBlanc, *Colorado Potato Beetle Life Stages.*

29 Rachel Carson, *Silent Spring,* 209; R.J. Milner, *History of Bacillus Thuringiensis,* 9–13; I. Watkinson, "Global View of Present and Future Markets for Bt Products," 3–7.

30 McGaughey and Whalon, "Managing Insect Resistance to Bacillus Thuringiensis Toxins," 145–5.

31 Ibid.

32 AAFC, *Determination of Environmental Safety of NatureMarks Potatoes.*

33 McGaughey, "Insect Resistance to Bacillus Thuringiensis Toxins," 193–5.

34 See H.D. Burges, "Possibilities for Pest Resistance to Microbial Control Agents," 445–57.

35 For both of these points see D.N. Ferro, "Potential for Resistance to Bacillus Thuringiensis," 38–44.

36 McGaughey, "Insect Resistance to the Biological Insecticide Bacillus Thuringiensis," 193–5.

37 D.L. Miller *et al.*, "Development of a Strain of Potato Beetle Resistant to the Delta-Endotoxin, 25."

38 Whalon *et al.*, "Selection of a Colorado Potato Beetle," 226–33.

39 Ferro, "Potential for Resistance to Bacillus Thuringiensis," 38–44; McGaughey and Whalon, "Insect Resistance to Bacillus Thuringiensis Toxins," 145–5; McGaughey, "Problems of Insect Resistance to Bacillus

Thuringiensis," 95–102; Rahardja and Whalon, "Inheritance of Resistance," 22–6; Whalon *et al.*, "Selection of a Colorado Potato Beetle," 226–33.

40 Doug Saunders, "Genetically Altered Spud to Go on Sale in Spring," *Globe and Mail,* 26 January 1996, A1.

41 Anne Reifenberg and Rhonda L. Rundle, "Buggy Cotton May Cast Doubt on New Seeds," *Wall Street Journal,* 23 July 1996; Tim Beardsley, "Picking on Cotton," *Scientific American,* October 1996, 275, no. 4, 45. In this coverage one can find many references to the disparity between the careful statements in the company's technical documents and the unqualified enthusiasms in the media-based product advertisements.

42 Barnaby J. Feder, "Geneticists Arm Corn against Corn Borer but Pest May Still Win," *New York Times,* 23 July 1996.

43 *Information Systems for Biotechnology (ISB) News Report,* "Report from Bt Forum"; Nora Macaluso, "Bug Develops in Insect War: Resistance to Bacterium Targeted," *Bloomberg Business News,* 17 April 1996.

44 R. Bud, *The Uses of Life.*

45 Article: See D.E. Albrecht, *Public Perceptions of Agricultural Biotechnology,* chapters: U. Fleising, "Public Perceptions of Biotechnology," in *Biotechnology: The Science and the Business,* ed. V. Moses and R.E. Cape, 89–102; conferences: W.S. Burke (ed.) *Symbol, Substance, Science,* 28–29 June 1993; *A New Paradigm for Food, the Farm, and the Public,* 10–11 June 1993; MacDonald, J.F. (ed.), *Agricultural Biotechnology* 1993; D. Cabirac and R. Warmbrodt, *Biotechnology: Public Perception:* January 1985– December 1992; studies: Lacy *et al.*, "Public Perceptions of Agricultural Biotechnology," in *Agricultural Biotechnology: Issues and Choices,* ed. B.R. Baumgardt and M.A. Martin; R. Kemp, "Social Implications and Public Confidence," in *The Release of Genetically Modified Microorganisms,* ed. D.E.S. Stewart-Tull and M. Sussman; books: L.R. Batra and W. Klassen, *Public Perceptions of Biotechnology.* An entire website is devoted to public perceptions of biotechnology: C. Hagedorn and S. Allender-Hagedorn, "Public Perceptions in Agricultural and Environmental Biotechnology: A Study of Public Concerns" (http://fbox.vt.edu:10021/cals/cses/chagedor/index.html).

46 There have been many surveys of public perception of biotechnology: W.K. Hallman and J. Metcalfe, *Public Perceptions of Agricultural Biotechnology: A Survey of New Jersey Residents;* T.J. Hoban and P.A. Kendall, *Consumer Attitudes about the Use of Biotechnology in Agriculture and Food Production;* J.D. Miller, *The Public Understanding of Science and Technology in the United States;* Hoban, *Agricultural Biotechnology: Public Attitudes and Educational Needs;* R.J. Berrier, "Public Perceptions of Biotechnology," in *Public Perceptions of Biotechnology,* ed. R. Batra and W. Klassen; Russell *et al.*, *The Novo Report;* U.S. Office of Technology Assessment, *New Developments in*

Biotechnology: Public Perceptions of Biotechnology, P. Lasley and G. Bultena, "Farmers' Opinions about Third-Wave Technologies," 122–6. For a review, see Zechendorf, "What the Public Thinks about Biotechnology," 870–5.

47 See P. Sparks and R. Shepherd, "Public Perceptions of the Potential Hazards Associated with Food Production," 799–806; Sparks *et al.*, "Gene Technology, Food Production and Public Opinion," 19–28.

48 J. Kelley, "Public Perceptions of Genetic Engineering." Several such surveys also were conducted in Canada: Powell and Griffiths, "Public Perceptions of Agricultural Biotechnology in Canada," and Optima Consultants, *Understanding the Consumer Interest in the New Biotechnology Industry.* Other regular surveys now include questions about biotechnology: e.g., Angus Reid Group, *Public Opinion on Food Safety and Biotechnology Applications in Agriculture;* CCGD, *Trends in Canada: Survey on Consumer Shopping.*

49 Hagedorn and Allender-Hagedorn, "Public Perceptions in Agricultural and Environmental Biotechnology."

50 R. Kemp, "Social Implications and Public Confidence," 99–114; Lacy *et al.*, "Public Perceptions of Agricultural Biotechnology," 139–61; McCabe and Fitzgerald, "Media Images of Environmental Biotechnology," 15–24; J.D. Miller, *The Public Understanding of Science and Technology in the United States.*

51 K. Hopkins, "Improving the Public Understanding of Science and Technology."

52 A. Lippman and P.L. Bereano, "Genetic Engineering: Cause for Caution," opinion page, *Globe and Mail,* 25 June 1993.

53 D.T. Dennis, "Canada Has a Stake in Designing a Better Tomato," opinion page, *Globe and Mail,* 4 May 1993.

54 Weart, *Nuclear Fear.*

55 A. Dubey, "Research Skewed," opinion page, *Kitchener-Waterloo Record,* 29 May 1933; M. Murray, "How to Build a Better Potato Chip," *Toronto Star,* 11 May 1993; D. Powell, "Invasion of the Mutant Tomatoes," *Globe and Mail,* 12 September 1992.

56 "Coffee Hottest Buzzword on Last Year's Food Scene," *Toronto Star,* 1 January 1997, B1.

57 Barnaby J. Feder, "Monsanto Chooses a Spinoff of Its Chemical Operations," 10 December 1996, *New York Times,* C4; Debora MacKenzie, "Europe Lets in American Supermaize," *New Scientist,* 4 January 97; "Greenpeace Stops Rhine Ship Bringing Soya to Swiss," *Reuters,* 12 December 1996; "Label Altered Food," *Calgary Herald,* 25 November 1996, A7.

58 David Graham, "Altering Food Called 'Dangerous Experiment,'" *Toronto Star,* 20 November 1996, E1.

59 Edmonds Institute, *The Puget Sound Workshop Biosafety Handbook*; PEER, *Genetic Genie*.

60 "1996 Risk Assessment Grants Announced," August 1996; *ISB News Report*. The Eighth Symposium on Environmental Releases of Biotechnology Products was held in June 1996 in Ottawa, Canada, where an estimated 250 participants heard data from research on the risks of biotechnology (C. Neal Stewart, Jr, "Risk Assessment of Transgenic Plants: Going beyond the Crossroads," *ISB News Report*, August 1996.)

61 P. Thompson, "Food Labels and Biotechnology."

62 *New York Times*, 31 July 1961, 18.

63 S. Hornig, "Reading Risk."

64 S. Priest, "Information Equity."

65 Simon Barber, personal communication, 10 September 1996.

66 Dittus and Hillers, "Consumer Trust and Behavior Related to Pesticides," 87–9.

67 E.O. van Ravenswaay, "Public Perceptions of Agrichemicals."

68 Frewer *et al.*, "What Determines Trust in Information about Food-Related Risks?" 473–86.

69 The characteristics of modernization risks have been discussed at length by authors such as Ulrich Beck and Anthony Giddens.

70 The three levels of uncertainty are adapted from S.O. Funtowicz and J.R. Ravetz, "Uncertainty, Complexity and Post-Normal Science," 1881–5.

71 This point is elaborated upon in chapter 7 and the references cited therein.

72 B. Wynne, "Uncertainty and Environmental Learning," 111–27.

CHAPTER EIGHT

1 Canadian Council of Resource and Environment Ministers (CCREM), *The PCB Story*.

2 Transformers convert electricity from one voltage to another, a process that creates a lot of heat. Capacitors stabilize disruptive variations in electric current to allow for the more efficient and economical use of electrical power. Capacitors can be found in large electrical generators as well as in fluorescent lamps and street lights. Many transformers and most capacitors manufactured between 1929 and 1978 used PCBs as an insulator and to prevent overheating (CCREM, *The PCB Story*, 24). PCBs were also an ideal fluid for heat exchange systems, many of which have been specifically designed around the use of PCBs (Burger, "A Case Study"). Heat exchange devices are used to "pasteurize" food material and, in the petroleum industry, to keep crude oil in a state of low viscosity to facilitate transportation. The 6,800 litres of askarel contained in the heating system of the Irving Whale recently salvaged from the bottom

of the Gulf of St Lawrence, for instance, served to keep four thousand
tonnes of bunker C oil from congealing.

3 Environment Canada, *PCBs: Question and Answer Guide.*
4 Goldman, "Controlling PCBs."
5 "Report of a New Chemical Hazard," 15 December 1966, *New Scientist,*
612; and Jensen, "The PCB Story," 123–31.
6 See National Swedish Environment Protection Board, *PCB Conference;*
Interdepartmental Task Force on PCBs, *Polychlorinated Biphenyls and the
Environment;* National Institute of Environmental Health Sciences "Meeting on Polychlorinated Biphenyls (PCBs)"; Selikoff, "Polychlorinated
Biphenyls – Environmental Impact." For a detailed chronology of the
United States' regulatory response to the PCB threat between 1970 and
1972, see Burger, "A Case Study," 187–201.
7 Burger, "A Case Study."
8 Safe, "PCBs and Human Health."
9 Burger, "Health As a Surrogate for the Environment," 133–53.
10 Barrie *et al.,* "Arctic Contaminants."
11 Organization for Economic Co-operation and Development (OECD),
PCB Seminar.
12 World Health Organization (WHO), *Polychlorinated Biphenyls and Terphenyls.*
13 Environment Canada, *Options for the Treatment.*
14 Environment Canada, *National Inventory of PCBs.*
15 In the following two weeks, more than one hundred articles appeared
in the press on the subject. See, for instance: "Deadly Spill in Kenora,"
Winnipeg Free Press, 14 April 1985, 1; "PCB Spill Sparks Cross-Country
Controversy," *Vancouver Sun,* 20 April 1985, B3; "The Big PCB Scare: A
Chain of Destruction," *Toronto Star,* 20 April 1985, A5; "Nordair Cargo
Workers Upset about PCBs," *Halifax Chronicle Herald,* 22 April 1985, 5;
"Truck Carrying PCBs Heads for Alberta Escorted by RCMP," *Globe and
Mail,* 24 April 1985, M6; "Spilling Dread on Highway 1," *Alberta Report,*
29 April 1985, 15; and "Politicians Scramble for Cover after PCB Spill,"
Montreal Gazette, 1 May 1985, B3.
16 For a sample of the press coverage of the incident, see "Properties of
PCBs Like Jekyll and Hyde," *Montreal Gazette,* 25 August 1988, and "How
a Toxic Firestorm Is Terrifying the Residents of a Quebec Town,"
Maclean's, 5 September 1988, 41. The latter refers to PCBs as "substances
that can cause several types of cancer, liver disorders, spontaneous abor-
tions and birth defects." For a critical evaluation of journalists' characterization of the risks posed by the fire, see "PCB Risk Was Exaggerated,
Some Scientists Say," *Montreal Gazette,* 3 September 1988, A7, and "For-
getting the Facts," *Content,* Nov-Dec. 1989, 17–18. See also "Ottawa Plays
Catch-up As PCB Worry Spreads," *Calgary Herald,* 3 September 1988, A5,

and "Opening Eyes to Pollution: Lobbyists Have Made the Environment the Top Issue in the Polls," *Globe and Mail*, 3 September 1988, D2. For an in-depth analysis of the organizational factors that led to a communication breakdown between government offficials, scientific experts, and the lay public, see Hélène Denis, *La gestion de la catastrophe: Le cas d'un incendie à St-Basile-le-Grand.* The detailed account of the toxicological investigation and public health monitoring of the incident are available in Stéphane Groulx, *Le suivi et la surveillance de la santé humaine après l'incendie de biphényles polychlorés (*BPC*) de St-Basile-le-Grand.* Rapport synthèse du Réseau de la Santé et des Services Sociaux du Québec, Département de Santé Communautaire, Hôpital Charles Lemoyne, 1992.

17 See "Shipping PCBs to Wales Decried," *Globe and Mail*, 2 August 1989, A2; "Canada Taking Heat for PCB Shipment," *Calgary Herald*, 13 August 1989, C6; "Not in Our Backyard, You Don't," *Montreal Gazette*, 20 August 1989, A5; "Residents Keep Vigil over PCBs to Prevent Removal from Dock," *Globe and Mail*, 25 August 1989, A5; and "Police Crash through PCB Protest," *Montreal Gazette*, 30 August 1989, A1.

18 The significance of the Kenora, St-Basile, and Baie Comeau incidents can be assessed by the amount of press coverage these episodes generated. A search for press reports on PCBs in Canadian data bases for the years 1985, 1988, and 1989 yielded a total of approximately 330, 400, and 535 articles respectively. (The data bases searched – *Canadian Business and Current Affairs, Canadian Periodical Index, Actualité Québec,* and *Repères* – include articles in both English and French languages.) In contrast, the number of entries found in bordering years was much lower: 1984 (25 articles), 1986 (45), 1987 (40), and 1990 (92). For the years 1991, 1992, and 1993, the number of entries was 43, 62, and 67 respectively, testifying to a steady level of audience interest in PCB-related stories. The higher number of press articles found in 1994 (114) results mostly from a PCB fire in Nova Scotia, use of the Swan Hills facility for the destruction of non-Alberta PCBs, and a series of public hearings initiated by the Quebec government to site a mobile incinerator in that province. The controversy over the marine salvage of the Irving Whale accounted for a further increase in the number of PCB articles published in 1995 (150). The actual lifting of the Whale, problems plaguing PCB disposal facilities in Quebec and Alberta, and proposed modifications to PCB export regulations all contributed to the high number of press reports on PCBs (200) again in 1996.

19 Parkinson *et al.*, "Toxic Effects of PCBs," 49–75.

20 Selikoff, "Polychlorinated Biphenyls – Environmental Impact," 249–362; Jensen, "Background Levels in Humans," 345–80; Skerfving *et al.*, "Exposure to Mixtures and Congeners of Polychlorinated Biphenyls," 1409–15.

21 Parkinson and Safe, "Mammalian Biologic and Toxic Effects of PCBs."

22 Most PCB mixtures have much lower toxicities than dioxins (PCDDs) and furans (PCDFs); in short-term toxicity tests, however, a few individual co-planar PCB congeners have toxic potencies up to 10 per cent of that of TCDD. However, because of species differences and additive and antagonistic interactions observed with PCB mixtures, "considerable caution" must be exerted in using this approach to predict the toxicity of PCBs (Safe, "Polychlorinated Biphenyls: Environmental Impact.")

23 Hayes, "Carcinogenic and Mutagenic Effects of PCBs"; Abelson, "Excessive Fear of PCBs," 361.

24 Idler, *PCBS: The Current Situation*; Kimbrough, "Polychlorinated Biphenyls (PCBs) and Human Health."

25 Parkinson and Safe, "Mammalian Biologic and Toxic Effects of PCBs"; World Health Organization (WHO), *Polychlorinated Biphenyls and Terphenyls.*

26 Kimbrough *et al.*, "Induction of Liver Tumors in Sherman Strain Female Rats by Polychlorinated Biphenyl Arochlor 1260"; Norback *et al.*, "Hepatocellular Carcinoma in the Sprague-Dawley Rat," 97–105.

27 Hayes, "Carcinogenic and Mutagenic Effects of PCBs," 77–95; World Health Organization (WHO), *Polychlorinated Biphenyls and Terphenyls*; Comité de Santé Environnementale (CSE), *L'Oncogénèse environnementale au Québec.*

28 Jacobson *et al.*, "Effects of Exposure to PCBs," 319–26; Rogan and Gladen, "PCBs, DDE and Child Development," 407–15.

29 Kimbrough, "Polychlorinated Biphenyls (PCBs) and Human Health."

30 Idler, *PCBs: The Current Situation*; Health and Welfare Canada, *PCBs,* 59–64; Comité de Santé Environnementale (CSE), *L'Oncogénèse environnementale au Québec*; Kimbrough, "The Human Health Effects of Polychlorinated Biphenyls," 211–28; Kimbrough, "Polychlorinated Biphenyls (PCBs) and Human Health."

31 World Health Organization (WHO), *Polychlorinated Biphenyls and Terphenyls.*

32 WHO, ibid.; Safe, "PCBs and Human Health," 133–45; Kimbrough, "The Human Health Effects of Polychlorinated Biphenyls"; Comité de Santé Environnementale (CSE), *L'Oncogénèse environnementale au Québec*; E. Dewailly *et al.*, "Polychlorinated Biphenyl (PCB) and Dichlorodiphenyl Dichloroethylene (DDE) Concentrations in the Breast Milk of Women in Quebec."

33 Jensen, "Background Levels in Humans," 345–80; Mes *et al.*, "Specific Polychlorinated Biphenyl Congener Distribution in Breast Milk of Canadian Women."

34 Strachan, *Polychlorinated Biphenyls: Fate and Effects in the Canadian Environment.*

35 Dewailly *et al.*, "High Levels of PCBs in Breast Milk of Inuit Women from Arctic Quebec"; Dewailly *et al.*, "PCB Exposure for Communities Living along the Gulf of St Lawrence," 1251–55; Dewailly *et al.*, "Inuit Exposure to Organochlorines," 618–20.

36 Grondin *et al.*, "Santé publique et environnement au Nunavik."

37 Ayotte *et al.*, "Health Risk Assessment for Inuit Newborns,"; Dewailly *et al.*, "Polychlorinated Biphenyl (PCB) and Dichlorodiphenyl Dichloroethylene (DDE) Concentrations in the Breast Milk of Women in Quebec," 1241–46.

38 Kinloch *et al.*, "Inuit Foods and Diet"; Dewailly *et al.*, *Breast Milk Contamination in Nunavik*; Ayotte *et al.*, "Health Risk Assessment for Inuit Newborns."

39 CCREM, *The PCB Story*; Kimbrough, "The Human Health Effects of Polychlorinated Biphenyls," 211–28.

40 Environment Canada, *National Inventory of Concentrated PCB (Askarel) Fluids*.

41 Strachan, *Polychlorinated Biphenyls (PCBs): Fate and Effects in the Canadian Environment*.

42 Abelson, "Excessive Fear of PCBs," 361.

43 Hansen, "Environmental Toxicology of PCBs"; Murray and Shearer, *Northern Contaminants Program*.

44 Health and Welfare Canada (HWC), PCBs; Mes *et al.*, "Specific Polychlorinated Biphenyl Congener Distribution in Breast Milk of Canadian Women," 555–65; Newsome *et al.*, "PCB and Organochlorined Pesticides in Canadian Human Milk," 2143–53.

45 Burger, "A Case Study," 187–201.

46 U.S. Environmental Protection Agency, *National Conference on Polychlorinated Biphenyls*.

47 Goldman, "Controlling PCBs," 345–71.

48 Buxton *et al.*, *The PCB Problem*; Environment Canada, *Background to the Regulation of Polychlorinated Biphenyls (PCB) in Canada*.

49 The first step towards controlling PCBs in Canada was actually a Notice to Disclose requiring Canadian industries as well as private and public institutions to report all PCBs in use or in storage for disposal. This information permitted the development of a national inventory on the basis of which the PCB Regulations were developed and implemented (Environment Canada, *National Inventory of Concentrated PCB (Askarel) Fluids*).

50 Environment Canada, *Handbook on PCBs in Electrical Equipment*. The fact that both American and Canadian governments fell short of a total ban on PCB uses reflects both the demonstrated usefulness of the chemical and the regulators' conviction that, once restricted to closed, electrical applications, PCBs' contribution to environmental distribution would be minimal.

51 Besides PCBs being regulated under the ECA (now the Canadian Environment Protection Act – CEPA) and the TDGA, some dispositions contained in the Fisheries Act, the Ocean Dumping Control Act, and the Canadian Coast Guard Regulations also apply to PCBs (Canadian Council of Resource and Environment Ministers (CCREM), *The PCB Story*).

52 In 1975, for instance, Health and Welfare Canada set a guideline specifying a maximum limit for PCB residues in the edible portion of commercial fish. The administration of this guideline involved the cancellation of commercial fishing licences for fish suspected to contain PCB residues in excess of 2mg/kg. As most chemical residue analyses of commercial fish in Canada are performed by the federal Department of Fisheries and Oceans (DOFO), cooperation between DOFO and the provincial deparments with jurisdiction over commercial fishing was required. (Grant, "PCBs in Canada," 383–92.)

53 CCREM, *The PCB Story*.

54 For instance, Health and Welfare Canada has set an interim "tolerable" exposure level to PCBs of 1 ug/kg-bw day. National guidelines regarding tolerable PCB concentrations in blood and breast-milk are also available (Kinloch *et al.*, 1992). In addition, several provinces have established voluntary standards recommending maximum PCB concentrations in various foods and feed, in ambient air, water, soil and wastes, or in regard to occupational exposure to PCBs. These guidelines do not have the force of regulation but rather serve as "rules of thumb" for guiding risk management decision in regards to PCBs (Environment Canada, *Summary of Environmental Criteria for Polychlorinated Biphenyls (PCBs)*).

55 Two methods have received regulatory approval in Canada for the treatment and destruction of PCB wastes. Electrical equipment and mineral oils with low PCB concentrations can be decontaminated through chemical treatment processes. Once decontaminated, oils and other materials (e.g., metals) can be recovered and reused. Chemical treatment technologies have been in operation in several provinces since the early 1980s, resulting in a substantial reduction in the volume of wastes in storage (Environment Canada, "Options for the Treatment/Destruction of Polychlorinated Biphenyls (PCBs) and PCB-contaminated Equipment"). For PCB liquids (i.e., askarels) and other materials contaminated with high concentrations of PCBs, high temperature incineration is the only approved method of disposal. The system must show a minimum PCB destruction and removal efficiency of 99.9999%. Compounds that can be formed as by-products of combustion are removed by air pollution control devices and disposed of in secure landfills. (Performance standards for incinerators and chemical treatment systems are specified in the Federal Mobile PCB Treatment and Destruction Regulations implemented in 1990 under CEPA.)

56 Environment Canada, *Federal PCB Destruction Program,* 5.
57 Canadian Broadcasting Corporation (CBC), "Public Enemy No. 1."
58 See "The Media's Eco-failure," *Globe and Mail,* 18 December 1991, A20, and "The PCB Bogeyman," 21 July 1994, A16.
59 Freudenburg *et al.,* "Media Coverage of Hazard Events."
60 Canadian Environmental Advisory Council (CEAC), *PCBs: A Burning Issue.*
61 Environment Canada, *Federal PCB Destruction Program Proceedings.*
62 Environment Canada, *Evaluation for a Mobile PCB Destruction Facility,* 10–11.
63 For examples of these criticisms, see Environment Canada, *Federal PCB Destruction Program Proceedings:* 5.
64 See "Federal PCBs Going to Alberta," *Montreal Gazette,* 13 May 1995, A5. There is also an indigenous Canadian technology for the destruction of PCBs using chemical processes instead of incineration (article by Geoffrey Rowan, *Globe and Mail,* 9 October 1996, B11). So far as we know, Environment Canada has made no effort to date to determine through public consultation whether using this technology would be both intrinsically acceptable to the public and also preferable to incineration.
65 The *Interim Order* made 20 November 1995, by then Environment minister Sheila Copps, extended the dispositions contained in the 1990 *PCB Waste Export Regulations.* These regulations, passed shortly after the Baie Comeau incident, only prohibited the *overseas* export of PCBs.
66 Environment Canada, "Canada to Allow PCB Exports to the United States for Destruction," news release, Ottawa, 26 September 1996.
67 John Frank and Jack Newman, "Breast-Feeding in a Polluted World," 33–7; Ayotte *et al.* "Health Risk Assessment for Inuit Newborns," 531–42; Ayotte *et al.,* "Arctic air pollution," 529–37.
68 Proulx, "Health and Well-Being in Nunavik," 1–15.
69 Usher *et al., Communicating about Contaminants.*
70 E. Dewailly, in Usher, *The Northern Food Dilemma.*
71 Ayotte *et al.,* "Arctic Air Pollution," 529–37.
72 Kuhnlein and Kinloch, "PCB's and Nutrients in Baffin Island Inuit," 155–8; Kinloch *et al.,* "Inuit Foods and Diet:," 247–78; Dewailly *et al.,* "Contaminants," 75–107; Dewailly *et al.,* "Evaluation of Health Risks for Infants."
73 Kinloch *et al.,* "Inuit Foods and Diet"; Usher *et al., Communicating about Contaminants.*
74 Kuhnlein *et al.,* "PCB's and Nutrients in Baffin Island Inuit"; Frank *et al.,* "Breast-Feeding in a Polluted World," 33–7; Ayotte *et al.,* "Arctic Air Pollution and Human Health," 529–37; Dewailly *et al.,* "Evaluation of Health Risks for Infants."
75 Grondin *et al.,* "Santé publique et environnement au Nunavik," 225–51.
76 Ibid.

77 Ibid.
78 See in particular Mireille Jetté, ed., *Report of the Santé Québec Health Survey*, 3 vol.
79 Usher *et al.*, *Communicating about Contaminants*.
80 Kinloch *et al.*, "Inuit Foods and Diet."
81 Ibid.
82 Ibid., 275.
83 *Globe and Mail*, 15 December 1988, A1.
84 *Globe and Mail*, 6 September 1989, A8.
85 Richard Allen, "Community Consequences," 22–4.
86 Usher *et al.*, *Communicating about Contaminants*.
87 Dewailly *et al.*, "High Levels of PCBs," 641–6.
88 Dewailly *et al.*, "Evaluation of Health Risks in Infants. "
89 Dewailly *et al.*, "Inuit Exposure to Organochlorines," 618–20.
90 Dewailly *et al.*, "Evaluation of Health Risks for Infants," 56.
91 Ibid.
92 Bruneau and Grondin, "Activities and Research in Nunavik," 356–8; Grondin *et al.*, *Health Advisories in Nunavik from 1978 to 1995*.
93 Bruneau *et al.*, "Activities and Research in Nunavik"; Wormworth, "The Impact of Food-Chain Contamination."
94 Dewailly *et al.*, "Contaminants," 75–107.
95 Usher *et al.*, *Communicating about Contaminants*.
96 Proulx, "Health and Well-Being in Nunavik"; Wenzel, "Environmentalism and Canadian Inuit."
97 Usher, "Research Relationships in the North"; Usher *et al.*, *Communicating about Contaminants*.
98 Usher *et al.*, *Communicating about Contaminants*.
99 Murray and Shearer, "1994/95 Northern Contaminants Program."
100 Suzanne Bruneau *et al.*, "Activities and Research in Nunavik," 356–8.
101 Usher *et al.*, *Communicating about Contaminants*, 204.
102 O'Neil, "Understanding of Risk Perceptions and Risk Acceptability."
103 Usher *et al.*, *Communicating about Contaminants*.
104 Ibid.
105 Bielawski, "Knowledge and Science in the Arctic."
106 O'Neil, "Understanding of Risk Perceptions and Risk Acceptibility," 357.
107 Freeman, "Nature and Utility of Traditional Ecological Knowledge."
108 Grondin *et al.*, "Santé publique et environnement au Nunavik"; Usher *et al.*, *Communicating about Contaminants*.
109 Archibald and Kosatsky, "Managing Risks to the James Bay Cree," 22–6.
110 Frank *et al.*, "Breast-Feeding in a Polluted World."
111 Usher *et al.*, *Communicating about Contaminants*.
112 Bruneau *et al.*, "Activities and Research in Nunavik."
113 John Stager, ed., *Canada and Polar Science*.

114 Ibid., 156–61.
115 *Communicating about Contaminants*, 64, 68, 215. Usher *et al.* have published the allegation that the "leaks" to the southern media were done with the deliberate intent to raise public concern and political alarm so as to ensure that major government funding for follow-up studies would be available. The authors of those passages told us that these allegations were made in confidence but that they believe them to be true.
116 Dr David Kinloch, cited in an article by Hugh Winsor, *Globe and Mail*, 6 September 1989.

CHAPTER NINE

1 The lessons we draw from our cases may be compared with the conclusions drawn in other published studies. In our opinion the best earlier collection of case studies is Krimsky and Plough, *Environmental Hazards*. We also recommend two studies on Yucca Mountain: Flynn *et al.*, "The Nevada Initiative"; and Flynn and Slovic, "Yucca Mountain."
2 Two recent cases of the last-mentioned type, involving Canadian chemical firms, are briefly described in Leiss, "Three Phases in the Evolution of Risk Communication Practice," 91–3; cf. the two studies by Caron Chess and colleagues (Chess, 1992; Chess, 1995).
3 One of us has been training a few young professionals in the area of risk communication for some years now; so far there are no positions open for them.
4 See Camille Limoges, "Expert Knowledge and Decision-Making in Controversy Events," 417–26.
5 The newspaper coverage we surveyed in chapter 3 is full of such statements, throughout the 1970s and 1980s, whenever concerns about the health effects of exposure to industrial chemicals were raised, especially about pesticides, and throughout the long controversy over 2,4,5-T in particular.
6 S. 64 of the new *Canadian Environmental Protection Act*, tabled in the House of Commons on 10 December 1996, which defines virtual elimination as "below any measurable quantity," adds the supplementary proviso "and that ... results or may result in a harmful effect on the environment or human life or health." However, for any substance already designated as "toxic" within the meaning of the act, as dioxins and furans are, the finding of harm has already been made, and so the supplementary proviso is not a limiting factor. This is a consequence of the fact that the definition of toxic in the act confuses hazard and risk (see Leiss, "Governance and the Environment," 153–9).
7 See generally Weinstein and Sandman, "Some Criteria for Evaluating Risk messages," 103–14, and Rohrmann, "The Evaluation of Risk Communication Effectiveness," 169–92.

8 *Biotechnology and the Convention on Biological Diversity*, 1994, 5pp.; *Genetically Engineered Plants: Releases and Impacts on Less Developed Plants*, 1994, 44pp.; *Environmental Risks of Genetically Engineered Organisms and Key Regulatory Issues*, 1994, 15pp; *Genetically Engineered Food: An Experiment with Nature*, pamphlet, 1996. There is a growing list of short papers on the Greenpeace International website. A number of the publications listed above are authored by recognized university-based researchers and issued under Greenpeace's auspices.

9 Soby *et al.*, "Integrating Public and Scientific Judgements into a Toolkit for Managing Food-Related Risks, Stage 1."

CHAPTER TEN

1 Speech to meeting of the Pacific Northwest Economic Region, as reported by Kate McNamara, *National Post*, 15 July 2003, A4. The North American beef market is highly integrated as between Canada and the United States, and thus BSE risk is properly treated in this way (as is shown by the second case, a Canadian-born cow which had been in the U.S. for years before being slaughtered). However, Canadian farmers faced a far higher risk relative to BSE, as will be shown.

2 Serecon Management Consulting Inc., "Economic Implications of BSE in Canada," November 2003, estimating $3.3 billion in direct economic costs and $1.8 billion in secondary impacts as of that month. http://www.animalhealth.ca/bse_info.htm

3 The best overview is Ridley and Baker, *Fatal Protein*. Two good websites are: http://www-micro.msb.le.ac.uk/3035/prions.html and http://www.priondata.org/

4 There is also a rare familial form of CJD, caused by a gene mutation that makes it more likely that the abnormal protein will appear and cause the disease by late middle age.

5 Ridley and Baker, 135.

6 "Risk Assessment of Transmissable Spongiform Encephalopathies in Canada." Draft Report – 30 June 2000. Prepared by Joan Orr, M.SC. and Mary Ellen Starodub, M.SC. for the Health Canada Science Team on TSEs (unpublished). The study was never completed and this draft report was never released to the public (it was obtained under a freedom-of-information request). Andrew Nikiforuk first revealed it in his article in *Business Edge* magazine, "Mad-cow crisis continues to spiral to new lows." 18 March 2004. http://www.businessedge.ca/viewnews.asp?id=5455

7 Interview with Bob Church, *Alberta Beef* magazine, March 2004 issue. Church is both a beef farmer and an authority on veterinary medicine.

8 The extraordinary attention to detail in the Health Canada draft report is revealed best in its comprehensive exposure pathway analysis diagram, Figure 3.2.1, "Overview of Canadian animal-based feeding

practices (since ruminant feeding ban August, 1997)." Exposure pathway analysis is one of the keys to a proper risk assessment: after one has identified the nature of the hazard (bovine materials potentially infected with BSE), one needs to know how consumers might come into contact with that hazard. This is what the pathway analysis seeks to do. Once that is done, the quantitative estimation of risk (hazard plus exposure) for the population as a whole, as well as discrete population segments, can be carried out.

9 "Report on the Assessment of the Geographical BSE-Risk (GBR) of Canada," Part II, 33; http://europa.eu.int/comm/food/fs/sc/ssc/out131_en.pdf

10 J.T. Cohen and George M. Gray, "Evaluation of the Potential Spread of BSE in Cattle and Possible Human Exposure following Introduction of Infectivity into the United States from Canada," nd [2003]. http://www.aphis.usda.gov/lpa/issues/bse/harvard_10-3/text_wrefs.pdf

11 Morley et al., "Assessment of the risk factors related to bovine spongiform encephalopathy," 157–78. This article concludes its summary as follows (http://www.oie.int/eng/publicat/rt/2201/a_r22110.htm): "The risk estimate ... indicates a negligible probability that BSE was introduced and established in Canada; nevertheless, the economic consequences would have been extreme." Subsequent events have shown that the second part of that statement, at least, was brutally accurate.

12 Quoted in an article by Joe Paraskevas, "Japan refuses to lift import ban on beef," *Ottawa Citizen*, 13 July 2003, A3.

13 http://www.inspection.gc.ca/english/corpaffr/newcom/2001/20010223e.shtml
The conditions imposed by Canada on Brazil as a condition of our lifting of the ban:

> Upon reviewing the data, the tripartite countries were assured that Brazil has taken sound measures to prevent BSE and that the suspension on imports should be lifted. There are three conditions that imports of Brazilian beef products must meet to enter the respective countries:
> 1 shipments must be certified as containing beef products from cattle that were born and raised in Brazil and not from any imported sources of beef;
> 2 the beef must come from cattle born after Brazil enacted its 1996 ruminant-to-ruminant feed ban; and
> 3 shipments must have a statement accompanying them that certify the cattle used in the products were exclusively grass-fed and not fed any animal proteins.

Most interesting: Canadian beef cattle certainly are not "exclusively grass-fed."

14 http://www.inspection.gc.ca/english/anima/heasan/disemala/bseesb/
bsefaqe.shtml

> Canada does not import commodities which are known to pose a risk
> of BSE from any country not known to be free of BSE, including
> Germany, France, Portugal, Denmark, Spain and Italy, which recently
> declared cases of BSE. Canada only allows the importation of live
> ruminants and their meat and meat products from countries free of
> BSE. Canada also has additional import controls in place for other
> animal products and by-products from countries which have
> confirmed BSE in native animals.

15 Remarks made by CFIA official Claude Lavigne just after the U.S. ban on
Japanese beef in September 2001 suggest a *de facto* rather than a *de jure*
Canadian ban on Japanese beef. "Lavigne said … [that the CFIA] is able
to screen for imports of cattle and beef from Japan through its permit
process. The agency hasn't had any permit requests of that nature
involving Japan." (Ian Bell, *Western Producer,* 27 September 2001.) In
other words, Japan has not requested import permits because it is aware
of Canada's general policy (see further below) of banning imports of
beef from any country having even a single reported case of BSE.

16 http://www.inspection.gc.ca/english/anima/heasan/policy/
ie-2001–17–4e.shtml

17 Because a list of such countries cannot be found in any CFIA document,
one has to infer that the list is the one maintained by OIE (see the following pages in the text). The USFDA lists thirty-four countries either as
having reported cases of BSE or as "considered to have a substantial risk
associated with BSE" (May 2003).

> These countries are: Albania, Austria, Belgium, Bosnia-Herzegovina,
> Bulgaria, Croatia, Czech Republic, Denmark, Federal Republic of
> Yugoslavia, Finland, France, Germany, Greece, Hungary, Ireland,
> Israel, Italy, Liechtenstein, Luxembourg, Former Yugoslavia Republic
> of Macedonia, The Netherlands, Norway, Oman, Poland, Portugal,
> Romania, Slovak Republic, Slovenia, Spain, Sweden, Switzerland,
> Japan, and United Kingdom (Great Britain including Northern
> Ireland and the Falkland Islands).

> Canada has recently been added to this list of countries from which
> imports are restricted.
> http://vm.cfsan.fda.gov/~comm/bsefaq.html

18 "Canadian Bovine Spongiform Encephalopathy (BSE) Import Policies.
Last Revised June 16th, 2003." http://www.inspection.gc.ca/english/
anima/heasan/policy/ie-2001–17–4e.shtml

> The alternative conditions are that any cases are non-indigenous, i.e.,
> imported from another country. This is OIE "category 1" status (see
> further n53).

19 Only "indigenous" cases are counted in my totals; cases in animals that were imported from another country, which are counted separately by OIE, are excluded (which is why Canada is 1). I have added up the totals, since the grand total for each country is not given on the OIE table. http://www.oie.int/eng/info/en_esbmonde.htm

20 http://www.oie.int/eng/info/en_esbincidence.htm

21 http://www.ca.emb-japan.go.jp/BSEdoc.html

22 "Japan defends prohibition on Canadian beef," *National Post*, 16 July 2003, A6.

23 Ian Bell, article in the *Western Producer*, 27 September 2001. http://www.producer.com/articles/20010927/news/ 20010927news05.html

24 Why would M. Lavigne make that last comment? The answer lies in one of the most disgraceful episodes in the entire history of the BSE episode: Britain's export of infected feed to eighty countries, including many in Asia, between 1980 and 1996. (Debora MacKenzie, "Have contaminated feed exports spread BSE across the globe?" *New Scientist*. http://www.newscientist.com/hottopics/bse/bse.jsp?id=22771200 (10 February 2001). The following quotation is from the briefing to U.K. Agriculture Minister John Gummer by one of his civil servants in July 1989:
> There has been criticism about the fact that we continue to permit the export of meat and bone meal even though it is banned from use in ruminants in this country. However it has been emphasised that importing countries have been made fully aware about BSE and its probable cause and it is, therefore, up to them to decide whether to import and under what conditions.

The BSE Inquiry (London, 16 vols., 2000), vol. 10, 70.

25 Editorial writers at the *National Post* also appear to believe it: "And a handful of infections in Japan itself set off a major panic [in 2001] (which caused various nations, including Canada, to embargo Japan's niche beef products)." 17 July 2003, A13.

26 http://www.inspection.gc.ca/english/anima/heasan/cahcc/cahcc2002/ dcac-app-a-e.shtml and http://www.inspection.gc.ca/english/sci/ahra/ bseris/bserisce.shtml

27 It is possible that the CFIA exercise (n26) did not use as complete an exposure pathway analysis as did the Health Canada team (n6); or did not characterize fully the uncertainties across many dimensions; or made assumptions about compliance with policy measures that were unwarranted. All of these and other factors can have large impacts on the final risk estimation.

28 http://bmj.bmjjournals.com/cgi/content/full/315/7113/939

29 http://www4.nationalacademies.org/news.nsf/isbn/ POD375?OpenDocument

30 Morley *et al.*, 170–1.
31 http://www.nrc.gov/reading-rm/doc-collections/nuregs/staff/sr0933/sec1/2-cr3.html
32 See http://www.systemsafety.com/examples/e_riskrating.pdf
   This scheme was developed by System Safety, Inc.
   (http://www.systemsafety.com/), which provides safety engineering
   expertise to the medical and process industry sectors.
33 http://www.inspection.gc.ca/english/anima/heasan/disemala/bseesb/internate.shtml
34 Kim Lunman, "Expect more BSE, expert says," *Globe and Mail*, 10 June
   2003, A9.
35 Cited in an article by Shawn McCarthy and Daniel Leblanc, "Chrétien
   pressures Japanese over beef," *Globe and Mail*, 2 July 2003.
36 http://www.eurocjd.ed.ac.uk/lancet5.html
   See also http://www.mrc.ac.uk/txt/index/public-interest/
   public-press_office/public-press_releases_2001/public-14_may_2001.htm
37 http://www.fda.gov/bbs/topics/NEWS/2003/NEW00924.html
   http://seattlepi.nwsource.com/business/cows26.shtml
38 *Kyodo News*, "Japan rejects request for early lifting of ban on Canada
   beef," 13 July 2003. http://asia.news.yahoo.com/030713/kyodo/
   d7s8bcdg3.html
39 The argument in support of this case was well presented by Andrew
   Nikiforuk, "Our beef is with bureaucrats," *Globe and Mail*, 29 May 2003, A21.
40 Barry Wilson, "Beef exports up, but clouds loom," *Western Producer*,
   20 February 2003.
41 The first set of changes has been announced (Patrick Brethour, "Tough
   rules in works for mad-cow testing," *Globe and Mail*, 18 July 2003, A1,
   A7) – but Canada still has a long way to go.
42 Renata D'Aliesio, "Show us the mad cow plan, Japan says," *Edmonton
   Journal*, 16 July 2003.
43 Marcus Doherr, veterinary epidemiologist at the University of Bern,
   Switzerland, as quoted by Alan Freeman, "Ban dangerous feed, experts
   say," *Globe and Mail*, 29 May 2003, A8. The CFIA risk assessment (n23)
   includes elaborate calculations on the cross-contamination risk.
44 The CFIA subjected its risk estimation to external peer review, and the
   reviewers asked some tough questions about the animal feed policy. But
   the CFIA's essential complacency about BSE risk is evident in one of the
   agency's answers to the peer reviewers: "However, there is a negligible
   likelihood of BSE in Canada. There is, currently, no scientific evidence
   showing that blood products represent a significant risk. Accordingly,
   the CFIA has not banned the use of blood meal as a protein source for
   ruminants." http://www.inspection.gc.ca/english/sci/ahra/bseris/
   revexae.shtml

45 Two excellent articles (both from the *Toronto Star*) are: Sandro Contenta, "Canada can learn from U.K. errors," 24 May 2003; Stuart Laidlaw, "Complacency is real killer in mad cow," 26 May 2003.

46 The delay was due in part to closing of provincial labs and in part to the mysterious Alberta policy of assigning a higher priority to the testing of elk: Deborah Yedlin, "Meat testing backlog created by cutbacks," *Globe and Mail*, 23 May 2003. http://www.globeandmail.com/servlet/ArticleNews/TPStory/LAC/20030523/RWEST_2/TPBusiness/TopStories

47 Debora MacKenzie, "BSE crosses the Atlantic," *New Scientist*, 31 May 2003. http://www.newscientist.com/hottopics/bse/bse.jsp?id=23970300

48 In 2001 Canada had 12.4 million head of beef cattle: *Risk Assessment on Bovine Spongiform Encephalopathy in Cattle in Canada, Part A: Evaluation of Risk Factors*, Section 3 and Table 1. http://www.inspection.gc.ca/english/sci/ahra/bseris/bserisa1e.shtml#A3

49 Quoted by Charles Gillis, "Canada told to start mass mad-cow tests," *National Post*, 3 June 2003, A7 (on Doherr, see n43).

50 "Report on the Assessment of the Geographical BSE-Risk (GBR) of Canada," Part II, 33. http://europa.eu.int/comm/food/fs/sc/ssc/out131_en.pdf. See generally D. Heim and U. Kihm, "Risk management of transmissible spongiform encephalopathies in Europe" (2003): http://www.oie.int/eng/publicat/rt/2201/11.%20Heim.pdf

51 "Is industry in safe hands?" *Calgary Herald*, 21 May 2003, A1, A2.

52 See the story of Donna and Bryan Babey, whose small cattle herd in Lloydminster, Sask. was taken away for slaughter, in Charles Gillis, "Lessons not learned," *National Post*, 31 May 2003, A9.

53 See http://www.oie.int/eng/normes/mcode/a_00068.htm for the OIE's "Terrestrial Animal Health Code 2003," article 2.3.13.2 and following. (Renata D'Aliesio of the *Edmonton Journal* called my attention to these OIE policy statements.) The OIE has the following categories: (1) "BSE free country or zone," (2) "BSE provisionally free country or zone," (3) "Country or zone with a minimal BSE risk," (4) "Country or zone with a moderate BSE risk," (5) "Country or zone with a high BSE risk." By my reckoning Canada currently falls in OIE category 4; provided that no other indigenous cases are found, we would have to wait until the year 2010 to qualify for category 3 status.
Category 3 ("minimal BSE risk") applies to countries where:
the last indigenous *case* of BSE has been reported less than 7 years ago, and the BSE incidence rate, calculated on the basis of indigenous *cases*, has been less than one case per million during each of the last four consecutive 12-month periods within the cattle population over 24 months of age in the country or zone … and: i) the ban on feeding ruminants with *meat-and-bone meal* and *greaves* derived from ruminants has been effectively enforced for at least 8 years. (article 2.3.13.5)

54 Quoted in Kelly Cryderman and Renata D'Aliesio, "More mad cow tests coming," *Edmonton Journal,* 7 January 2004.

55 J. T. Cohen *et al.,* "Evaluation of the Potential for Bovine Spongiform Encephalopathy in the United States," 26 November 2001. http://www.hcra.harvard.edu/pdf/madcow.pdf; additional information at: http://www.aphis.usda.gov/lpa/issues/bse/bse-riskassmt.html J. T. Cohen and George M. Gray, "Evaluation of the Potential Spread of BSE in Cattle and Possible Human Exposure following Introduction of Infectivity into the United States from Canada," nd [2003]. http://www.aphis.usda.gov/lpa/issues/bse/harvard_10-3/text_wrefs.pdf (the USDA website (http://www.usda.gov/Newsroom/0373.03.html) has a transcript of a news conference with George Gray, dated 31 October 2003).

56 http://www.inspection.gc.ca/english/anima/heasan/disemala/bseesb/ minrisexece.shtml

57 http://www.inspection.gc.ca/english/anima/heasan/policy/ ie-2001-17-4e.shtml

58 The CFIA's spokesman on BSE, chief veterinarian Brian Evans, said after confirmation that the second cow came from Canada: "With the results of our previous investigation, we have always accepted the reality that a small number of additional cases could not be ruled out over the next 18-month period." Quoted in Lisa Schmidt, "DNA proves mad cow was Canadian," *Ottawa Citizen,* 7 January 2004, A1. To the best of my knowledge, this concession had never been made publicly by the CFIA before these remarks appeared.

59 http://www.foodstandards.gov.uk/bse/facts/cattletest Breakdowns on testing on a country-by-country basis (fifteen countries) are given for the period January – November 2003, during which time 8 million tests were carried out; 248 cases were positive and 122 tests are pending. An additional 400,000 tests were done in Poland and the Slovak Republic during the same period. The numbers "do not include BSE suspect animals ... nor 'at risk' animals (defined as those found dead-on-farm; emergency slaughtered animals; and those sent for normal slaughter but found to be sick at ante-mortem inspection)." See also: http://europa.eu.int/comm/food/fs/bse/testing/bse_results_en.html

60 Sandra Blakeslee, "Jumble of tests may slow mad cow solution," *New York Times,* 4 January 2004.

61 See Hrudey and Leiss, "Risk Management and Precaution: Insights on the Cautious Use of Evidence," for a recent discussion of the issue of false positives and false negatives. http://www.leiss.ca/articles/126

62 http://www.aphis.usda.gov/lpa/issues/bse/bse-surveillance.html (nd). See also the useful pieces from the *New York Times:* Michael Moss *et al.,* "Mad cow forces beef industry to change course," 5 January 2004; Eric Schlosser, "The cow jumped over the USDA," 2 January 2004; and Verlyn

Klinkenborg, "Holstein dairy cows and the inefficient efficiencies of modern farming," 5 January 2004. In early January the U.S. invited an international panel to review its policies, and the panel took direct issue with the Harvard risk assessments relied on by USDA (emphasis in original):

> However, the Committee cannot adequately resolve the differing BSE risk assessment presented by the Subcommittee as compared to the assessment by Harvard University. A major discrepancy exists with the Subcommittee's conclusions that BSE continues to circulate, or even amplify, in the US and North America, when compared with the Harvard risk assessment. The Committee must have this issue of risk resolved prior to completing its recommendations to the Secretary.
> *It is imperative that the Secretary has the best available science and more precise risk assessments in order to make appropriate regulatory decisions.*

http://www.aphis.usda.gov/lpa/issues/bse/US_BSE_Report.pdf (2 February 2004). The interim USDA response may be found at: http://www.aphis.usda.gov/lpa/issues/bse/bse_responsetorep.pdf

63 http://www.inspection.gc.ca/english/anima/heasan/disemala/bseesb/ bseesbsurvfse.shtml

64 http://vm.cfsan.fda.gov/~comm/bsefaq.html

65 Dr David Westaway, a molecular biologist and specialist on prion diseases at the University of Toronto, reacted as follows to our most recent announcement about increasing testing to 8,000 annually: "Whoop-de-do. Eight thousand a day would be good. They've got to find the other animals [with BSE]. They can't just leave things in limbo, and they're not going to find the rest of the other animals by screening 8,000." Quoted in Kelly Cryderman, "Test plan gets mixed reviews," *Edmonton Journal,* 9 January 2004. For additional background on this point see the important article by Andrew Nikiforuk, "Diagnosing BSE: An issue comes to a head," *Globe and Mail,* 8 January 2004, A17.

66 It is often alleged that such a policy would be prohibitively costly. Here is one estimate: "Testing all the animals in Canada's herd would cost $30 million to $60 million annually, according to Canadian beef industry officials." (Gina Teel, "More testing urged to fight mad cow," *Calgary Herald/Canwest News Service,* 4 January 2004.) By way of offering some perspective on the numbers, economic losses to Canada from the first case already total over $5 billion, and that figure is still rising.

67 Readers unfamiliar with this subject can consult the following web-essay on scientific methods for rapid BSE testing by Mike Tyshenko, "BSE Risk in Canada, Part 2: Methods of Testing for Bovine Spongiform Encephalopathy" (14 January 2004). http://www.leiss.ca/bse/142

68 Donald McNeil Jr, "Mad cow case may bring more meat testing," *New York Times,* 26 December 2003.

69 Donald G. McNeil Jr, "U.S. Won't Let Company Test All Its Cattle for Mad Cow," *New York Times,* 10 April 2004. The Canadian Cattlemen's Association (CCA) takes a similar stance, in the process insulting those who want to do more testing: "Overreacting by introducing testing that goes way beyond what is necessary based on science would encourage other countries to continue to react in an irrational manner." This sentence occurs shortly after one that notes that Canada will increase its testing from under 4,000 animals in 2002 to 30,000 sometime in the future – of course, the previous number was described at the time as being "based on science." Not to put too fine a point on the matter, remarks such as these by the CCA are just plain stupid, as well as being deeply offensive to our trading partners, who must be persuaded at some point to reopen their borders to Canadian beef. http://www.cattle.ca/newsroom/NewsCurrent/ BSE%20Surveillance%20and%20Testing%20FAQJan04.pdf (January 2004, "FAQs on Surveillance and Testing").

70 http://www.fda.gov/cvm/index/updates/bse72001.htm (6 July 2001); "U.S. Department of Justice Files Consent Decree Of Permanent Injunction Against X-Cel Feeds, Inc. Based on Violations of FDA's 1997 Animal Feed Rule," 11 July 2003. http://www.fda.gov/bbs/topics/NEWS/2003/NEW00924.html

71 Chad Skelton, "Plant probed for mad-cow link had labeling problems," *National Post,* 2 January 2004, A4; Jason Markusoff, "Investigators draw possible link between 2 mad cow cases," *Edmonton Journal,* 31 December 2003. The reporters have commented on the lack of responsiveness, on the part of both federal regulators and industry personnel, to requests for a more detailed accounting of feed-mill practices.

72 On 16 January 2004 the *Globe and Mail* ("U.S. cites six plants in Canada for feed violations," A6) reported that the USFDA had added six more Canadian animal feed plants – to the list of eight cited earlier – to its "import alert" list. The FDA statement said that the "firms listed ... have attempted to import feed products containing animal material of indeterminate origin."

73 Bill Curry, "Food agency doubted disease could hit humans," *National Post,* 29 August 2003, A8.

74 http://www.hhs.gov/news/press/2004pres/20040126.html

75 Joe Paraskevas, "Officials plan foot and mouth defence," *Ottawa Citizen,* 3 January 2004, A6.

76 For the U.S., see the carefully detailed section 9 in the web-essay by Peter M. Sandman and Jody Lanard, "Misleading toward the truth: The

U.S. Department of Agriculture mishandles mad cow risk communication" (18 March 2004): http://www.psandman.com, which tracks in excruciating detail the terminological games played with the concept of "sound science" by federal officials in that country. On 2 January 2004 the U.S. announced a set of major new risk management policies of a more precautionary nature (http://www.usda.gov/Newsroom/ 0457.04.html), never once conceding that the previous set was inadequate. This happened again, on 15 March 2004, with the announcement of an enhanced surveillance program. http://www.usda.gov/ Newsroom/0105.04.html

77 http://www.hhs.gov/news/press/2004pres/20040126.html

CHAPTER ELEVEN

1 Intergovernmental Panel on Climate Change. *Climate change 2001.*
2 See, for example, this statement supporting the IPCC: Joint Statement by 17 National Academies of Science (2001).
3 Society of Environmental Toxicology and Chemistry (SETAC) (1999). Sound Science Technical Issue Paper.
4 Ziman, *Reliable knowledge: an exploration of the grounds for belief in science.*
5 Ziman, *Real science: what it is, and what it means,* 255.
6 Robert B. Peterson, past Chairman, President, and Chief Executive Officer, Imperial Oil Limited. Remarks to Imperial Oil Annual General Meeting, 24 April 2001. Available at: http://www.imperialoil.ca/Canada-English/News/Issues/N_I_KyotoRBP.asp (accessed 12 March 2004).
7 Essex and McKitrick. *Taken by storm: the troubled science, policy and politics of global warming.*
8 Edwards and Schneider. "Self-governance and peer review in Science-for-Policy."
9 For more information, see The Royal Society of Canada's Expert Panels: Manual of Procedural Guidelines at www.rsc.ca/english/ expert_manual_intro.html (accessed 15 March 2004).
10 In 2001, the U.S. White House asked the National Academy of Sciences to outline the key uncertainties of climate science and to assess whether there were any substantive differences between the IPCC reports and their respective summaries. See National Academy of Sciences, *Climate Change Science.*
11 "The Science of Climate Change: What do we know?" *Isuma: Canadian Journal of Policy Research,* vol. 2, no. 4 (Winter 2001). www.isuma.net.
12 There is direct evidence of our complicity in these upward trends. This is based on chemical analysis of the different isotopes of carbon in the atmosphere, through which the signature of old carbon from long-buried fossil fuels and burned since the beginning of the Industrial

Revolution can be differentiated from carbon emitted through natural cycles.

13 See chapter 3, "The Carbon Cycle and Atmospheric Carbon Dioxide," *Climate change 2001.*

14 Ibid. See especially the relevant work on scenarios of projected emissions (SRES).

15 See chapter 6, "Radiative Forcing of Climate Change," *Climate change 2001.*

16 For a more complete description of Pascal's wager see Leiss, *In the Chamber of Risks,* 261–2. Pascal's wager has also been described as the Maximin Rule in decision theory and readers seeking further information on this should see Lemons, ed., *Scientific Uncertainty and Environmental Problem Solving,* 23–8.

17 National Research Council (U.S.). Committee on Abrupt Climate Change. *Abrupt climate change: inevitable surprises.*

18 For one recent perspective on the risks of rapid deglaciation, see Hansen, "Defusing the global warming time bomb." Hansen feels that "the highest prudent level of additional global warming [should] not [be] more than about one degree C" (75) to deal with the risks of substantial deglaciation.

19 Reduction in greenhouse gases emissions can, under the Kyoto Protocol, be made to any of six different greenhouse gases (carbon dioxide, methane, nitrous oxide, hydrofluorocarbons, perfluorocarbons, sulphur hexafluoride), although carbon dioxide is the most important of these gases to climate change.

20 Environment Canada. *Climate Change Plan for Canada.*

21 Toulin, "UN Pokes Holes in Kyoto Plan."

22 The authoritative view on emissions scenarios can be found in Nakicenovic and Swart, *Emissions Scenarios. Special Report of the Intergovernmental Panel on Climate Change.* A very readable overview of emissions scenarios that will lead to stabilized concentrations can be found in Wigley, *Stabilization of greenhouse gas concentrations.*

23 Prediction of business-as-usual emissions is, as with any forecast, uncertain. Canada's Third National Report on Climate Change, updated from the second report in 1997, has changed 57 Mt CO_2e to the 2010 business-as-usual prediction because of changes in assumptions such as activity in specific industrial sectors and economic forecasts.

24 The Kyoto Protocol to the United Nations Framework Convention on Climate Change. Article 25, paragraph 1. www.unfccc.org. The 55/55 hurdle became even more daunting with the withdrawal of the U.S., the world's largest single nation emitter of greenhouse gases.

25 Environment Canada, "Major Agreement Achieved on Kyoto Protocol," Government of Canada press release, 10 November 2001. www.ec.gc.ca/Press/2001/011110_n_e.htm

26 Environment Canada. *Climate Change Plan for Canada.*
27 The website for the Large Industrial Emitters group is
   http://www.nrcan-rncan.gc.ca/lfeg-ggef/
28 Drexhage, "Still up in the air."
29 Calamai, "Kyoto plan falls short of targets, Ottawa told."
30 Perrin Beatty, "Our climate change strategy must reflect Canadian
   realities," *National Post*, 27 February 2002, FP15.
31 David Anderson, "Notes for an address on the occasion of a panel
   discussion on climate change," University of Victoria, 9 January 2003.
   http://www.ec.gc.ca/minister/speeches/2003/030109_s_e.htm
32 Kate Jaimet, "Kyoto would 'shut down' economy: Oil, gas, electricity to
   be the hardest hit Chamber of Commerce official warns," *Ottawa Citizen*,
   25 November 2001, A6.
33 Lily Nguyen, "'Agnostic' oil patch seeks Kyoto clarity: Some firms don't
   see climate treaty as a threat," *Globe and Mail*, 16 March 2002, B1.
34 Tom Spears, "Oil industry scoffs at plan to cut gases: Petroleum makers
   slam government's 'blind approach' to global warming," *Ottawa Citizen*,
   28 November 2001, A8.
35 Ian Jack and Carol Howes, "Ottawa thinking twice about Kyoto:
   Goodale," *National Post*, 29 November 2001, FP2.
36 Brent Jang, "Imperial Oil executives mince no words on Kyoto or
   anything else," *Globe and Mail*, 13 March 2002, B9.
37 Ross McKitrick, "Kyoto's real cost: While there is little chance the Kyoto
   Protocol will improve the environment, it will definitely hurt the
   economy, possibly even triggering another recession," *National Post*,
   26 February 2002, FP17.
38 Canadian Manufacturers and Exporters. "Pain without gain: Canada and the
   Kyoto protocol." February 2002. 21 pp. www.cme-mec.ca/kyoto/index.html
   Although they indicate that the cost prediction in their report comes
   from the Climate Change Secretariat (Analysis & Modelling Group,
   November 2000 report), the CME stresses that, "The economic analysis
   and modelling exercises undertaken by the Canadian government and
   Canada's Climate Change Secretariat seriously underestimate the costs
   that would be involved in Kyoto compliance."
39 Alberta. "Albertans & climate change."
   The bulk of the cost estimates are contained in appendix A. Within the
   report, the Alberta government states: "Single point forecasts ignore the
   real range of uncertainties and risks. Only by being explicit about risks
   and uncertainties can we identify, consult and agree on the policies
   needed to minimize costs and manage risks" (10). This is sound advice
   but hardly reflected in the tone of the Alberta government press release
   and its single point forecast accompanying the report, titled "Kyoto
   could cost Canada up to $40 billion, study shows."

40 Nancy Hughes Anthony, "Climate Change – A National Issue Affecting All Canadians" Notes for an address by the President and CEO of the Canadian Chamber of Commerce, 4 March 2002. www.chamber.ca/public_info/2002/speeches/speech020304.pdf.

41 Environment Canada, "Costs of Kyoto – What we know." 2002. www.ec.gc.ca/minister/speeches/2002/020318_t_e.htm.

42 Randall Wigle, "Sector impacts of Kyoto compliance." Working Paper Number 34. Industry Canada Research Publications Program. March 2001. strategis.ic.gc.ca/SSG/ra01796e.html

43 M.G.J. den Elzen, and A.P.G. de Moor. *The Bonn Agreement and Marrakesh Accords: An updated analysis,* RIVM report 728001017/2001. Dutch Ministry of Environment, 2002.

44 National Climate Change Process, Analysis and Modeling Group (see generally http://www.nccp.ca/NCCP/national_process/issues/analysis_e.html); "An Assessment of the Economic and Environmental Implications for Canada of the Kyoto Protocol," November 2000. http://www.nccp.ca/NCCP/pdf/AMG_finalreport_eng.pdf

45 Diane Francis, "Kyoto Accord a bad deal for Canada." *National Post,* 19 February 2002, FP3. Francis was so impressed with these numbers, which were provided to her by Bob Peterson of Imperial Oil and the CEO Council according to her response to our e-mail inquiry, she repeated them verbatim a second time in her column on 12 March 2002.

46 Boustie, Raynolds, *et al., How Ratifying the Kyoto Protocol Will Benefit Canada's Competitiveness.* 50.

47 Baillie, Bernow, *et al., The Bottom Line on Kyoto: Economic Benefits of Canadian Action.*

48 Anil Markandya, Kirsten Halsnaes, *et al.,* "Costing Methodologies," chapter 7 from Working Group III of the IPCC Third Assessment Report. Cambridge, U.K.: Cambridge University Press, 2001.

49 An authoritative and readable book on predicting the costs of greenhouse gas reductions in Canada is Jaccard, Nyboer, *et al. The cost of climate policy.*

50 Canadian Manufacturers and Exporters. "Pain without gain," 10.

51 More information can be found at www.nccp.ca

52 We ignore for the time being the ongoing debate regarding the merits of using the GDP to measure human welfare. Many environmentalists argue the metric is flawed and should be replaced by some form of green GDP. See www.rdprogress.org and www.nrtee-trnee.ca/indicators for more information.

53 Environment Canada. "Costs of Kyoto – What we know."

54 Weyant, *An introduction to the economics of climate change policy.*

55 Wigle, "Sector impacts of Kyoto compliance."

56 Jaccard, "Costing greenhouse gas abatement: Canada's technological and behavioural potential," 47.

57 These models include the MARKAL (operated by McGill) and CIMS (developed at Simon Fraser University) energy-technology models, the CASGEM (developed by Department of Finance), and the Infometrica Model. The former two models are more closely aligned with bottom-up and hybrid approaches, while the latter two models are top-down models. In the AMG process, the CIMS and MARKAL models provided input to the Informetrica Model while the CASGEM used other input assumptions.

58 The most recent projections are available within Canada's Third National Report on Climate Change. www.climatechange.gc.ca/english/3nr/index.html

59 Drexhage, "Still up in the air."

60 This last factor is defined by a coefficient referred to as the Autonomous Energy Efficiency Improvement (AEEI). (Markandya, Halsnaes, et al., "Costing Methodologies.") The presumed AEEI in any model will be crucial in setting the base-case scenario.

61 Markandya, Halsnaes, et al., "Costing Methodologies."

62 Alberta, Albertans & climate change.

63 Brethour, "Russia can't ratify Kyoto."

64 Many people in Russia retain a preference for central control over markets and would be hesitant to allow the government to sell credits. As well, Russia may want to hold on to its credits for the next Kyoto compliance period (i.e., post 2012) when the U.S. could be back in an international market. See Robert A. Reinstein, "The outlook for International GHG Credits." Background paper prepared for the Canadian Chamber of Commerce. 10 February 2002. www.chamber.ca/public_info/2002/reinstein.pdf

65 Chase, "Canada plans to stick to Kyoto, minister says."

66 This was noted by Maclean's backpage columnist Paul Wells. See http://www.macleans.ca/paulwells/archives/week_2004_03_14-2004_03_20.asp#000195 for more detail. Accessed 23 March 2004.

67 Environment Canada. Climate Change Plan for Canada. See in particular chapter 3.

68 National Post columnist Andrew Coyne suggests that the worst case scenario (i.e., 3 per cent forgone GDP, or roughly C$40 billion) is much less than the possible consequences of climate change. "The Canadian Chamber of Commerce, whose president says Kyoto would 'cripple our economy,' puts the damage at $30 billion. With a little more ingenuity, the Canadian Manufacturers and Exporters managed to produce a figure of $40 billion. True, that's twice as much as the government estimates. But on a $1.4 trillion economy, both are essentially rounding errors." Coyne, "What is the cost of 'hot air'?"

69 Dr James E. Hansen, Head, NASA Goddard Institute for Space Studies. Statement before the Committee on Commerce, Science and Transportation, United States Senate. May 2001. 2. www.senate.gov/~commerce/ hearings/0501han.pdf.

70 For one example, see Hubert, "Climate Change and Canadian Sovereignty in the Northwest Passage."

71 Robust economic growth makes it easier to meet an intensity target (since the denominator is growing quickly). The corollary of this is that a severe recession would make it virtually impossible to meet a greenhouse gas intensity target. This problem is particularly acute for developing nations that experience economic readjustment because of foreign debt loads.

72 See Matthew Bramley, *An Assessment of Alberta's Climate Change Action Plan.*

73 For example, at the website of the Canadian Coalition for Responsible Environmental Solutions (CCRES) – the public relations front group for industry's anti-Kyoto lobby effort – you can find this statement about the merits of international trading: "If Canada ratifies the Kyoto Protocol, any greenhouse gas emissions created by residents or businesses in this country that exceed Kyoto's aggressive target will have to be paid for by purchasing 'emissions credits' from other countries. These credits are essentially transfers of money out of Canada to other jurisdictions – many of whom will have excess emissions capacity to sell since they have no targets to meet. This transfer of wealth could instead be spent in Canada, developing technologies that fight greenhouse gases and that can be sold around the world." http://www.canadiansolution.com/ backgrounders.asp

74 Quoted from CBC online, www.cbc.ca, 29 March 2001.

75 Text of a letter from the President to Senators Hagel, Helms, Craig, and Roberts. www.whitehouse.gov/news/releases/2001/03/20010314.html

76 Paul Cellucci, "Washington's better idea," *Globe and Mail,* 19 March 2002, A17.

77 Bramley, *A comparison of current government action on climate change in the U.S. and Canada.*

78 www.bp.com/centres/press/stanford/index.asp

79 For example: Alberta Premier Ralph Klein was highly critical of Jean Chrétien's understanding of Kyoto: "Does he really understand what this is all about? When I try to talk to the Prime Minister about it, it's not a very intelligent conversation. It isn't. It's not intelligent from my end because I get so frustrated, wrapped up in trying to talk to him about this." globeandmail.com, 29 October 2002.

80 Mackay, "Firing public health MD."

81 The 2004 federal budget announced the government's intention to sell their shares in Petro-Canada within the 2004 fiscal year and to invest

this money in Kyoto-related technology development. The proceeds are estimated to be approximately C$2 billion. More information can be found at the budget website: http://www.fin.gc.ca/budtoce/2004/budliste.htm

82 In Spring 2001 President George W. Bush asked his NAS to tell him whether the IPCC reports fairly represent the prevailing consensus of scientists on the issue of climate forcing. He also asked whether the IPCC's "summary for policy makers" could be trusted (http://books.nap.edu/books/0309075742/html/index.html). The answer to both questions was: Yes. The Royal Society provided a similar answer to its government and the British public: http://www.royalsoc.ac.uk/policy/climate_report.pdf Unfortunately for the Canadian citizen, the Government of Canada did not request a similar report from its own Royal Society.

CHAPTER TWELVE

1 There is an excellent commentary by Harold Bloom in the Signet Classic edition and a full contextual analysis in Susan J. Wolfson's more recent edition.

2 *The Guardian*. Philip Angell, U.S. director of corporate communications for agro-chemical corporation Monsanto: "This technology might prove attractive." He added that it was "not very different from 'hybrid' crops, which do not reproduce." http://users.westnet.gr/~cgian/guardian.htm (accessed 16 March 2004).

3 Nobel Prize-winning scientist James Watson, who co-discovered the structure of DNA, admitted that his reaction to the cloning of Dolly was surprise that she had been cloned from an adult cell. The Science Show, http://www.abc.net.au/rn/science/ss/stories/s10969.htm (accessed 11 March 2004); and John Carey, "Cloning's strange past – and stranger future." http://www.businessweek.com/1998/05/b3563047.htm (accessed 16 March 2004).

4 "The next big thing – Cloning." http://www.open2.net/nextbigthing/cloning/story_so_far/story_so_far.htm (accessed 15 March 2004).

5 Cloning of various animals as reviewed in: Shin *et al.*, "A cat cloned by nuclear transplantation."

6 K. H. Campbell *et al.*, "Sheep cloned by nuclear transfer from a cultured cell line."

7 New Scientist, "One giant leap into the unknown." http://www.newscientist.com/hottopics/cloning/cloning.jsp?id=20710300 (accessed 16 March 2004); BBC news, "The race to clone the first human." http://news.bbc.co.uk/1/hi/sci/tech/158526.stm (accessed 16 March 2004).

8 CNN, "Clone report sparks fresh debate." http://www.cnn.com/2004/ HEALTH/02/13/science.clone/index.html (accessed 8 March 2004).

9 Nic Robertson, "Scientists: Cloned sheep Dolly has 'old' DNA." 26 May 1999. http://edition.cnn.com/NATURE/9905/26/dolly.clone.02/ index.html (accessed 11 March 2004).

10 CNN, "First cloned sheep Dolly dies at 6." http://www.cnn.com/2003/ WORLD/europe/02/14/cloned.dolly.dies/ (accessed 12 March 2004); BBC, "Dolly the sheep clone dies young." http://news.bbc.co.uk/1/hi/ sci/tech/2764039.stm (accessed 12 March 2004).

11 "Bioinformatics – a definition." http://www.pasteur.fr/recherche/unites/ Binfs/definition/bioinformatics_definition.pdf (accessed 11 March 2004).

12 "NCBI Genbank statistics." http://www.ncbi.nlm.nih.gov/Genbank/ genbankstats.html (accessed 25 January 2004).

13 Genovations, "Physicians Guide to Clinical Genomics." http://www.genovations.com/clinician_overview.html (accessed 16 March 2004).

14 U.S. Department of Energy – Office of Science, "What is Pharmacogenomics?" http://www.ornl.gov/sci/techresources/Human_Genome/ medicine/pharma.shtml#whatis (accessed 11 March 2004).

15 Sachidanandam et al., "A map of human genome sequence variation containing 1.42 million single nucleotide polymorphisms."

16 TIGR's Minimal Genome Project, "How Many Genes Are Necessary To Sustain Life?" http://www.biosino.org/bioinformatics/20020408–3.htm (accessed 8 March 2004).

17 Human Genome Project, "Gene testing, Pharmacogenomics, and Gene Therapy." http://www.ornl.gov/sci/techresources/Human_Genome/ publicat/primer2001/6.shtml (accessed 8 March 2004).

18 Human Genome Project, "Medicine and the new genetics, Genomics and its impact on science and society: The human genome project and beyond." http://www.ornl.gov/sci/techresources/Human_Genome/ publicat/judicature/article3.html#box6 (accessed 7 March 2004).

19 "The central dogma of biology." http://web.mit.edu/esgbio/www/ dogma/dogma.html (accessed 15 March 2004).

20 "Transcriptomics." http://www.biochem.mpg.de/oesterhelt/overview/ transcriptomics.html (accessed 13 January 2004).

21 The human genome U133 (HG-U133) set consists of two gene chip arrays representing more than 39,000 transcripts derived from approximately 33,000 well-substantiated human genes. This set design uses sequences selected from large DNA databases (GenBank, dbEST, and RefSeq). Affymetrix Gene Chip Arrays. http://www.affymetrix.com/ products/arrays/specific/hgu133.affx (accessed 15 March 2004).

22 EMBL-EBI, Microarray databases. http://www.ebi.ac.uk/Databases/ microarray.html (accessed 13 January 2004).

23 Bio-Sino, "Use of Genomic Data in Risk Assessment."
http://www.biosino.org/bioinformatics/20020408–3.htm (accessed
13 January 2004).

24 The National Center for Biotechnology Information (NCBI) was
established in 1988 as a national resource for molecular biology
information. NCBI maintains public genome databases,
http://www.ncbi.nlm.nih.gov/; TrEMBL and Swiss-Prot have been incorporated into the Universal Protein Resource or UniProt database maintained by the European Bioinformatics Institute. http://www.ebi.ac.uk/
swissprot/ (accessed 12 March 2004).

25 "Proteomics." http://www.biochem.mpg.de/oesterhelt/overview/
proteomics.html

26 Casey, "Genes, Dreams and Reality: The promise and risks of the new
genetics." http://www.ornl.gov/sci/techresources/Human_Genome/
publicat/judicature/article3.html (accessed 13 March 2004).

27 See n23.

28 CDC, Laura M. Beskow, Marta Gwinn, and Mark A. Rothstein,
"Integrating Genomics into Public Health Policy and Practice."
http://www.cdc.gov/genomics/oldWeb01_16_04/info/books/beskow.htm
(accessed 11 March 2004).

29 ABC News, "Scientist: Bar mixed human-animals." 20 August 1999.
http://abcnews.go.com/sections/science/DailyNews/chmera0402.html.
(accessed 16 March 2004).

30 Biospace. Jim Kling, "When it absolutely, positively has to be there!
Making Gene Therapy Deliver." http://www.biospace.com/articles/
063099.cfm (accessed 10 March 2004).

31 Genethics, "Eugenics: A brief history." http://home.earthlink.net/
~johnmur/walker/history.html (accessed 4 March 2004).

32 Genetics Science Research Center, University of Utah, "Gene
enhancement and science fiction." http://gslc.genetics.utah.edu/units/
genetherapy/gtenhance/ (accessed 4 March 2004).

33 National Human Genome Research Institute, Kathi E. Hanna, "Genetic
Enhancements." http://www.21stcenturyhgh.com/hgh-nih-hgh-
research.htm (accessed 4 March 2004).

34 Lee et al., "Viral expression of insulin-like growth factor-I enhances
muscle hypertrophy in resistance-trained rats."

35 Times Online, Mark Henderson, "Gene doping is 'new frontier' for
sports cheats." 16 February 2004. http://www.timesonline.co.uk/article/
0,,1-1004273,00.html (accessed 5 March 2004).

36 Genetics and Public Policy Center, "Gene enhancements."
http://www.dnapolicy.org/genetics/enhancement.jhtml (accessed
11 March 2004).

37 Human Genome Project. http://www.ornl.gov/sci/techresources/
Human_Genome/medicine/genetherapy.shtml

38 PBS, Gene Therapy. http://www.pbs.org/newshour/bb/health/
jan-june00/gene_therapy_2-2.html (accessed 16 March 2004).

39 Human Genome Project. http://www.ornl.gov/sci/techresources/
Human_Genome/publicat/primer2001/6.shtml (accessed 4 March
2004).

40 *The Journal of Gene Medicine*, September 1999 update.
http://www.wiley.co.uk/genetherapy/clinical/countries.html#2 (accessed
4 March 2004).

41 BRAVO Canada – Gene Therapy. http://strategis.ic.gc.ca/epic/internet/
inbravo-canada.nsf/vwapj/whnewgenether.html/$FILE/
whnewgenether.html (accessed 11 March 2004).

42 Epistatis occurs when one gene interferes with the expression of
another. "Gene Interactions." http://www.emc.maricopa.edu/faculty/
farabee/BIOBK/BioBookgeninteract.html (accessed 18 March 2004).

43 Pleiotropic gene: A gene that has multiple, apparently unrelated,
phenotypic manifestations. An example is the "frizzle-trait" in chickens.
The primary effect of this gene is the production of defective feathers,
secondary effects include increased metabolic rate, decreased egg-laying,
changes in organs (heart, kidney, and spleen). Pleiotropic gene is
synonymous with polyphenic gene.

44 Biotechnology Industry Organization, "The Value of Therapeutic
Cloning for Patients." http://www.bio.org/bioethics/tcloning.asp
(accessed 11 March 2004).

45 "Therapeutic cloning. How it is done; possible benefits."
http://www.religioustolerance.org/clo_ther.htm (accessed 11 March 2004).

46 Daar and Sheremeta, "The Science of stem cells: Some implications for
law and policy."

47 "The science involving stem cells." http://www.bereskinparr.com/
publications/art_html/biotech-stemcell-nador.html#Patent%20Law
(accessed 11 March 2004).

48 This is Francis Bacon's idea. See Leiss, *The Domination of Nature*,
chapter 3.

49 Dennis, "The Bugs of War."

50 The best example is the fate of the International Convention on
Biological and Toxic Weapons, which came into force in 1974 but
remains a "dead letter" because it has no inspection and verification
protocol. Full information is available at: http://www.bradford.ac.uk/
acad/sbtwc/ (accessed 16 March 2004).

51 This ugly episode is related and documented in Glantz *et al.*, *The
Cigarette Papers*, chapter 8.

52 For an overview see Leiss, *In the Chamber of Risks.*

53 BBC News, "Women at higher risk of lung cancer." http://news.bbc.co.uk/ 1/hi/health/2542725.stm (accessed 17 March 2004); WomenOf.com, "Women at higher risk of lung cancer." http://www.womenof.com/ Articles/hc0117002.asp (accessed 17 March 2004).

54 Saying "smoking is a risk factor for lung cancer" can be confusing to some people because it is not the only risk factor for this disease, although it happens to be the overwhelmingly predominant one. The statements (1) "smoking accounts for 30 per cent of cancer deaths," (2) "10 per cent of regular smokers will get lung cancer," and (3) "smoking causes 75–85 per cent of lung cancers," are all accurate.

55 Brad Evenson, "U.S. scientists aim to build new life in a test tube," *National Post,* 22 November 2002, A3.

56 This quote is from a website sponsored by the U.S. Department of Energy Office of Science, Office of Biological and Environmental Health and Human Geneome Program. GeneTherapy, http://www.ornl.gov/sci/ techresources/Human_Genome/medicine/genetherapy.shtml (accessed 15 March 2004).

57 The University of Michigan, "The process of speciation." http://www.globalchange.umich.edu/globalchange1/current/lectures/ speciation/speciation.html (accessed 16 March 2004).

58 Alan P. Agins, "Quitting Time: Pharmacological Approaches to Weight Loss, Alcohol Cessation and Smoking Cessation." http://www.aanp.org/ NR/rdonlyres/ez3hfkuvppgt3kopceek7hcalyzm4cdjvpmjkro23y6zpavo7 d7fsk4gfq3vderhzv4ovielrfvpag/1%252e4%252e68agins.pdf; USA Today, "Researchers say stem cells could one day help cure baldness." http://www.usatoday.com/news/health/2004-03-14-bald-cure_x.htm; *Baltimore Sun,* 16 February 2004, "Interest growing in natural remedies." http://www.qctimes.com/internal.php?story_id=1024293&t=Health&c= 9,1024293 (accessed 16 March 2004).

59 Gardner, "Can human genetic enhancement be prohibited?" (accessed 11 March 2004).

60 An allele is defined as one of an array of possible mutational forms of a given gene. For example, two different individuals may have a single base nucleotide difference at the same position when the same gene is compared nucleotide for nucleotide. Thus we would say that for this gene there are two different gene alleles. A gene may have one or several allele forms in a population of individuals.

61 Samson *et al.,* "Resistance to HIV-1 infection in Caucasian individuals bearing mutant alleles of the CCR-5 chemokine receptor gene."

62 InterPress Third World News Agency. 1998. As quoted in Danielle Knight, "New Seed Technology Threatens Farmers." http://users.westnet.gr/~cgian/knight.htm (accessed 14 March 2004).

63 "Genetic Seed Sterilization is 'Holy Grail' for Ag Biotechnology Firms. New Patents for 'Suicide Seeds' Threaten Farmers and Food Security Warns RAFI." http://www.etcgroup.org/article.asp?newsid=129 (accessed 16 March 2004).

64 For an excellent overview of the terminator technology see: Martha L. Crouch, Indiana University, "How the terminator terminates: an explanation for the non-scientist of a remarkable patent for killing second generation seeds of crop plants." The Edmonds Institute Occasional Paper Series, 1998. http://www.psrast.org/terminexpl.htm (accessed 16 March 2004).

65 Action aid, May 2003. www.actionaid.org/resources/pdfs/gatg.pdf (accessed 16 March 2004).

66 BBC news, "Action to tackle antibiotic resistance." 24 July 2001. http://news.bbc.co.uk/1/hi/health/1454198.stm (accessed 16 March 2004).

67 Action aid, May 2003. www.actionaid.org/resources/pdfs/gatg.pdf (accessed 16 March 2004).

68 Ibid.

69 The Winds Consulting, "Seed Sterilization Has Profound Implications." 1998. http://members.aol.com/poesgirl/seed.htm (accessed 12 March 2004).

70 Organic Consumers Association, "Syngenta Goes Forward on Terminator Gene." http://www.organicconsumers.org/patent/junkieplant.cfm (accessed 15 March 2004).

71 BBC news, sci/tech, "Terminator gene halt a 'major U-turn.'" http://news.bbc.co.uk/1/hi/sci/tech/465222.stm (accessed 16 March 2004).

72 PBS, "Plague war." Interviews section. http://www.pbs.org/wgbh/pages/frontline/shows/plague/ (accessed 12 March 2004).

73 Richard Preston, "Annals of warfare, the bioweaponeers," New Yorker, 9 March 1998: 52–65.

74 Ricki Lewis, "Bioweapons research proliferates," The Scientist, 27 April 1998.

75 Cole, "The Specter of Biological Weapons."

76 Finkel, "Engineered Mouse Virus Spurs Bioweapon Fears."

77 Bostrom, "Existential Risks: Analyzing human extinction scenarios and related hazards."

78 The GBMC fertility clinic, "Technologies and procedures." http://www.gbmc.org/fertilitycenter/procedures.cfm (accessed 16 March 2004).

79 Human Genome Project, "Gene testing." http://www.ornl.gov/sci/techresources/Human_Genome/medicine/genetest.shtml (accessed 16 March 2004).

80 Tasca and McClure, "The Emerging Technology and Application of Preimplantation Genetic Diagnosis."

81 Paunesku *et al.*, "Biology of TiO2-oligonucleotide nanocomposites."

82 Tsukamoto *et al.*, "Gene transfer and expression in progeny after intravenous DNA injection into pregnant mice."

83 Crooke, "Basic principles of antisense therapeutics."

84 Campbell *et al.*, "Homologous recombination involving small single-stranded oligonucleotides in human cells."

85 Brain briefings, 1994, "The Opiate Receptor." http://web.sfn.org/content/Publications/BrainBriefings/opiate.html (accessed 17 March 2004)

86 Cannabis news, Toni Baker, "Researchers Study Brain Receptors Linked To Memory." http://www.cannabisnews.com/news/thread7994.shtml (accessed 18 March 2004).

87 CNN health, Elizabeth Cohen, "Link found between obesity and brain receptors." http://www.cnn.com/2001/HEALTH/02/01/obesity.dopamine/ (accessed 17 March 2004).

88 U.S. Census Bureau, Total Midyear Population for the World: 1950–2050. http://www.census.gov/ipc/www/worldpop.html (accessed 17 March 2004).

89 http://www-genome.wi.mit.edu/media/2003/pr 03 leighsynd.html; Carolyn Abraham, "Rogue gene found in rare Quebec illness," *Globe and Mail,* 14 January 2003, A1, A8.

90 Stephen Scherer (University of Toronto), "The Human Genome Project." Presentation to the Queen's Public Executive Program, 1 October 2001, "Twin Studies of Personality Traits," showing the possible proportion of genetic factors in explaining various personality traits and outcomes in specific populations.

91 "I smell a cloned rat," *Globe and Mail,* 4 January 2003, A15. Bill C-13 passed as Bill C-6 (*Assisted Human Reproduction Act*) in March 2004: 3rd Session, 37th Parliament, 52-53 Elizabeth II, 2004 House of Commons of Canada BILL C-6, http://www.parl.gc.ca/37/3/parlbus/chambus/house/bills/government/C-6/C-6_3/90187bE.html

92 "Cloning for stem cell research unnecessary and dangerous," *Hill Times,* 3 February 2003.

93 Lois Rogers (*Times,* London), "Chinese claim first human embryo clone," *Calgary Herald,* 26 January 2003, A6.

94 "Cloning surprise sparks raging controversy." *Singapore Straits Times.* 14 February 2004. http://www.genetics-and-society.org/resources/items/20040214_straitstimes.html (accessed 16 March 2004).

95 Gina Kolata, "Researchers Find Big Risk of Defect in Cloning Animals," *New York Times,* 25 March 2001. http://www.mindfully.org/GE/Cloning-Defect.htm (accessed 17 March 2004).

96 Gardner, "Can human genetic enhancement be prohibited?"
97 *Frankenstein or the Modern Prometheus*, Wolfson ed., 185.

APPENDIX

1 Consumers' Association of Canada, *Food Safety in Canada*, 22; Nelkin, *Selling Science.*
2 Slovic *et al.*, *Health Risk Perception in Canada.*
3 D. Nelkin, *Selling Science.*
4 U.S. National Research Council (1989).
5 Kone and Mullet, "Societal Risk Perception and Media Coverage," 21–4.
6 As summarized in Krippendorff, *Content Analysis.*
7 Gamson, " A Constructionist Approach to Mass Media."
8 Krippendorff, *Content Analysis.*
9 Berelson and Lazarsfeld, *The Analysis of Communication Content.*; I.L. Janis, "Validating Content Analysis," 55–82; K. Krippendorff, *Content Analysis.*
10 C.L. Coleman, "The Influence of Mass Media."
11 For example, see Liu and Smith, "Risk Communication and Attitude Change," 331–49.
12 T. Gitlin, *The Whole World Is Watching,* 7.
13 McCombs and Shaw, "The Agenda-Setting Function of the Mass Media," 176–87.
14 Shaw and Martin, "The Function of Mass Media Agenda Setting," 902–20.
15 Fan *et al.*, "Prediction of the Public Agenda," 163–78.
16 A. Mazur, "Media Coverage and Public Opinion," 106–15.
17 Austin and Dong, "Source v. Content," 973–83.
18 G. Miller, "The Magical Number Seven, Plus or Minus Two," 81–97.
19 Hertog *et al.*, "Media Coverage of AIDS, Cancer, and Sexually Transmitted Diseases," 291–304.
20 Gibson and Zillmann, "Exaggerated versus Representative Exemplification," 603–24; Brosius and Bathelt, "The Utility of Exemplars in Persuasive Communications," 48–78.
21 Zillmann *et al.*, "Impression-Formation Effects of Printed News Varying in Descriptive Precision and Exemplification," 168–85.
22 Griffin *et al.*, "Public Reliance on Risk Communication Channels."
23 Frewer *et al.*, "Modelling the Media"; Nelkin, *Selling Science.*
24 Nelkin, *Selling Science.*
25 Ibid.
26 DiBella *et al.*, "Scientists' Reasons for Consenting to Mass Media Interviews," 740–9.

27 Dunwoody and Ryan, "Scientific Barriers to the Popularization of Science," 26–42.

28 M.E. Newman, "Electromagnetic Fields," 164–5.

29 S. Biagi, *Media Impact.*

30 Nelkin, "AIDS and the News Media," 293–307; Squires, "The Gatekeepers of Medical News," 8–9.

31 T.F. Kirn, "Networks, Local Stations Providing Air Time for Physicians," 2169–71.

32 A.S. Relman, "Reporting the Aspirin Study," 918–20.

33 E. Singer, "A Question of Accuracy," 102–16.

34 Layoff and Johnson, *Metaphors We Live By.*

35 Nelkin, *Selling Science.*

36 Ibid.

37 Ibid.

38 *New York Times,* 16 March 1985.

39 Priest and Talbert, "Mass Media and the Ultimate Technological Fix," 76–85.

40 Scientists' Institute for Public Information, *The Public's Interest in News about Science.*

41 Chew *et al.,* "Sources of Information and Knowledge about Health and Nutrition," 17–29.

42 Schanne and Meier, *Media Coverage of Risk in Biotechnology in Public.*

43 U.S. National Research Council, *Improving Risk Communication.*

44 E. Groth, "Communicating with Consumers about Food Safety and Risk Issues."

45 F. Molitor, "Accuracy in Science News Reporting by Newspapers," 209–24.

46 Protess *et al.,* "The Impact of Investigative Reporting," 166–85.

47 S. Dunwoody, *Telling Public Stories about Risk in Agricultural Biotechnology,* 97–106.

48 Atman *et al.,* "Designing Risk Communications," 779–88; Bostrom *et al.,* "Evaluating Risk Communications," 789–99; Frewer and Shepherd, "Attributing Information to Different Sources," 385–401; McCallum *et al.,* "Communicating about Environmental Risks," 349–61.

49 Johnson *et al.,* "Testing the Role of Technical Information," 341–64.

50 Johnson *et al.,* "Presenting Uncertainty in Health Risk Assessment," 485–94.

51 Burns *et al.,* "Incorporating Structural Models into Research," 611–23.

52 Sandman *et al.,* "Agency Communication, Community Outrage and Perception of Risk," 585–98; Kraus *et al.,* "Intuitive Toxicology," 215–32.

53 Hornig, "Reading Risk," 95–109.

54 Nelkin, "AIDS and the News Media," 293–307.

55 E.F. Einsiedel, "Portrayals of Science and Technology in the Canadian Press"; Nelkin, *Selling Science*.
56 M. Neuzil, "Gambling with Databases," 44–54; C. Zollars, "The Perils of Periodical Indexes," 698–716.
57 D.W. Smythe, "Some Observations on Communications Theory," 248–60.
58 K. Krippendorff, *Content Analysis*.
59 Evans and Priest, "Science Content and Social Context," 327–40.

Bibliography

Abelson, Philip H. "Excessive Fear of PCBs." *Science* 253, 5018 (1991): 361.

Agriculture and Agri-food Canada. *Agenda; Jobs and Growth.* Ottawa: AAFC 1995.

– "All about Canada's Vegetable Industry." http://aceis/agr.ca/cb/facts/fao14e.html. Accessed 2 January 1997.

– Plant Biotechnology Office. *Assessment Criteria for Determining Environmental Safety of Plants with Novel Traits.* Regulatory Directive 94-08, Ottawa: AAFC 1994.

– Plant Biotechnology Office. *The Biology of Brassica Napus L. (Canola).* Regulatory Directive 94-09, Ottawa: AAFC 1994.

– Plant Biotechnology Office. *The Biology of Solanum Tuberosum L. (Potato),* Regulatory Directive T-1-09-96, Ottawa: AAFC 1996.

– *Biotechnology in Agriculture and Agri-Food: General Information.* Ottawa: AAFC 1996.

– *Determination of Environmental Safety of Monsanto Canada Inc.'s Roundup Tolerant Brassica Napus Canola Line GT73.* Decision Document DD 95-02, Ottawa: AAFC 1995.

– Plant Biotechnology Office. *Determination of Environmental Safety of Nature-Marks Potatoes' Colorado Potato Beetle (CPB) Resistant Potato.* Decision Document DD96-09, Ottawa Plant Biotechnology Office: AAFC 1996.

– *Field Testing Genetically Modified Plants in Canada.* Ottawa: AAFC 1994.

– "Field Trials." http://aceis.agr.ca/fpi/agbiotec/fieldt96.html. Accessed 4 January 1997.

– *Workshop on Food Biotechnology: An Information Session to Increase Awareness of Food Biotechnology within Agriculture Canada.* Ottawa: Agri-Food Safety and Strategies Division, AAFC 1993.

Agriculture Canada. *Report to Federal Ministers of the Federal-Provincial Agriculture Committee on Environmental Sustainability.* Ottawa: Government of Canada 1990.

Alberta. *Albertans & climate change: a strategy for managing environmental & economic risks.* Edmonton: Government of Alberta 2002. 39 leaves. http://www3.gov.ab.ca/env/climate/actionplan/docs/strategy.pdf

Albrecht, D.E. *Public Perceptions of Agricultural Biotechnology: An Overview of Research to Date.* College Station, TX: Center for Biotechnology Policy and Ethics 1992.

Allen, Richard W. "Research: Thinking about Community Consequences." In *Nuna Med' 91 – En Gronlandsmedicinsk Konference,* ed. P. Kern and T. Cordtz, 22–4. Nuuk: Gronlandmedicinsk Selskab et Gronlands Laegekredsforening 1991.

Anderson, R.M., et al. "Transmission Dynamics and Epidemiology of BSE in British Cattle," *Nature* 382 (29 August 1996): 779–88.

Angell, Marcia. "Do Breast Implants Cause Systemic Disease? Science in the Courtroom." *New England Journal of Medicine* 330, no. 24 (16 June 1994): 1748–9.

– *Science on Trial: The Clash of Medical Evidence and the Law in the Breast Implant Case.* New York: W.W. Norton 1996.

Angus Reid Group. *Public Opinion on Food Safety and Biotechnology Applications in Agriculture.* Winnipeg 1995.

"Another Herbicide on the Blacklist." *Nature* 226 (25 April 1970): 309–10.

Archibald, Chris P., and Tom Kosatsky. "Public Health Response to an Identified Environmental Toxin: Managing Risks to the James Bay Cree Related to Cadmium in Caribou and Moose." *Canadian Journal of Public Health* 82 (January/February 1991): 22–6.

Atman, C.J., A. Bostrom, B. Fischhoff, and G.M. Morgan. "Designing Risk Communications: Completing and Correcting Mental Models of Hazardous Processes." Part 1. *Risk Analysis* 14 (1994): 779–88.

Austin, E.W., and Q. Dong. "Source v. Content Effects on Judgements of News Believability." *Journalism Quarterly* 71 (1994): 973–83.

Ayotte, P., E. Dewailly, S. Bruneau, H. Careau, and A. Vezina. "Arctic Air Pollution and Human Health: What Effects Should Be Expected?" *Science of the Total Environment* 160/161 (1995): 529–37.

Ayotte, P., G. Carrier, and E. Dewailly. "Health Risk Assessment for Inuit Newborns Exposed to Dioxin-Like Compounds through Breast Feeding." *Chemosphere* 32, no. 3 (1996): 531–42.

Baillie, A., S. Bernow, et al. *The Bottom Line on Kyoto: Economic Benefits of Canadian Action.* Vancouver, B.C.: David Suzuki Foundation 2002. http://www.davidsuzuki.org/files/kyotoreport.pdf

Ball, N. "Essential Connections: Past and Future, Technology and Society." In *Beyond the Printed Page: Online Documentation,* 11–28. Proceedings of the Second Conference on Quality in Documentation, Waterloo, ON: University of Waterloo 1992.

Barrie, L.A., D. Gregor, B. Hargrave, R. Lake, D. Muir, R. Shearer, B. Tracey, and T. Bidleman. "Arctic Contaminants: Sources, Occurrence and Pathways." *Science of the Total Environment* 122 (1992): 1–74.

Batra, L.R., and W. Klassen. *Public Perceptions of Biotechnology.* Bethesda, MD: Agricultural Research Institute 1987.

Bauman, D.E. "Bovine Somatotropin: Review of an Emerging Animal Technology." *Journal of Dairy Sciences* 75 (1992): 3432–51.

Bauman, D.E., B.W. McBride, J.L. Burton, and K. Sejrsen. "Somatotropin (BST): International Dairy Federation Technical Report." *Bulletin of the IDF* 293 (1994): 2.

Bayerische Rück, ed. *Risk Is a Construct.* Munich: Knesebeck 1993.

Berelson, B., and P.F. Lazarsfeld. *The Analysis of Communication Content.* Chicago and New York: University of Chicago Press 1948.

Berrier, R.J. "Public Perceptions of Biotechnology." In *Public Perceptions of Biotechnology,* ed. R. Batra and W. Klassen, 37–52. Bethesda, MD: Agricultural Research Institute 1987.

Bertazzi, P.A., *et al.* "Cancer Incidence in a Population Accidentally Exposed to 2,3,7,8-tetrachlorodibenzo-para-dioxin." *Epidemiology* 4, no. 5 (1993): 398–406.

Biagi, S. *Media Impact: An Introduction to Mass Media.* Belmont, CA: Wadsworth 1990.

Bielawski, Ellen. "Inuit Indigenous Knowledge and Science in the Arctic." In *Human Ecology and Climate Change – People and Resources in the Far North,* ed. D.L. Peterson and D.R. Johnson, 219–27. Washington, DC: Taylor & Francis 1995.

Boiteau, G., and J.P.R. Le Blanc. *Colorado Potato Beetle Life Stages.* Ottawa: Agriculture Canada 1992.

Bostrom, A., C.J. Atman, B. Fischhoff, and G.M. Morgan. "Evaluating Risk Communications: Completing and Correcting Mental Models of Hazardous Processes." Part 2. *Risk Analysis* 14 (1994): 789–99.

Bostrom, Nick. "Existential Risks. Analyzing human extinction scenarios and related hazards." *Journal of Evolution and Technology,* vol. 9, March 2002.

Boustie, S., M. Raynolds, *et al. How Ratifying the Kyoto Protocol will Benefit Canada's Competitiveness.* Drayton Valley, Alberta: Pembina Institute for Appropriate Development 2002.
http://www.pembina.org/pdf/publications/competitiveness_report.pdf

Bradley, R., and J. Wilesmith. "Epidemiology and Control of Bovine Spongiform Encephalopathy (BSE)." *British Medical Bulletin* 49 (1993): 932–59.

Bramley, Matthew. *An Assessment of Alberta's Climate Change Action Plan.* Drayton Valley, Alberta: Pembina Institute for Appropriate Development September 2002. http://www.pembina.org/publications_item.asp?id-138

Bramley, M., K. Hamilton, *et al. A comparison of current government action on climate change in the U.S. and Canada.* Drayton Valley, Alberta: Pembina Institute for Appropriate Development 2002: 53.

Brandner, S., S. Isenmann, A. Raeber, M. Fischer, A. Sailer, Y. Kobayashi, S. Marino, C. Weismann, and A. Aguzzi. "Normal Host Prion Protein Necessary for Scrapie-Induced Neurotoxicity." *Nature* (25 January 1996): 339–43.

Brethour, P. "Russia can't ratify Kyoto, official says." *Globe and Mail.* 26 February 2004: B2.

Brosius, H., and A. Bathelt. "The Utility of Exemplars in Persuasive Communications." *Communications Research* 21, no. 1 (1994): 48–78.

Bruneau, Suzanne, and Jacques Grondin. "Development of Risk Communication Activities and Research in Nunavik." *Arctic Medical Research* 53, suppl. 2 (1994): 356–8.

Bryne, John A. *Informed Consent.* New York: McGraw-Hill 1996.

Brzuzy, L., and R. Hites. "Global Mass Balance for Polychlorinated Dibenzo-p-dioxins and Dibenzofurans." *Environmental Science and Technology* 30 (1996): 1797–1804.

Bud, R. *The Uses of Life: A History of Biotechnology.* Cambridge: Cambridge University Press 1993.

Burger, Edward J. "A Case Study: Polychlorinated Biphenyls." In *Protecting the Nation's Health: The Problems of Regulations,* 187–201. Lexington, MA: Lexington Books 1976.

– "Health as a Surrogate for the Environment." *Daedalus* 119, no. 4 (1990): 133–53.

Burges, H.D. "Possibilities for Pest Resistance to Microbial Control Agents." In Burges, H.D., and N.W. Hussey, eds. *Microbial Control of Insects and Mites,* 445–57. New York: Academic Press 1971.

Burke, W.S., ed. *Symbol, Substance, Science: The Societal Issues of Food Biotechnology.* North Carolina Biotechnology Centre, 28–29 June 1993. Research Triangle Park, NC: Institute for Science in Society 1993.

Burns, W.J., P. Slovic, R.E. Kasperson, J.X. Kasperson, O. Renn, and S. Emani. "Incorporating Structural Models into Research on the Social Amplification of Risk: Implications for Theory Construction and Decision Making." *Risk Analysis* 13 (1993): 611–23.

Burton, J.L., and B.W. McBride. "Recombinant Bovine Somatotropin (rBST): Is There a Limit for Biotechnology in Applied Animal Agriculture?" *Journal of Agricultural Ethics* 2 (1989): 129–59.

Burton, J.L., B.W. McBride, E. Block, D.R. Glimm, and J.J. Kennelly. "A Review of Bovine Growth Hormone." *Canadian Journal of Animal Science* 74 (1994): 167–201.

Butler, Declan. "Panel Urges Precautionary Approach." *Nature* (17 October 1996): 99.

Buxton, G.V., D.B.W. Robinson, and M.F. Millson. *The PCB Problem: A Background Paper for Policy Consideration.* Report EPS-7-72-1. Ottawa: Minister of Supply and Services 1972.

Cabirac, D., and R. Warmbrodt. *Biotechnology: Public Perception: January 1985–December 1992.* QB93-15. Beltsville, MD: U.S. National Agricultural Library 1993.

Calamai, P. "Kyoto plan falls short of targets, Ottawa told: Audit reveals little progress in cuts to greenhouse gases." *Toronto Star.* 5 April 2004.

Caldwell, R.B., and L.H. Duke. *The Regulation of Plant Biotechnology in Canada.* Part 1. Ottawa: Agriculture Canada 1988.

Campbell, C.R., W. Keown, L. Lowe, D. Kirschling, and R. Kucherlapati. "Homologous recombination involving small single-stranded oligonucleotides in human cells." *New Biology* 1(2) (1989): 223–7.

Campbell, K.H., J. McWhir, W.A. Ritchie, and I. Wilmut. "Sheep cloned by nuclear transfer from a cultured cell line." *Nature* 380 (1996): 64–6.

Canadian Broadcasting Corporation (CBC). "Public Enemy No. 1." *Fifth Estate,* 10 October 1989.

Canadian Council of Resource and Environment Ministers (CCREM). *The PCB Story.* N.p. 1986.

– *Dioxins and Furans: The Canadian Perspective.* N.p., n.d.

Canadian Environmental Advisory Council (CEAC). *PCBs: A Burning Issue – On the Siting of a Mobile PCB Incinerator.* Report to the Federal Minister of the Environment, 2 January 1989.

Canadian Council of Grocery Distributors. *Trends in Canada: Survey on Consumer Shopping.* CCGD 1993.

– *Trends in Canada: Survey on Consumer Shopping.* CCGD 1995.

Canola Council of Canada. *The Canola Growers Manual,* by P. Thomas. Winnipeg, MB: Canola Council of Canada 1996.

Carson, R. *Silent Spring.* Cambridge, MA: Riverside Press 1962.

Carter, C.D., R.D. Kimbrough, J.A. Liddle, R.E. Cline, M.M. Zack, and W.F. Barthel. "Tetrachlorodibenzodioxin: An Accidental Poisoning Incident in Horse Arenas." *Science* 188 (1974): 738–40.

Casey, Denise K. "Genes, Dreams and Reality: The promise and risks of the new genetics." *Judicature,* vol. 83, no. 3 (November 1999). http://www.ornl.gov/sci/techresources/Human_Genome/publicat/judicature/article3.html

Chase, S. "Canada plans to stick to Kyoto, minister says." *Globe and Mail.* 30 September 2003: A9.

Chess, Caron, M. Greenberg, M. Tamuz, and A. Saville. "The Organizational Links between Risk Communication and Risk Management: The Case of Sybron Chemicals, Inc." *Risk Analysis* 12 (1992): 431–8.

Chess, Caron, M. Tamuz, and M. Greenberg. "Organizational Learning about Environmental Risk Communication: The Case of Rohm and Haas' Bristol Plant." *Society and Natural Resources* 8 (1995): 57–66.

Chew, F., S. Palmerand, and S. Kim. "Sources of Information and Knowledge about Health and Nutrition: Can Viewing One Television Programme Make a Difference?" *Public Understanding of Science* 4 (1995): 17–29.

Cohn, M.B., and R.A. Giannella. "Hemorrhagic Colitis Associated with *Escherichia Coli* O157:H7." *Advances in International Medicine* 37 (1992): 173–95.

Cole, Leonard A. "The Specter of Biological Weapons." *Scientific American* 275 (December 1996): 60–4.

Coleman, C.L. "The Influence of Mass Media and Interpersonal Communication on Societal and Personal Risk Judgement." *Communications Research* 20 (1993): 611–28.

Collinge, J., K.C.L. Sidle, J. Meads, J. Ironside, and A. Hill. "Molecular Analysis of Prion Strain Variation and the Aetiology of 'New Variant' CJD." *Nature* 383 (24 October 1996): 685–90.

Comité de Santé Environnementale (CSE). *L'Oncogénèse environnementale au Québec.* Québec: Comité de Santé Environnementale 1995.

Consumers' Association of Canada. *Food Safety in Canada.* Ottawa: Consumers' Association of Canada 1990.

Coulston, F., and F. Pocchari, eds. *Accidental Exposure to Dioxins – Human Health Aspects.* New York: Academic Press 1983.

Council for Agricultural Science and Technology (CAST). *Foodborne Pathogens: Risks and Consequences.* Ames, IA: CAST 1994.

Covello, V.T. "The Perception of Technological Risks: A Literature Review." *Technical Forecasting of Social Change* 23 (1983): 285–97.

Covello, Vincent, Detlof von Winterfeldt, and Paul Slovic. *Risk Communication.* Washington, DC: Conservation Foundation 1987.

Coyne, A. "What is the cost of 'hot air'?" *National Post.* 17 May 2002.

Crawley, M.J., and S.L. Brown. "Seed Limitation and the Dynamics of Feral Oilseed Rape on the M25 Motorway." *Proceedings of the Royal Society of London British Sciences* 259, no. 1354 (1995): 49–54.

Creative Research International. *Consumer Environment Study.* Ottawa 1993.

Crooke, Stanley T. "Basic principles of antisense therapeutics." In Crooke, S.T., ed., *Antisense research and application.* Berlin: Springer Publisher 1998: 1–50.

Daar, A.S., and L. Sheremeta. "The science of stem cells: Some implications for law and policy." *Health Law Review* 11 (2002): 5–13.

Darmency, H., A. Fleury, and E. Lefol. "Effect of Transgenic Release on Weed Biodiverisity: Oilseed Rape and Wild Radish." Brighton Crop Protection Conference (1995): 433–8.

Daughaday, W.H., and D.M. Barbano. "Bovine Somatotropin Supplementation of Dairy Cows: Is the Milk Safe?" *Journal of the American Medical Association* 264 (1990): 1003–5, 1028.

Davis, B. *The Genetic Revolution: Scientific Prospects and Public Perceptions.* Baltimore, MD: Johns Hopkins University Press 1991.

Denis, Hélène. *La gestion de la catastrophe: Le cas d'un incendie à St-Basile-le-Grand.* Québec: Publications du Québec 1990.

Dennis, Carina. "The Bugs of War." *Nature* 114 (2001): 232–5.

DeVito, Michael J., and Linda S. Birnbaum. "Toxicology of Dioxins and Related Chemicals." In *Dioxins and Health*, ed. A. Schecter, 139–62. New York: Plenum Press 1994.

Dewailly, E., P. Ayotte, S. Bruneau, C. Laliberté, D.C.G. Muir, and R.J. Norstrom. "Inuit Exposure to Organochlorines through the Aquatic Food Chain in Arctic Québec." *Environmental Health Perspectives* 101, no. 7 (1993): 618–20.

Dewailly, E., P. Ayotte, C. Laliberté, Jean-Philippe Weber, S. Gingras, and A.J. Nantel. "Polychlorinated Biphenyl (PCB) and Dichlorodiphenyl Dichloroethylene (DDE) Concentrations in the Breast Milk of Women in Quebec." *American Journal of Public Health* 86, no. 9 (1996): 1241–6.

Dewailly, E., S. Bruneau, C. Laliberté, and S. Gingras. *Breast Milk Contamination in Nunavik: Evaluation of Health Risks for Infants*. Centre de Santé Publique de Québec and Kativik Regional Board of Health and Social Services, Québec 1994.

Dewailly, E., S. Bruneau, C. Laliberté, G. Lebel, S. Gingras, J. Grondin, and P. Levallois. "Contaminants." In *A Health Profile of the Inuit: Report of the Santé Québec Health Survey among the Inuit of Nunavik*, vol. 1, ed. M. Jetté, 75–107. Québec: Gouvernement du Québec 1992.

Dewailly, E., C. Laliberté, L. Sauvé, L. Ferron, J.J. Ryan, S. Gingras, and P. Ayotte. "Sea-Bird Consumption As a Major Source of PCB Exposure for Communities Living along the Gulf of St Lawrence." *Chemosphere* 25 (1992): 1251–5.

Dewailly, E., A. Nantel, J.P. Webber, and F. Meyer. "High Levels of PCBs in Breast Milk of Inuit Women from Arctic Quebec." *Bulletin of Environmental Contamination and Toxicology* 43, no. 5 (1989): 641–6.

DiBella, S.M., A.J. Ferri, and A.B. Padderud. "Scientists' Reasons for Consenting to Mass Media Interviews: A National Survey." *Journalism Quarterly* (Winter 1991): 740–9.

Dittus, K.L., and V.N. Hillers. "Consumer Trust and Behavior Related to Pesticides." *Food Technology* 47, no. 7 (1993): 87–9.

Dow Corning Canada Inc. "Detailed Background on 1970 Dog Study." *Dow Corning Corporation and the Silicone Breast Implant Issue: Case Study Source Materials* (1996).

– "Dow Corning's Disclosure of Gel-Breast Implant Complications, 1960s – 1985." *Dow Corning Corporation and the Silicone Breast Implant Issue: Case Study Source Materials* (1996).

– *Facts You Should Know about Your New Look*. Brochure, n.p., 1970, 1972, 1976, 1980.

Doyle, M.P., and J.L. Schoeni. "Survival and Growth of *Escherichia Coli* Associated with Hemorrhagic Colitis." *Applied and Environmental Microbiology* 48, no. 4 (1984): 855–6.

Drexhage, J. "Still up in the air." *Carbon Finance.* 2004: 16–17.

Duarte-Davidson, R., A. Sewart, R.E. Alcock, I.T. Cousins, and K.C. Jones. "Exploring the Balance between Sources, Deposition, and the Environmental Burden of PCDD/FS in the U.K. Terrestrial Environment." *Environmental Science and Technology* 31 (1997): 1–11.

Dunwoody, S. *Telling Public Stories about Risk in Agricultural Biotechnology: A Public Conversation about Risk.* Ithaca, NY: National Agricultural Biotechnology Council 5 1993.

Dunwoody, S., and M. Ryan. "Scientific Barriers to the Popularization of Science in the Mass Media." *Journal of Communications* 35 (1985): 26–42.

Durant, J., ed. *Biotechnology in Public: A Review of Recent Research.* London: Science Museum 1992.

Eckert, J.E. "The Flight Range of the Honeybee." *Journal of Agricultural Research* 47 (1933): 257–85.

Ecobichon, Donald J. "Toxic Effects of Pesticides." In *Casarett and Doull's Toxicology: The Basic Science of Poisons,* ed. Curtis D. Klaasen, Mary O. Amdur, and John Doull, 643–89. New York: McGraw-Hill 1996.

Edmonds Institute. *Assessment of Genetically Engineered Organisms in the Environment: The Puget Sound Workshop Biosafety Handbook.* Seattle, WA: Edmonds Institute 1996.

Edwards, P.N., and S.H. Schneider. "Self-governance and peer review in Science-for-Policy." In *Changing the atmosphere: Expert knowledge and environmental governance.* C.A. Miller and P.N. Edwards. Cambridge, MA: The MIT Press 2001: 219–46.

Ehsan, Masood. "BSE Transmission Data Pose Dilemma for UK Scientists." *Nature* (8 August 1996).

Einsiedel, E.F. "Portrayals of Science and Technology in the Canadian Press." Paper presented to the American Association for the Advancement of Science, San Francisco, CA, 14–19 January 1989.

Ellstrand, N.C. "Pollen As a Vehicle for the Escape of Engineered Genes?" *Trends in Ecology and Evolution* 3, no. 4 (1988): S30–S32.

Environment and Health Canada. *Priority Substances List Assessment Report No. 1.* Ottawa, n.d.

Environment Canada. *Background to the Regulation of Polychlorinated Biphenyls (PCB) in Canada.* Technical Report 76-1 of the Task Force on PCB, 1 April 1976, to the Environmental Contaminants Committee of Environment Canada and Health and Welfare Canada 1976.

– "Canada to Allow PCB Exports to the United States for Destruction." News release, Ottawa, 26 September 1996.

– *Climate Change Plan for Canada.* Ottawa: Government of Canada 2002. http://www.climatechange.gc.ca/plan_for_canada/index.html

– *Federal PCB Destruction Program: Proceedings, National Stakeholder Workshop.* Edmonton, AB, 22 November 1989.

– *Handbook on PCBs in Electrical Equipment.* Ottawa: Minister of Supply and Services Canada 1988.
– *Managing PCBs.* Ottawa: Minister of Supply and Services Canada 1987.
– *National Inventory of Concentrated PCB (Askarel) Fluids* (1985 Summary Update). EPS 5/HA/4. Ottawa: Minister of Supply and Services Canada 1986.
– *National Inventory of PCBs in Use and PCB Wastes in Storage in Canada – 1993 Annual Report.* Ottawa: Hazardous Waste Management Branch, Environmental Protection Service 1993.
– *Options for the Treatment/Destruction of Polychlorinated Biphenyls (PCBs) and PCB-contaminated Equipment.* EPS 2/HA/1. Ottawa: Minister of Supply and Services Canada 1991.
– *PCBs: Question and Answer Guide Concerning Polychlorinated Biphenyls.* EN40-335. Ottawa: Minister of Supply and Services Canada 1986.
– *Report of the Independent Review Committee on the Initial Environmental Evaluation for a Mobile PCB Destruction Facility.* N.p. 24 June 1994.
– *Strategy of the Federal PCB Destruction Program.* Ottawa: Conservation and Protection Branch, October 1990.
– *Summary of Environmental Criteria for Polychlorinated Biphenyls (PCBs).* EPS 4/HA/1. Ottawa: Minister of Supply and Services Canada 1987.
Environment Canada, ARET (Accelerated Reduction and Elimination of Toxics) Secretariat. *Environmental Leaders 1: Voluntary Commitments to Action on Toxics through ARET.* Ottawa: March 1995.
Essex, C., and R. McKitrick. *Taken by storm: the troubled science, policy and politics of global warming.* Toronto: Key Porter Books 2002.
Evans, W., and Priest S. Hornig. "Science Content and Social Context." *Public Understanding of Science* 4 (1995): 327–40.
Fan, D.P., H.B. Brosius, and H.M. Kepplinger. "Prediction of the Public Agenda from Television Coverage." *Journal of Broadcasting Electronic Media* 38 (1994): 163–78.
Feder, J. Barnaby. "Picking on Cotton." *Scientific American* 275, no. 4 (October 1996).
Felix, O. "O157:H7 Outbreak Creates New Cooking Standard." *Food Protection Report* 9, no. 2 (1993): 1.
Ferro, D.N. "Potential for Resistance to Bacillus Thuringiensis: Colorado Potato Beetle (Coleoptera: Chrysomelidae) – A Model System." *American Entomologist* 39, no. 1 (1993): 38–44.
Fingerhut, M.L., *et al.* "Cancer Mortality in Workers Exposed to 2,3,7,8-tetra-chlorodibenzo-p-dioxin." *New England Journal of Medicine* 324, no. 4 (1991): 212–18.
Finkel, A.M. "Dioxin: Are We Safer Now Than Before?" *Risk Analysis* 8 (1988): 161–5.
Finkel, Elizabeth. "Engineered Mouse Virus Spurs Bioweapon Fears." *Science* 291 (2001): 585.

Fleising, U. "Public Perceptions of Biotechnology." In *Biotechnology: The Science and the Business*, ed. V. Moses and R.E. Cape, 89–102. Chur, Switzerland: Harwood Academic Publishers 1991.

Flynn, J., and P. Slovic. "Yucca Mountain: A Crisis for Policy." *Annual Review of Energy and Environment* 20 (1995): 83–118.

Flynn, J., P. Slovic, and C.K. Mertz. "The Nevada Initiative: A Risk Communication Fiasco." *Risk Analysis* 13 (1993): 497–502.

Food Marketing Institute (FMI). *Trends, Consumer Attitudes and the Supermarket.* Washington, DC: Food Marketing Institute 1994.

Foster, E.M. "A Half Century of Food Microbiology – And a Glimpse at the Years Ahead." *Dairy and Food Sanitation* 8, no. 11 (1988): 586–92.

Foulke, J.E. "How to Outsmart Dangerous E. Coli Strain." *FDA Consumer* (January/February 1994).

Fowler, C., and P. Mooney. *Shattering: Food, Politics and the Loss of Genetic Diversity.* Tucson, AZ: University of Arizona Press 1991.

Frank, John W., and Jack Newman. "Breast-Feeding in a Polluted World: Uncertain Risks, Clear Benefits." *Canadian Medical Association Journal* 149, no. 1 (1993): 33–7.

Frankton, C., and G.A. Mulligan. *Weeds of Canada.* Ottawa: Department of Agriculture 1980.

Freeman, Milton. "The Nature and Utility of Traditional Ecological Knowledge." *Northern Perspectives* 20, no. 1 (1992): 9–12.

Freudenburg, W.R., C.-L. Coleman, J. Gonzales, and C. Helgeland. "Media Coverage of Hazard Events: Analyzing the Assumptions." *Risk Analysis* 16, no. 1 (1996): 31–42.

Frewer, L.J., and R. Shepherd. "Attributing Information to Different Sources: Effects on the Perceived Qualities of Information, on the Perceived Relevance of Information, and on Attitude Formation." *Public Understanding of Science* 3 (1994): 385–401.

Frewer, L.J., C. Howard, D. Hedderley, and R. Shepherd. "What Determines Trust in Information about Food-Related Risks? Underlying Psychological Constructs." *Risk Analysis* 16 (1996): 473–86.

Frewer, L.J., M.M. Raats, and R. Shepherd. "Modelling the Media: the Transmission of Risk Information in the Quality British Press." *Journal of the Institute of Mathematics and Its Applications to Industry* 5 (1993/4): 235–47.

Fumento, Michael. "A Confederacy of Boobs: How Special Interests, Assorted Ideologues, and a Sensationalist Press Torpedoed Breast Implants – and Now Threaten Other Medical Devices." *Reason* (October 1995): 36–43.

Funtowicz, S.O., and J.R. Ravetz. "Uncertainty, Complexity and Post-Normal Science." *Environmental Toxicology and Chemistry* 13, no. 12 (1994): 1881–5.

Gabriel, Sherine E., *et al.* "Risk of Connective-Tissue Diseases and Other Disorders after Breast Implantation." *New England Journal of Medicine* 330, no. 24 (16 June 1994): 1697–702.

Gamson, W.A. "The 1987 Distinguished Lecture: A Constructionist Approach to Mass Media and Public Opinion." *Symbolic Interaction* 11 (1987): 161–74.

Gardner, W. "Can human genetic enhancement be prohibited?" *Journal of Medicine and Philosophy*, 20 (1995): 4–5. http://research.mednet.ucla.edu/pmts/Germline/Therapy%20verus%20Enhancement?tewg4.htm

Garthright, W.E., D.L. Archer, and J.E. Kvenberg. "Estimates of Incidence and Costs of Intestinal Infectious Diseases in the United States." *Public Health Report* 103 (1988): 107–15.

Genigeorgis, C. "Problems Associated with Perishable Processed Meats." *Food Technology* 40, no. 4 (1986): 150–4.

Gibson, R., and D. Zillmann. "Exaggerated Versus Representative Exemplification in News Reports." *Communication Research* 21 (1994): 603–24.

Gitlin, T. *The Whole World Is Watching.* Berkeley, CA: University of California Press 1980.

Glantz, Stanton A. *et al. The Cigarette Papers.* Berkeley: University of California Press 1996.

Glass, K.A., J.M. Loeffelholz, J.P. Ford, and M.P. Doyle. "Fate of *Escherichia Coli* O157:H7 As Affected by pH or Sodium Chloride in Fermented, Dry Sausage." *Applied Environmental Microbiology* 58 (1992): 2513–16.

Goldman, Abe. "Controlling PCBs." In *Perilous Progress – Managing the Hazards of Technology,* ed. R.W. Kates, C. Hohenemser, and J.X. Kasperson, 345–71. Boulder and London: Westview Press 1984.

Gough, Michael. *Dioxin, Agent Orange – The Facts.* New York: Plenum Press 1986.

– 1991. "Human Health Effects: What the Data Indicate." *Science of the Total Environment* 104: 129–58.

Government of Ontario. *Biotechnology in Ontario – Growing Safely.* Government of Ontario 1989.

Grant, Donald D. "Regulation of PCBs in Canada." In *PCBs: Human and Environmental Hazards,* ed. F.M. D'Itri and M.A. Kamrin, 383–92. Boston: Butterworth Publishers 1983.

Greenpeace. *Achieving Zero Dioxin,* by Joe Thornton. Washington, DC: Greenpeace USA 1994.

– *Alternatives to PVC Products.* Vienna: Greenpeace Austria 1995.

– *Biotechnology and the Convention on Biological Diversity,* by Isabelle Meister and Cathy Fogel. Amsterdam: Greenpeace International 1994.

– *Body of Evidence: The Effects of Chlorine on Human Health.* Amsterdam: Greenpeace International 1995.

– *Comments on U.S. EPA Dioxin Reassessment,* by Joe Thornton. Washington, DC: Greenpeace USA 1995.

– *Dioxin and the Failure of Canadian Public Health Policy,* by Jay Palter. Toronto: Greenpeace Canada 1994.

– *Dioxin and Human Health: A Public Health Assessment of Dioxin Exposure in Canada,* by Tom Webster. N.p., Greenpeace Canada 1995.

– *Dioxin Factories: A Study of the Creation and Discharge of Dioxins and Other Organochlorines from the Production of PVC.* Amsterdam: Greenpeace International 1993.
– *Dow Brand Dioxin.* Edited by Jack Weinberg. N.p. 1995.
– *Environmental Risks of Genetically Engineered Organisms and Key Regulatory Issues,* by Peter Kareiva and Ingrid Parker. Amsterdam: Greenpeace International 1994.
– *Genetically Engineered Food: An Experiment with Nature.* Amsterdam: Greenpeace International 1996.
– *Genetically Engineered Plants: Releases and Impacts on Less Developed Countries,* by Isabelle Meister and Sue Mayer. Amsterdam: Greenpeace International 1994.
– *Hazardous Waste Incineration: Impacts on Agriculture,* by Joe Thornton. Washington, DC: Greenpeace USA 1993.
– *No Margin of Safety,* by Carol Van Strum and Paul Merrell. Washington, DC: Greenpeace USA 1987.
– *Polyvinyl Chloride (PVC) Plastic: Primary Contributor to the Global Dioxin Crisis,* by Bonnie Rice. N.p. 1995.
– *PVC at the Hospital: Use, Risks, and Alternatives in the Health Care Sector.* Vienna: Greenpeace Austria 1995.
– *Taking Back our Stolen Future: Hormone Disruption and PVC Plastic.* Amsterdam: Greenpeace International 1996.
Gregory, Robin, James Flynn, and Paul Slovic. "Technological Stigma." *American Scientist* 83 (1995): 220–3.
Griffin, P.M. "*Escherichia Coli* O157:H7 and Other Enterohemorrhagic *Escherichia Coli.*" In *Infections of the Gastrointestinal Tract,* ed. M.J. Blaser, P.D. Smith, J.I. Ravdin, H.B. Greenberg, and R.I. Guerrant, 739–61. New York: Raven Press 1995.
Griffin, P.M., and R.V. Tauxe. "The Epidemiology of Infections Caused by *Escherichia Coli* O157:H7, Other Enterohemorrhagic *E. Coli,* and the Associated Hemolytic Uremic Syndrome." *Epidemiology Review* 13 (1991): 60–98.
Griffin, R.J., S. Dunwoody, F. Zabala, and M. Kamerick. "Public Reliance on Risk Communication Channels in the Wake of a Cryptosporidium Outbreak." Presented to the Society for Risk Analysis annual meeting, Baltimore, MD 1994.
Griffiths, A. "Implementation of Biotechnology Research and Development Policy: Implications for Sustainable Agriculture." Doctoral thesis, University of British Columbia 1996.
Griffiths, M.W. "The Role of ATP Bioluminescence in the Food Industry: New Light on Old Problems." *Food Technology* 50, no. 6 (1996): 62–72.
Grondin, J., S. Hodgins, J.-F. Proulx, and C. Blanchette. *A Review of Environmental Health Advisories in Nunavik from 1978 to 1995.* Québec Centre for Public Health and Nunavik Regional Board of Health and Social Services 1996.

Grondin, J., J.-F. Proulx, S. Bruneau, and E. Dewailly. "Santé publique et environnement au Nunavik." *Etudes/Inuit/Studies* 18, 1–2 (1994): 225–51.

Groth, E. "Communicating with Consumers about Food Safety and Risk Issues." *Food Technology* 45, no. 5 (1991): 248–53.

Groulx, Stéphane. *Le suivi et la surveillance de la santé humaine après l'incendie de biphényles polychlorés (BPC) de St-Basile-le-Grand.* Rapport synthèse du Réseau de la Santé et des Services Sociaux du Québec, Département de Santé Communautaire, Hôpital Charles Lemoyne 1992.

Grover, R. "Boxed in at Jack-in-the-Box." *Business Week* (15 February 1993): 40.

Hagedorn, C., and S. Allender-Hagedorn. "Public Perceptions in Agricultural and Environmental Biotechnology: A Study of Public Concerns." Virginia Polytechnic Institute and State University, Public Perceptions of Biotechnology web page (http://fbox.vt.edu:10021/cals/cses/chagedor/index.html) 1995.

Hallman, W.K., and J. Metcalfe. *Public Perceptions of Agricultural Biotechnology: A Survey of New Jersey Residents.* New Jersey: Rutgers University 1994.

Hansen, J. "Defusing the global warming time bomb." *Scientific American* March 2004: 68–77.

Hansen, L.G. "Environmental Toxicology of PCBs." in *PCBs: Mammalian and Environmental Toxicology,* ed. S. Safe and O. Hutzinger, 77–95. Environmental Toxin Series 1, New York: Springer-Verlag 1987.

Harris, M.K. "Bacillus Thuringiensis and Pest Control." *Science* 253 (1991): 1075.

Harrison, Kathryn, and George Hoberg. *Risk, Science and Politics.* Montréal: McGill-Queen's University Press 1994.

Harvard Report on Cancer Prevention, Harvard School of Public Health, Boston, MA, November 1996.

Hayes, M.A. "Carcinogenic and Mutagenic Effects of PCBs." In *PCBs: Mammalian and Environmental Toxicology,* ed. S. Safe and O. Hutzinger, 77–95. Environmental Toxin Series 1, New York: Springer-Verlag 1987.

Hayes, W.J., Jr. *Pesticides Studied in Man.* Baltimore and London: Williams and Wilkins 1993.

Health and Welfare Canada (HWC). "PCBs." In *A Vital Link,* 59–64. Health and Welfare Canada, Ottawa: Minister of Supply and Services 1992.

Health Canada. *Dioxins and Furans.* Ottawa: Health Protection Branch 1988.

Hecht, D.W. "Bovine Somatotropin Safety and Effectiveness: An Industry Perspective." *Food Technology* 45, no. 4 (1991): 120–6.

Hennekens, Charles H., I-Min Lee, Nancy R. Cook, Patricia R. Hebert, Elizabeth W. Karleson, Fran LaMotte, JoAnn E. Manson, and Julie E. Buring. "Self-Reported Breast Implants and Connective-Tissue Diseases in Female Health Professionals: A Retrospective Cohort Study." *Journal of the American Medical Association* 1275, no. 8 (28 February 1996): 616–21.

Hertog, J.K., J.R. Finnegan, Jr., and E. Kahn. "Media Coverage of AIDS, Cancer, and Sexually Transmitted Diseases: A Test of the Public Arenas Model." *Journalism Quarterly* 71 (1994): 291–304.

Hoban, T.J. *Agricultural Biotechnology: Public Attitudes and Educational Needs.* Raleigh, NC: North Carolina State University 1990.

Hoban, T.J., and P.A. Kendall. *Consumer Attitudes about the Use of Biotechnology in Agriculture and Food Production.* Raleigh, NC: North Carolina State University 1992.

Hobbelink, H. *Biotechnology and the Future of World Agriculture.* London, U.K.: Zed Books 1991.

Holloway, Marguerite. "A Great Poison." *Scientific American* 263 (November 1990).

Hopkin, K. "Improving the Public Understanding of Science and Technology." *Science* 259 (1993): 697–8.

Hornig, S. "Reading Risk: Public Response to Print Media Accounts of Technological Risk." *Public Understanding of Science* 2 (1993): 95–109.

Hotchkiss, J.H. "How Safe? A Tale of Two Food Supplies." *New York's Food Life Sciences Quarterly* 19 (1989): 2–4.

House of Commons Standing Committee on Environment and Sustainable Development. *It's About Our Health! Towards Pollution Prevention: CEPA Revisited.* Ottawa: Government of Canada 1995.

"How BSE Crisis Forced Europe out of Its Complacency," *Nature* (2 January 1997): 6–7.

Hrudey, S.E., and D. Krewski. "Is There a Safe Level of Exposure to a Carcinogen?" *Environmental Science and Technology* 29 (1995): 370–5.

Hrudey, S.E., and W. Leiss. "Risk Management and Precaution: Insights on the Cautious Use of Evidence." *Environmental Health Perspectives* 111, 13 (October 2003): 1577–81.

Hsu, Chen-Chin *et al.* "The Yu-cheng Rice Oil Poisoning Incident." In *Dioxins and Health*, ed. A. Schecter, 661–84. New York: Plenum Press 1994.

Hubert, R. "Climate Change and Canadian Sovereignty in the Northwest Passage." *Isuma* 4 (2) 2001: 86–94.
http://www.isuma.net/v02n04/huebert/huebert_e.pdf

Idler, K.L. *PCBs: The Current Situation.* Hamilton, ON: Canadian Centre for Occupational Health and Safety, Ministry of Labour 1986.

Industry Science and Technology Canada. *Biotechnology Public Awareness Workshop: Summary of Proceedings.* Ottawa: Industry, Science and Technology Canada 1993.

Institute of Food Technologists. *Assessing the Optimal System for Ensuring Food Safety: A Scientific Consensus.* A report of a workshop sponsored by the Institute of Food Technologists, Chicago, IL 1990.

Interdepartmental Task Force on PCBs. *Polychlorinated Biphenyls and the Environment.* COM-72-10419. Washington, DC, May 1972, National Technical Information Service, U.S. Department of Commerce, Springfield, VA.

Intergovernmental Panel on Climate Change. *Climate change 2001: the scientific basis: contribution of Working Group I to the third assessment report of the*

Intergovernmental Panel on Climate Change. New York: Cambridge University Press 2001.

Jaccard, Mark. "Costing greenhouse gas abatement: Canada's technological and behavioural pattern." *Isuma* (Winter 2001). http://www.isuma.net

Jaccard, M.K., J. Nyboer, *et al. The cost of climate policy.* Vancouver: UBC Press 2002.

Jacobson, J.L, S.W. Jacobson, and H.E.B. Humphrey. "Effects of Exposure to PCBs and Related Compounds on Growth and Activity in Children." *Neurotoxicology and Teratology* 12 (1990): 319–26.

Janis, I.L. "The Problem of Validating Content Analysis." In *Language of Politics,* ed. H.D. Lasswell *et al.,* 55–82. Cambridge, MA: MIT Press 1965.

Jensen, A.A. "Background Levels in Humans." In *Halogenated Biphenyls, Terphenyls, Naphtalenes, Dibenzodioxins and Related Products,* ed. R.D. Kimbrough and A.A. Jensen, 345–80. Amsterdam: Elsevier 1989.

Jensen, Sören. "The PCB Story." *Ambio* 1, no. 4 (1972): 123–31.

Jetté, Mireille, ed. *A Health Profile of the Inuit: Report of the Santé Québec Health Survey among the Inuit of Nunavik.* 3 vol. Québec: Gouvernement du Québec 1992.

Johnson, B.B., and P. Slovic. "Presenting Uncertainty in Health Risk Assessment: Initial Studies of Its Effects on Risk Perception and Trust." *Risk Analysis* 15 (1995): 485–94.

Johnson, B.B., P.M. Sandman, and P. Miller. "Testing the Role of Technical Information in Public Risk Perception." *Risk: Issues in Health and Safety* 3 (1992): 341–64.

Johnson, R.P., R.C. Clarke, J.B. Wilson, S.C. Read, Kris Rahn, S.A. Renwick, K.A. Sandhu, David Alves, M.A. Karmali, Herme Lior, S.A. McEwen, J.S. Spika, and C.L. Gyles. "Growing Concerns and Recent Outbreaks Involving Non-O157H7 Serotypes of Verotoxigenic *Escherichia Coli.*" *Journal of Food Protection* 59, no. 10 (1996): 1112–22.

Johnson, R.W. "Microbial Food Safety." *Dairy and Food Sanitation* 7, no. 4 (1987): 174–6.

Joint Statement by 17 National Academies of Science. "The Science of Climate Change." *Science* 292(5520) 2001: 1261–.

Juskevich, J.C., and Guyer, C.G. "Bovine Growth Hormone: Human Food Safety Evaluation." *Science* 249 (1990): 875–84.

Kalous M.J., and L.H. Duke. *The Regulation of Plant Biotechnology in Canada, part 2: The Environmental Release of Genetically Altered Plant Material.* Ottawa: Agriculture Canada 1989.

Kasperson, R.E., O. Renn, P. Slovic, *et al.* "The Social Amplification of Risk." *Risk Analysis* 8, no. 2 (1988): 177–87.

Kavlock, Robert J., and Gerald T. Ankley. "A Perspective on the Risk Assessment Process for Endocrine-Disruptive Effects on Wildlife and Human Health." *Risk Analysis* 16, no. 6 (1996): 731–9.

Kelley, J. "Public Perceptions of Genetic Engineering: Australia 1994." Canberra: Australian Department of Industry, Science and Technology (http://www.das.gov.au/~dist/home.html) 1995.

Kemp, R. "Social Implications and Public Confidence: Risk Perception and Communication." In *The Release of Genetically Modified Microorganisms*, ed. D.E.S. Stewart-Tull and M. Sussman, 99–114. New York: Plenum Press 1992.

Kenney, M. "The University in the Information Age: Biotechnology and the Less Developed Countries." *Development* 4 (1987): 60–7.

Kimbrough, Renate D. "The Human Health Effects of Polychlorinated Biphenyls." In *Phantom Risk – Scientific Inference and the Law*, ed. K.F. Foster, D.E. Bernstein, and P.W. Huber, 211–28. Cambridge, MA: MIT Press 1994.

– "Polychlorinated Biphenyls (PCBs) and Human Health: An Update." *Critical Reviews in Toxicology* 25, no. 2 (1995): 133–63.

Kimbrough, R.D., R.A. Squire, R.E. Linder, J.D. Strandberg, R.J. Montali, and V.W. Burst. "Induction of Liver Tumors in Sherman Strain Female Rats by Polychlorinated Biphenyl Arochlor 1260." *Journal of the National Cancer Institute* 55 (1975): 1453–9.

Kinloch, D., H. Kuhnlein, and D.C.G. Muir. "Inuit Foods and Diet: A Preliminary Assessment of Benefits and Risks." *Science of the Total Environment* 122 (1992): 247–78.

Kirn, T.F. "Networks, Local Stations Providing Air Time for Physicians to Report, Advise." *Journal of the American Medical Association* 258 (1987): 2169–71.

Klaasen, Curtis D., Mary O. Amdur, and John Doull, eds. *Casarett and Doull's Toxicology: The Basic Science of Poisons.* New York: McGraw-Hill 1996.

Klein, K.K., J.E. Hobbs, and W.A. Kerr. "Farmer Acceptance of Biotechnology and Marketing Strategies: Implications for Agribusiness from Surveys in Western Canada." *Journal of International Food and Agribusiness Marketing* 6, no. 1 (1993): 71–88.

Kone, D., and E. Mullet. "Societal Risk Perception and Media Coverage." *Risk Analysis* 14 (1994): 21–4.

Kraus, N., T. Malmfors, and P. Slovic. "Intuitive Toxicology: Expert and Lay Judgements of Chemical Risks." *Risk Analysis* 12 (1992): 215–32.

Krimsky, Sheldon. *Biotechnics and Society: The Rise of Industrial Genetics.* New York: Praeger 1991.

Krimsky, S., and A. Plough. *Environmental Hazards: Communicating Risks as a Social Process.* Dover, MA: Auburn House 1988.

Krimsky, Sheldon, and Roger Wrubel. *Agricultural Biotechnology and the Environment.* Urbana, IL: University of Illinois Press 1996.

Krippendorff, K. *Content Analysis: An Introduction to Its Methodology.* London: Sage Publications 1980.

Kuhnlein, H.V., and D. Kinloch. "PCB's and Nutrients in Baffin Island Inuit Foods and Diets." *Arctic Medical Research* 47, suppl. 1 (1988): 155–8.

Kvenberg, J.E., and D.L. Archer. "Economic impact of colonization control on foodborne disease." *Food Technology* 41, no. 7 (1987): 77–98.

Lacey, W.B., L. Busch, and L.R. Lacy. "Public Perceptions of Agricultural Bio-technology." In *Agricultural Biotechnology: Issues and Choices*, ed. B.R. Baum-gardt and M.A. Martin, 139–61. West Lafayette, IN: Purdue University Agricultural Experiment Station 1991.

Langeried, J.P.M., and M.A. Smits. "BSE Researchers Bemoan 'Ministry Secrecy.'" *Nature* (10 October 1996).

Lasley, P., and G. Bultena. "Farmers' Opinions about Third-Wave Technolo-gies." *American Journal of Alternative Agriculture* (Summer 1986): 122–6.

Layoff, G., and M. Johnson. *Metaphors We Live By*. Chicago: University of Chicago Press 1980.

Lee, K. "Food Neophobia: Major Causes and Treatments." *Food Technology* 43, no. 12 (1989): 62–73.

Lee, S., E.R. Barton, H.L. Sweeney, and R.P. Farrar. "Viral expression of insu-lin-like growth factor-I enhances muscle hypertrophy in resistance-trained rats." *Journal of Applied Physiology* 96, 3 (2004): 1097–104.

Leiss, W. *In the Chamber of Risks*. Montreal: McGill-Queen's University Press 2001.

– "Biotechnology in Canada Today: Not More Regulation, but More Credible Regulation." Presentation to the House of Commons Standing Committee on Environment and Sustainable Development, June 1996.

– "'Down and Dirty': The Use and Abuse of Public Trust in Risk Communi-cation." *Risk Analysis* 15 (1995): 685–92.

– "Governance and the Environment." In *Policy Frameworks for a Knowledge Economy*, ed. T. Courchene, 121–63. Kingston, ON: John Deutsch Institute, Queen's University 1996.

– "On the Vitality of Our Discipline: New Applications of Communications Theory." *Canadian Journal of Communication* 16 (1991): 291–305.

– "Three Phases in the Evolution of Risk Communication Practice." In *New Directions in Risk Management*, ed. H. Kunreuther and P. Slovic, Special Issue, *The Annals of the American Academy of Political and Social Science* 545 (May 1996): 85–94.

– *The Domination of Nature*. Reprint. Montreal: McGill-Queen's University Press 1994 (first edition 1972).

Leiss, W., and C. Chociolko. *Risk and Responsibility*. Montreal: McGill-Queen's University Press 1994.

Lemons, John, ed. *Scientific Uncertainty and Environmental Problem Solving*. Cambridge, Massachusetts: Blackwell Science 1996.

Levitt, A. "The Flap over Bovine Growth Hormone." *Prepared Foods* 159, no. 3 (1990): 21.

Limoges, C. "Expert Knowledge and Decision-Making in Controversy Events." *Public Understanding of Science* 2 (1993): 417–26.

Limoges, C., *et al.* "Les risques associés au largage dans l'environnement d'organismes génétiquement modifiés: analyse d'une controverse." *Cahiers de recherche sociologique* 21 (1993): 17–52.

Line, J.E., A.R. Fain, A.B. Moran, L.M. Martin, R.V. Lechowich, J.M. Carosella, and W.L. Brown. "Lethality of Heat to *Escherichia Coli* O157:H7: D-Value and Z-Value Determinations in Ground Beef." *Journal of Food Protection* 54 (1991): 762–6.

Lior, H. "*Escherichia Coli* O157:H7 and Verotoxigenic *Escherichia Coli* (VTEC)." *Dairy Food Environment Sanitation* 14 (1994): 378–82.

Liu, J.T., and V.K. Smith. "Risk Communication and Attitude Change: Taiwan's National Debate over Nuclear Power." *Journal of Risk and Uncertainty* 3 (1990): 331–49.

Long, J.R., and D.J. Hanson. "Dioxin Issue Focuses on Three Major Controversies in U.S." *Chemical and Engineering News* (6 June 1983): 23–36.

Lowrance, William W. *Of Acceptable Risk*. Los Altos, CA: William Kaufmann 1976.

Lutman, P.J.W. "The Occurrence and Persistence of Volunteer Oilseed Rape (Brassica napus)." *Aspects of Applied Biology* 35 (1993): 29–36.

MacDonald, J.F., ed. *Agricultural Biotechnology: A Public Conversation about Risk*. National Agricultural Biotechnology Council (NABC) Report 5, Ithaca, NY 1993.

MacDonald, K.L., and M.T. Osterholm. "The Emergence of *Escherichia Coli* O157:H7 Infection in the United States: The Changing Epidemiology of Foodborne Disease." *Journal of the American Medical Association* 269, no. 17 (1993): 2264.

MacDonald, K.L., M.J. O'Leary, M.L. Cohen, *et al.* "*Escherichia Coli* O157:H7, an Emerging Gastrointestinal Pathogen: Results of a One-Year Prospective Population-Based Study." *Journal of the American Medical Association* 259 (1988): 3567–70.

Mackay, B. "Firing public health MD over pro-Kyoto comments a no-no, Alberta learns." *Canadian Medical Association Journal* 167(10) 2002: 1156a.

Marquart, J., G.J. O'Keefe, and A.C. Gunther. "Believing in Biotech: Farmers' Perceptions of the Credibility of BGH Information Sources." *Science Communication* 16, no. 4 (1995): 388–402.

Masuda, Yoshito. "The Yusho Rice Oil Poisoning Incident." In *Dioxins and Health*, ed. A. Schecter, 633–59. New York: Plenum Press 1994.

Mazur, A. "Media Coverage and Public Opinion on Scientific Controversies." *Journal of Communication* (Spring 1981): 106–15.

McCabe, A.S., and M.R. Fitzgerald. "Media Images of Environmental Biotechnology: What Does the Public See?" In *Environmental Biotechnology for Waste Treatment*, ed. G.S. Sayler, R. Fox, and J.W. Blackburn. New York: Plenum Press 1991.

McCallum, D.B., S.L. Hammond, and V.T. Covello. "Communicating about Environmental Risks: How the Public Uses and Perceives Information Sources." *Health Education Quarterly* 18 (1991): 349–61.

McCombs, M.E., and D.L. Shaw. "The Agenda-Setting Function of the Mass Media." *Public Opinion Quarterly* 36 (1972): 176–87.

McGaughey, W.H. "Insect Resistance to the Biological Insecticide Bacillus Thuringiensis." *Science* 229 (1985): 193–5.

– "Problems of Insect Resistance to Bacillus Thuringiensis. *Agriculture, Ecosystems and Environment* 49 (1994): 95–102.

McGaughey, W.H., and M.E. Whalon. "Managing Insect Resistance to Bacillus Thuringiensis Toxins." *Science* 258 (1992): 1451–5.

McNamra, Kathy. "It Seemed We Had It All Wrong." *Forbes Media Critic* (Winter 1996).

Mes, J., D.J. Davies, J. Doucet, D. Weber, and E. McMullen. "Specific Polychlorinated Biphenyl Congener Distribution in Breast Milk of Canadian Women." *Environmental Technology* 14, 6 (1993): 555–65.

Mikkelsen, T.R., B. Andersen, and R.B. Jorgensen. "The Risk of Crop Transgene Spread." *Nature* 380 (1996): 31.

Miller, D.L., U. Rahardja, and M.E. Whalon. "Development of a Strain of Colorado Potato Beetle Resistant to the Delta-Endotoxin of Bt." *Pest Resistance Management* 2, no. 2 (1990): 25.

Miller, G. "The Magical Number Seven, Plus or Minus Two." *Psychology Review* 63 (1956): 81–97.

Miller, J.D. *The Public Understanding of Science and Technology in the United States, 1990.* Washington, DC: National Science Foundation 1992.

Milner, R.J. "History of Bacillus Thuringiensis." *Agriculture, Ecosystems and Environment* 49 (1994): 9–13.

Molitor, F. "Accuracy in Science News Reporting by Newspapers: The Case of Aspirin for the Prevention of Heart Attacks." *Health Communication* 5 (1993): 209–24.

Moore, John A., R. Kimbrough, and M. Gough. "The Dioxin TCDD." In *Keeping Pace with Science and Technology*, ed. Myron Uman, 221–42. Washington, DC: National Academy Press 1993.

Morley, R.S., *et al.* "Assessment of the risk factors related to bovine spongiform encephalopathy." *Rev. sci. tech. Off. Int. Epiz.*, 22 (1) 2003: 157–78.

Murray, J.L., and R.G. Shearer. *Synopsis of Research Counducted under the 1994/95 Northern Contaminants Program.* Environmental Studies No. 73, Northern Affairs Program, Indian Affairs and Northern Development, Ottawa 1996.

Nakicenovic, N., and R. Swart, eds. *Emissions Scenarios. Special Report of the Intergovernmental Panel on Climate Change.* Cambridge, U.K.: Cambridge University Press 2000.

National Academy of Sciences. *Climate Change Science: An Analysis of Some Key Questions.* Washington, D.C.: National Academy Press 2001.

National Breast Implant Task Force. *NBITF News*, 1, no. 1 (June-July-August, 1986): 6.

National Institute of Environmental Health Sciences. "Proceedings of meeting on Polychlorinated Biphenyls (PCBs), Rougemont, NC, Dec. 20–21, 1971." *Environmental Health Perspectives*, Experimental Issue No. 1. North Carolina: National Institute of Environmental Health Sciences, April 1972.

National Institutes of Health. *Bovine Somatotropin.* Technology Assessment Conference Statement. Washington, DC (Dec. 1990): 5–7.

National Research Council of Canada Associate Committee on Scientific Criteria for Environmental Quality. *Polychlorinated Dibenzo-p-dioxins: Criteria for Their Effect on Man and His Environment.* Ottawa 1981.

National Research Council (U.S.). Committee on Abrupt Climate Change. *Abrupt climate change: inevitable surprises.* Washington, D.C.: National Academy Press 2002.

National Swedish Environment Protection Board. *PCB Conference.* Research Secretariat, Wenner Gren Center, Stockholm, 29 September 1970.

Neill, M.A. "*E. Coli* O157:H7 Time Capsule: What Do We Know and When Did We Know It?" *Dairy Food Environmental Sanitation* 14 (1994): 374–7.

Nelkin, D. "AIDS and the News Media." *Millbank Quarterly* 69 (1991): 293–307.

– "Forms of Intrusion: Comparing Resistance to Information Technology and Biotechnology in the USA." In *Resistance to New Technology,* ed. M. Bauer, 379–90. Cambridge: Cambridge University Press 1995.

– *Selling Science: How the Press Covers Science and Technology.* New York: W.H. Freeman 1987.

Neuzil, M. "Gambling with Databases: A Comparison of Electronic Searches and Printed Indices." *Newspaper Research Journal* 15 (1994): 44–54.

Newman, M.E. "Electromagnetic Fields and Cancer – Media and Public Attention Affect Research." *Journal of the National Cancer Institute* 83 (1991): 164–5.

Newsome, W.H., D. Davies, and J. Doucet. "PCB and Organochlorined Pesticides in Canadian Human Milk." *Chemosphere* 30, no. 11 (1995): 2143–53.

Nocera, Joe. "Fatal Litigation." *Fortune* (16 October 1995).

Norback, D.H., and R.H. Weltman. "Polychlorinated Biphenyl Induction of Hepatocellular Carcinoma in the Sprague-Dawley Rat." *Environmental Health Perspective* 60 (1985): 97–105.

O'Neil, J. "A Study into the Social, Cultural, and Disciplinary Understanding of Risk Perceptions and Risk Acceptability of Contaminants in the Canadian Arctic." In *Synopsis of Research Conducted under the 1994/95 Northern Contaminants Program,* ed. J.L. Murray and R.G. Shearer, 355–59. Environmental Studies no. 73, Northern Affairs Program, Indian Affairs and Northern Development, Ottawa 1996.

Optima Consultants. *Understanding the Consumer Interest in the New Biotechnology Industry.* Ottawa: Industry Canada 1994.

Organization for Economic Cooperation and Development (OECD). "Biotechnology, Agriculture and Food." *Observer* (1992): 4–8.

– *PCB Seminar.* Scheveningen, The Hague, Netherlands, 28–30 September 1983.

Ouellet, Eric. "Organizational Analysis and Environmental Sociology: The Case of Greenpeace Canada." In *Environmental Sociology,* ed. M.D. Mehta and E. Ouellet, 321–38. North York, ON: Captus Press 1995.

Paneth, N. "Human Reproduction after Eating PCB Contaminated Fish." *Health and Environment Digest* 5 (1991): 4–6.

Park, A.J., J. Walsh, P.S.V. Reddy, V. Chetty, and A.C.H. Watson. "The Detection of Breast Implant Rupture Using Ultrasound." *British Journal of Plastic Surgery* 49 (1996): 299–310.

Parkinson, A., and S. Safe. "Mammalian Biologic and Toxic Effects of PCBs." In *PCBs: Mammalian and Environmental Toxicology*, ed. S. Safe and O. Hutzinger, 49–75. Environmental Toxin Series 1, New York: Springer-Verlag 1987.

Patino, M.M., J.-J. Liu, J.R. Glover, and S. Lindquist. "Support for the Prion Hypothesis for Inheritance of a Phenotypic Trait in Yeast." *Science* (2 August 1996): 622–6.

Paunesku, T., T. Rajh, G. Wiederrecht, J. Maser, S. Vogt, N. Stojicevic, M. Protic, B. Lai, J. Oryhon, M. Thurnauer, and G. Woloschak. "Biology of TiO2-oligonucleotide nanocomposites." *Nature Materials* 2, 5 (2003): 343–6.

Peters, W., E. Keystone, and D. Smith. "Factors Affecting the Rupture of Silicone-Gel Breast Implants." *Annals of Plastic Surgery* 32, no. 5 (May 1994): 449–51.

Pocchiari, F., A. Di Domenico, V. Silano, and G. Zapponi. "Environmental Impact of the Accidental Release of Tetrachlorodibenzo-p-dioxin (TCDD) at Seveso (Italy)." In *Accidental Exposure to Dioxins – Human Health Aspects*, ed. F. Coulston and F. Pocchari, 5–35. New York: Academic Press 1983.

Portier, C., A. Tritscher, M. Kohn, C. Sewall, G. Clark, L. Edler, D. Hoel, and G. Lucier. "Ligand/Receptor Binding for 2,3,7,8-TCDD: Implications for Risk Assessment." *Fundamental and Applied Toxicology* 20 (1993): 48–56.

Powell, D.A., and M.W. Griffiths. *Public Perceptions of Agricultural Biotechnology in Canada*. Institute of Food Technologists annual meeting, Atlanta, 25–29 June 1994.

Priest, Susanna H. "Information Equity, Public Understanding of Science, and the Biotechnology Debate." *Journal of Communication* 45 (1995): 39–54.

Priest, Susanna H., and J. Talbert. "Mass Media and the Ultimate Technological Fix: Newspaper Coverage of Biotechnology." *Southwestern Mass Communication Journal* 10 (1994): 76–85.

Protess, D.L., F.L. Cook, T.R. Curtin, M.T. Gordon, D.R. Leff, M.E. McCombs, and P. Miller. "The Impact of Investigative Reporting on Public Opinion and Policymaking." *Public Opinion Quarterly* 51 (1987): 166–85.

Proulx, Jean-François. "Introduction: Health and Well-Being in Nunavik, A Historical Overview." In *A Health Profile of the Inuit: Report of the Santé Québec Health Survey among the Inuit of Nunavik*, vol. 1, ed. M. Jetté, 1–15. Québec: Gouvernement du Québec 1992.

Prusiner, S. "The Prion Diseases." *Scientific American* 272, no. 1 (1995): 47–57.

Public Employees for Environmental Responsibility (PEER). *Genetic Genie: The Premature Commercial Release of Genetically Engineered Bacteria*. Washington, DC: PEER 1995.

Rahardja, U., and M. Whalon. "Inheritance of Resistance to Bacillus Thuringiensis Subsp. Tenebrionsis Cryiii Delta-Endotoxin in Colorado Potato Beetle (Coleoptera: Chrysomelidae)." *Journal of Economic Entomology* 88, no. 1 (1995): 22–6.

Rappe, C. "Sources and Environmental Concentrations of Dioxins and Related Compounds." *Pure and Applied Chemistry* 68, no. 9 (1996): 1781–9.

Rawls, Rebecca L. "Dioxin's Human Toxicity Is Most Difficult Problem." *Chemical and Engineering News* (6 June 1983): 37–48.

– "Dow Finds Support, Doubt for Dioxin Ideas." *Chemical and Engineering News* (12 February 1979): 23–8.

rBST Task Force. *Review of the Potential Impact of Recombinant Bovine Somatotropin (rBST) in Canada.* Ottawa 1995.

Relman, A.S. "Reporting the Aspirin Study." *New England Journal of Medicine* 318 (1988): 918–20.

Remis, R.S., K.L. MacDonald, L.W. Riley, et al. "Sporadic Cases of Hemorrhagic Colitis Associated with *Escherichia Coli* O157:H7." *Annals of Internal Medicine* 101 (1984): 624–6.

"Report of a New Chemical Hazard." *New Scientist* (15 December 1966): 612.

Ridley, R.M., and H.F. Baker. *Fatal Protein.* Oxford: Oxford University Press 1998.

Riley, L.W., R.S. Remis, S.D. Helgerson, et al. "Hemorrhagic Colitis Associated with a Rare *Escherichia Coli* Serotype." *New England Journal of Medicine* 308 (1983): 681–5.

Rissler, J., and M. Mellon. *The Ecological Risks of Genetically Engineered Crops.* Boston, MA: MIT Press 1996.

Roberts, Leslie. "Dioxin Risks Revisited." *Science* 251 (8 February 1991): 624–6.

Roberts, T. "Human Illness Costs of Food-Borne Bacteria." *American Journal of Agricultural Economics* 71 (1989): 468–74.

Roberts, T., and E. van Ravenswaay. "The Economics of Food Safety." *Food Review* 12, no. 3 (July/September 1989): 1–8.

Robertson, Gordon W., and Silas Braley. "Toxicologic Studies, Quality Control, and Efficacy of the Silastic Mammary Prosthesis." *Medical Instrumentation* 7 (1973): 100–3.

Robinson, O.G. Jr, E.L. Bradley, and D.S. Wilson. "Analysis of Explanted Silicone Implants: A Report of 300 Patients." *Annals of Plastic Surgery* 34, no. 1 (January 1995): 1–7.

Rodricks, Joseph V. *Calculated Risks.* Cambridge: Cambridge University Press 1992.

Rogan W.J., and B.C. Gladen. "PCBs, DDE and Child Development at 18 to 24 Months." *Annals of Epidemiology* 1 (1991): 407–15.

Rohrmann, Bernd, Peter Wiedemann, and Helmut Stegelmann, eds. *Risk Communication: An Interdisciplinary Bibliography.* 3rd edn. Jülich, Germany: Research Center Jülich GMBH 1990.

Rowe, William D. *An Anatomy of Risk*. New York: Wiley 1977.

Russell, V., R. Denny, S. Parnett, F. Walton, D. Merriam, and K. Barnes. *The Novo Report: American Attitudes and Beliefs about Genetic Engineering*. New York: Research and Forecasts, Inc. 1987.

Sachidanandam, R., D. Weissman, S. C. Schmidt, *et al.* "A map of human genome sequence variation containing 1.42 million single nucleotide polymorphisms." *Nature* 409 (2001): 928–33.

Safe, Stephen H. "Polychlorinated Biphenyls (PCBs): Environmental Impact, Biochemical and Toxic Responses, and Implications for Risk Assessment." *Critical Reviews in Toxicology* 24, no. 2 (1994): 87–149.

– "PCBs and Human Health." In *PCBs: Mammalian and Environmental Toxicology*, ed. S. Safe and O. Hutzinger, 133–145. Environmental Toxin Series 1, New York: Springer-Verlag 1987.

Salter, L. *Mechanisms and Practices for the Assessment of the Social and Cultural Implications of Science and Technology*. Occasional Paper No. 8, Ottawa: Industry Canada 1995.

Samson, M., F. Libert, B.J. Doranz, J. Rucker, C. Liesnard, C.M. Farber, S. Saragosti, C. Lapoumeroulie, J. Cognaux, C. Forceille, G. Muyldermans, C. Verhofstede, G. Burtonboy, M. Georges, T. Imai, S. Rana, Y. Yi, R.J. Smyth, R.G. Collman, R.W. Doms, G. Vassart, and M. Parmentier. "Resistance to HIV-1 infection in Caucasian individuals bearing mutant alleles of the CCR-5 chemokine receptor gene." *Nature* 382 (1996): 722–5.

Sanchez-Guerrero, Jorge, Graham A. Colditz, Elizabeth W. Karlson, David J. Hunter, Frank E. Speizer, and Matthew H. Liang. "Silicone Breast Implants and the Risk of Connective-Tissue Diseases and Symptoms." *New England Journal of Medicine* (22 June 1995): 1666–70.

Sandman, P.M., P.M. Miller, B.B. Johnson, and N.D. Weinstein. "Agency Communication, Community Outrage and Perception of Risk: Three Simulation Experiments." *Risk Analysis* 13 (1993): 585–98.

Schanne, M., and W. Meier. *Media Coverage of Risk in Biotechnology in Public: A Review of Recent Research*. London: Science Museum 1992.

Schecter, A. ed. *Dioxins and Health*. New York: Plenum Press 1994.

Scheer, Robert. "The Great American Breast Implant Hoax? A Shocking Look at the Real Story behind the Silicone Scare!" *Cosmopolitan* (September 1995): 232.

Scheffler, J.A., R. Parkinson, and P.J. Dale. "Frequency and Distance of Pollen Dispersal from Transgenic Oilseed Rape (Brassica Napus)." *Transgenic Research* 2 (1993): 356–64.

Scheffler, J., and P.J. Dale. "Opportunities for Gene Transfer from Transgenic Oilseed Rape (Brassica Napus) to Related Species." *Transgenic Research* 3 (1994): 263–78.

Schreuder, B.E.C., L.J.M. van Keulen, and M.E.W. Vromans. "Preclinical Test for Prion Diseases." *Nature* 381 (13 June 1996): 563.

Schuck, P.H. *Agent Orange on Trial – Mass Toxic Disasters in the Courts.* Cambridge, MA: Belknap Press of Harvard University Press 1986.

Science Council of Canada. *Biotechnology in Canada: Promises and Concerns.* Ottawa: Government of Canada 1980.

Scientists' Institute for Public Information. *The Public's Interest in News about Science: A Mandate for Increased Coverage.* Washington, DC 1993.

Selikoff, I.J., ed. "Polychlorinated Biphenyls-Environmental Impact: A Review by the Panel on Hazardous Trace Substances." *Environmental Research* 5 (1972): 249–362.

Shaw, D.L., and S.E. Martin. "The Function of Mass Media Agenda Setting." *Journalism Quarterly* 69, no. 4 (1992): 902–20.

Shelley, Mary W. *Frankenstein or the Modern Prometheus.* Signet Classic edition. New York: Penguin Books 1983.

– *Frankenstein or the Modern Prometheus.* ed. Susan J. Wolfson. New York: Longman 2003.

Shin T., D. Kraemer, J. Pryor, L. Liu, J. Rugila, L. Howe, S. Buck, K. Murphy, L. Lyons, and M. Westhusin. "A cat cloned by nuclear transplantation." *Nature* 415 (2002): 859.

Shrecker, T., C. Elliott, C.B Hohhmaster, and M.A. Somerville. *Ethical Issues Associated with the Patenting of Higher Life Forms.* McGill University 1994.

Siddall, Ernest, and Carl Bennett. "A People-Centred Concept of Society-Wide Risk Management." In *Environmental Health Risks: Assessment and Management,* ed. R. Stephen McColl. Waterloo, ON: University of Waterloo Press 1987.

Silverman, B.G., S.L. Brown, R.A. Bright, R.G. Kaczmarek, J.B. Arrowsmith-Lowe, and D.A. Kessler. "Reported Complications of Silicone Gel Breast Implants: An Epidemiologic Review." *Annals of Internal Medicine* 124, no. 8 (15 April 1996): 744–56.

Singer, E. "A Question of Accuracy: How Journalists and Scientists Report Research on Hazards." *Journal of Communication* 40 (1990): 102–16.

Skerfving, S., B.G. Svensson, L. Asplund, and L. Hagmar. "Exposure to Mixtures and Congeners of Polychlorinated Biphenyls." *Clinical Chemistry* 407, part 2 (1994): 1409–15.

Slovic, Paul, and Donald J. MacGregor. "The Social Context of Risk Communication." Unpublished paper, Decision Research, Eugene, OR, May 1994.

Slovic, P., J. Flynn, C.K. Mertz, and L. Mullican. *Health Risk Perception in Canada.* Ottawa: Health Canada 1993.

Smallwood, D. "Consumer Demand for Safer Foods." *National Food Review* 12 (1989): 9–11.

Smart, Tim. "Breast Implants: What Did the Industry Know, and When?" *Business Week* (10 June 1991): 94.

Smith, B.J., and R.H. Warland. "Consumer Responses to Milk from BST-Supplemented Cows." In *Bovine Somatotropin and Emerging Issues – An Assessment,* ed. M.C. Hallberg, 243–64. Boulder, CO: Westview Press 1992.

Smythe, D.W. "Some Observations on Communications Theory." *Audio Visual Communication Review* 2 (1954): 248–60.

Soby, B.A., A.C.D. Simpson, and D.P. Ives. "Integrating Public and Scientific Judgements into a Toolkit for Managing Food-Related Risks; Stage 1: Literature Review and Feasibility Study." *Research Report No. 16.* Environmental Risk Assessment Unit, University of East Anglia, U.K. 1993.

Society of Environmental Toxicology and Chemistry (SETAC). *Sound Science Technical Issue Paper.* Pensacola, FL. U.S. http://www.setac.org/sstip.html

Sparks, P., and R. Shepherd. "Public Perceptions of the Potential Hazards Associated with Food Production and Food Consumption: An Empirical Study." *Risk Analysis* 14 (1994): 799–806.

Sparks, P., R. Shepherd, and L.J. Frewer. "Gene Technology, Food Production and Public Opinion: A UK Study." *Agriculture and Human Values* 11 (1994): 19–28.

Squires, S. "The Gatekeepers of Medical News: Leading Journals Determine the Agenda." *Washington Post Health* (2 July 1986): 8–9.

Stager, John, ed. *Canada and Polar Science.* Proceedings of a conference sponsored by the Canadian Polar Commission, Yellowknife, NWT, May 17–19, 1994, Ottawa: Canadian Polar Commission 1994.

Statistics Canada. *Cereals and Oilseeds Review.* Ottawa: Government of Canada, 1994.

Strachan, W.M.J. *Polychlorinated Biphenyls (PCBs): Fate and Effects in the Canadian Environment.* EPS 4/HA/2. Ottawa: Minister of Supply and Services 1988.

Tasca, Richard J., and Michael E. McClure. "The Emerging Technology and Application of Preimplantation Genetic Diagnosis." *Journal of Law, Medicine and Ethics* 26, 1 (1998): 7–16.

Telling, Glenn C., Piero Parchi, Stephen J. DeArmond, Pietro Cortelli, Pasquale Montagna, Ruth Gabizon, James Mastrianni, Elio Lugaresi, Pierluigi Gambetti, and Stanley B. Prusiner. "Evidence for the Conformation of the Pathologic Isoform of the Prion Protein Enciphering and Propagating Prion Diversity." *Science* 274 (20 Dec. 1996): 2079–82.

Thiess, A.M., R. Frentzel-Beyme, and R. Link. "Mortality Study of Persons Exposed to Dioxin in a Trichlorophenol-Process Accident That Occurred in the BASF AG on November 17, 1953." *American Journal of Industrial Medicine* 3 (1982): 179–89.

Thomas, V., and T. Spiro. "The U.S. Dioxin Inventory: Are There Missing Sources?" *Environmental Science and Technology* 30 (1996): 82–5.

Thompson, Paul B. *Food Labels and Biotechology: The Ethics of Safety and Consent.* Discussion Paper 93-1. Center for Biotechnology Policy and Ethics, Texas A & M University, January 1993.

Tiedje, J.M., R.K. Colwell, Y.L. Grossman, R.E. Hodson, R.E. Lenski, R.N. Mack, and P.J. Regal. "The Planned Introduction of Genetically Engineered Organisms: Ecological Considerations and Recommendations." *Ecology* 70, no. 2 (1989): 298–315.

Todd, E.C.D. "Preliminary Estimates of Costs of Food-Borne Disease in United States." *Journal of Food Protection* 52 (1989): 595–601.
– "Preliminary Estimates of Costs of Foodborne Disease in Canada and Costs to Reduce Salmonellosis." *Journal of Food Protection* 52 (1989): 586–94.
Toulin, A. "UN Pokes Holes in Kyoto Plan." *National Post.* 20 March 2002: A1.
Tschirley, Fred H. "Dioxin." *Scientific American* 254, no. 2 (Feb. 1986): 29–35.
Tsukamoto, M., T. Ochiya, S. Yoshida, T. Sugimura, and M. Terada M. "Gene transfer and expression in progeny after intravenous DNA injection into pregnant mice." *Nature Genetics* 9 (1995): 243–8.
U.K. Institute of Food Science and Technology. *Bovine Spongiform Encephalopathy (BSE) Position Statement.* U.K. 22 November 1996.
Uman, Myron, ed. *Keeping Pace with Science and Technology.* Washington, DC: National Academy Press 1993.
United Nations Conference on Environment and Development (UNCED). *Report of the United Nations Conference on Environment and Development.* Rio de Janeiro: United Nations 1992.
United States. Department of Agriculture Food Safety and Inspection Service. *Report on the Escherichia Coli O157:H7 Outbreak in the Western States.* N.p., 21 May 1993.
United States. Environmental Protection Agency. *Estimating Exposure to Dioxin-like Compounds,* 3 vols. Washington, DC, June 1994.
– *Health Assessment Document for Polychlorinated Dibenzo-p-dioxins.* Washington, DC, September 1985.
– *Health Assessment Document for 2,3,7,8-Tetrachlorodibenzo-p-dioxin (TCDD) and Related Compounds,* 3 vols. Washington DC, June 1994.
– *Interim Report on Data and Methods for Assessment of 2,3,7,8-Tetrachlorodibenzo-p-dioxin Risks to Aquatic Life and Associated Wildlife.* Washington, DC, March 1993.
– *National Conference on Polychlorinated Biphenyls (Nov. 19–21, 1975, Chicago, Illinois).* Conference Proceedings, Office of Toxic Substances, EPA-560/6-75-004, March 1976.
United States. Executive Branch of the Federal Government. *Use of Bovine Somatotropin (BST) in the United States: Its Potential Effects.* Washington, DC 1994.
United States. National Institutes of Health. *Technology Assessment Conference Statement on Bovine Somatotropin.* Bethesda, MD: Department Human Health and Services 1990.
United States. National Research Council. *Improving Risk Communication.* Washington, DC: National Academy Press 1989.
United States. Office of Technology Assessment, U.S. Congress. *New Developments in Biotechnology: Public Perceptions of Biotechnology.* OTA-BP-BA-45. Washington, DC: U.S. Government Printing Office 1987.
Usher, Peter. *Negotiating Research Relationships in the North.* Background paper for a workshop on guidelines for responsible research, Yellowknife, 22–23 September 1993. Ottawa: Inuit Tapirisat of Canada 1993.

– *The Northern Food Dilemma.* Video, Taqmamiut Nipingat Inc., 2 February 1996.

Usher, Peter J., M. Baikie, M. Demmer, D. Nakashima, M.G. Stevenson, and M. Stiles. *Communicating about Contaminants in Country Food: The Experience in Aboriginal Communities.* Ottawa: Inuit Tapirisat of Canada 1995.

Van Ravensway, E.O. *Public Perceptions of Agrichemicals.* Ames, IA: Council for Agricultural Science and Technology 1995.

Waltner-Toews, D. *Food, Sex and Salmonella: The Risks of Environmental Intimacy.* Toronto: NC Press 1992.

Watkinson, I. "Global View of Present and Future Markets for Bt Products." *Ecosystems and Environment* 49 (1994): 3–7.

Weart, S.R. *Nuclear Fear: A History of Images.* Cambridge, MA: Harvard University Press 1988.

Webster, Thomas, and Barry Commoner. "Overview: The Dioxin Debate." In *Dioxins and Health,* ed. A. Schecter, 1–50. New York: Plenum Press 1994.

Weinstein, N.D., and P.M. Sandman. "Some Criteria for Evaluating Risk Messages." *Risk Analysis* 13 (1993): 103–14.

Weisman, Rebecca. "Reforms in Medical Device Regulation: An Examination of the Silicone Gel Breast Implant Debacle." *Golden Gate University Law Review* 23 (Summer 1993): 973–8.

Wenzel, George W. "Warming the Arctic: Environmentalism and Canadian Inuit." In *Human Ecology and Climate Change – People and Resources in the Far North,* ed. D. L. Peterson and D.R. Johnson, 169–84. Washington, DC: Taylor & Francis 1995.

Weyant, John P. *An Introduction to the Economics of Climate Change Policy.* Pew Centre on Global Climate Change July 2000.
http://www.pewclimate.org/projects/econ_introduction.pdf

Whalon, M.E., D.L. Miller, R.M. Hollingworth, E.J. Grafius, and J.R. Miller. "Selection of a Colorado Potato Beetle (Coleoptera: Chrysomelidae) Strain Resistant to Bacillus Thuringiensis." *Journal of Economic Entomology* 86, no. 2 (1993): 226–33.

Wigley, T.M.L. *Stabilization of greenhouse gas concentrations.* U.S. Policy on Climate Change: What Next? Aspen Environmental Policy Forum, Aspen Institute 2002: 15–34.

Wildavsky, Aaron. *But Is It True?* Cambridge, MA: Harvard University Press 1995.

Wilkinson, M.J., A.M. Timmons, Y. Charters, S. Dubbels, A. Robertson, N. Wilson, S. Scott, E. O'Brien, and H.M. Lawson. "Problems of Risk Assessment with Genetically Modified Oilseed Rape." *Brighton Crop Protection Conference* (1995): 1035–44.

Will, R.G., J.W. Ironside, M. Zeidler, S.N. Cousens, K. Estibeiro, A. Alperovitch, S. Poser, M. Pocchiari, A. Hofman, and P.G. Smith. "A New Variant of Creutzfeldt-Jakob Disease in the U.K." *Lancet* 347 (6 April 1996): 921–5.

Wolf, I.D. "Critical Issues in Food Safety, 1991–2001. "*Food Technology* 46, no. 1 (1992): 64–70.

World Health Organization (WHO). *Polychlorinated Biphenyls and Terphenyls.* 2nd ed. Environmental Health Criteria 140, Geneva: World Health Organization 1993.

Wormworth, Janice. "Toxins and Tradition: The Impact of Food-Chain Contamination on the Inuit of Northern Quebec." *Canadian Medical Association Journal* 152, no. 8 (1995): 1237–9.

Wynne, B. "Uncertainty and Environmental Learning." *Global Environmental Change* 2 (1992): 111–27.

Yonkers, R.D. "Potential Adoption and Diffusion of BST among Dairy Farmers." In *Bovine Somatotropin and Emerging Issues – An Assessment,* ed. by M.C. Hallberg, 177–92. Boulder, CO: Westview Press 1992.

Zechendorf, B. "What the Public Thinks about Biotechnology." *Biotechnology* 12 (1994): 870–5.

Zillmann, D., J.W. Perkins, and S.S. Sundar. "Impression-Formation Effects of Printed News Varying in Descriptive Precision and Exemplification." *Medienpsychologie* 3 (1992): 168–85.

Ziman, J.M. *Reliable knowledge: an exploration of the grounds for belief in science.* Cambridge, U.K.: Cambridge University Press 1978.

– *Real science: what it is, and what it means.* Cambridge, New York: Cambridge University Press 2000.

Zollars, C. "The Perils of Periodical Indexes: Some Problems in Constructing Samples for Content Analysis and Culture Indicators Research." *Communication Research* 16 (1994): 698–716.

Zook, D.R. and C. Rappe. "Environmental Sources, Distribution, and Fate of Polychlorinated Dibenzodioxins, Dibenzofurans, and Related Organochlorines." In *Dioxins and Health,* ed. A. Schecter, 84. New York: Plenum Press 1994.

ADDITIONAL REFERENCES TO CHAPTER TWO

The following are all from the U.K. Institute of Food Science and Technology (IFST) 1996. A selection of key references is given below. Reports and articles on BSE and other encephalopathies have appeared widely in the scientific literature.

An on-line outline of U.K. government program for the eradication of BSE may be found at <http://www.open.gov.uk/maff/bse/eradprog/eradprog.htm#top>.

Outlines of ongoing research projects on BSE at the Institute of Animal Health may be found at its World Wide Web addresses <http://www.iah.bbsrc.ac.uk/Institut/public/3wtse.htm> and <http://www.iah.bbsrc.ac.uk/Institut/public/reports/1995/3wtse.htm>. An archive of summaries of over three hundred BSE-related research papers may be found on the World Wide Web site of CAB International at <http://www.cabi.org/>.

A wealth of information relating to CJD may be accessed on the CJD Surveillance Unit's website at <http://www.cjd.ed.ac.uk/>. Another World Wide Web site with much useful information is at <http://http2.brunel.ac.uk: 8080/~hssrsdn/bse.htm>.

There are escalating numbers of websites in which organizations and individuals have compiled links with other websites. Often the links are assembled indiscriminately. Apart from the compilations being highly repetitious, some of the linked websites carry untrustworthy material (views of various pressure groups, uninformed opinions presented with an air of authority, and speculation and rumour presented as established fact). The same is true of some of the postings on Internet mailing lists and newsgroups.

UK Legislative Provisions Relating to BSE

The Bovine Spongiform Encephalopathy Order 1988. HMSO.
The Bovine Spongiform Encephalopathy (Amendment) Order 1988. HMSO.
The Bovine Spongiform Encephalopathy Compensation Order 1988. HMSO.
The Bovine Spongiform Encephalopathy (No. 2) Order 1988. HMSO.
The Bovine Offal (Prohibition) Regulations 1989. HMSO.
The Bovine Spongiform Encephalopathy Compensation Order 1990. HMSO
The Bovine Spongiform Encephalopathy (No. 2) (Amendment) Order 1990. HMSO.
The Bovine Animals (Identification, Marking and Breeding Records) Order 1990. HMSO.
The Bovine Spongiform Encephalopathy Order 1991. HMSO. †
The Bovine Spongiform Encephalopathy Compensation Order 1994. HMSO.
The Bovine Offal (Prohibition) Regulations 1994. HMSO.
The Bovine Offal (Prohibition) (Amendment) Regulations 1995. HMSO.
The Specified Bovine Offal Order 1995. HMSO.
The Specified Bovine Offal (Amendment) Order 1995. HMSO.
The Animal By-Products (Identification) Regulations 1995. HMSO.
The Beef (Emergency Control) Order 1996. HMSO. *
The Beef (Emergency Control) (Amendment) Order 1996. HMSO. *
The Beef (Emergency Control) (Amendment) (No. 2) Order 1996. HMSO. *
The Beef (Emergency Control) (Amendment) (No. 3) Order 1996. HMSO. *
The Bovine Spongiform Encephalopathy (Amendment) Order 1996. HMSO. †
The Specified Bovine Material Order 1996. HMSO.
The Fertilisers (Mammalian Meat and Bone Meal) Regulations 1996. HMSO.
The Fresh Meat (Beef Controls) Regulations 1996. HMSO. +
The Beef (Emergency Control)(Revocation) Order 1996. HMSO. (revoking those marked *).
The Fresh Meat (Beef Controls) (No 2) Regulations 1996. HMSO. (revoking that marked +).

HMSO. The Bovine Spongiform Encephalopathy Order 1996. (revoking those marked †).

The Heads of Sheep and Goats Order 1996. HMSO.

The Bovine Products (Despatch to other Member States) Regulations 1996. HMSO.

Index

AAFC (Agriculture and
Agri-Food Canada):
decision documents,
155, 164–5, RBST task
force, 138, 140, 141
adenovirus, 311
aflatoxin, 28
Agent Orange, 47–9, 56,
58, 66, 68, 143, 217
Ah receptor, 53–4
Alar, 84, 95
alcohol, risks, 28
Alibekow, Kanatjan, 326
Alvarez, Pierre, 274
American Association
for the Advancement
of Science, 296
American Meat Institute,
91
amyloid plaques, 231
Analysis and Modelling
Group (AMG), 279,
280, 281, 282
Anderson, David, 274, 281
Andrews, Dave, 22
Angell, Marcia, 101–2,
105, 116
animal feed, 258–9; blood
in, 258–9, 261; and
FDA, 247, 259

animal-health issues, 251,
259–60
anthrax, 325–6
Arctic, Canadian. See
Nunavik, Nunavimmuit
asbestos, 316
Ashdown, Keith, 132, 136
Asilomar conference,
154–5
askarel, 182, 264n2,
269n55. See also PCBS
AstraZeneca, 324
athletes: and gene ther-
apy, 296–7; and SNPs,
309
automobile-related fatalities, 28
avian flu, 259

Bachorik, Lawrence,
19–20
Bacillus amyloliquefaciens,
174–5
Bacillus thuringiensis (Bt),
166–72; foliar sprays
167–70; insect resis-
tance to, 168–9, 171–2
Bacon, Francis, 301
Baie Comeau, Quebec,
and PCB blockade,

187–8; and PCB incin-
eration, 192
Barnard, Neil, 129
BASF, 323
Bauman, Dale, 125, 146
Baxter International:
breast implants, 100,
120
Bayer Aventis, 323
Baylis, Françoise, 333,
337
Beatty, Perrin, 274
beef: in Alberta, 259;
consumption, 230, 242,
244; international
inspection, 251. See also
BSE
beef, banning of, 237,
246, 250–1; Brazilian,
236; British, 7, 8–9;
Japanese, 236, 238–9;
from schools, 8, 9, 10
beef, exporting of: by
Canada, 234, 245–6,
259; by Japan, 244; by
U.S., 244, 259
beef, importing of, 237–9,
246, 250–1, 254,
256–7; from Brazil,
236; from Japan, 236,

238–9; from U.K., 233; from U.S., 256
behaviour: genetic modification, 332, 333, 335t; risk-taking, 317
Ben and Jerry's, 149
Berg, Paul, 154
Bernays, Edward, 228
biochemical individuality, 303
biodiversity, reduction in, 321
bioinformatics, 302
biological weapons. See bioweapons
Biologics and Genetic Therapies Directorate (BGTD), 312
biotechnology: controversial nature of, 154–5, 180–1; defined by Canadian Environmental Protection Act, 153–4; and genetic engineering 154–9; government bias towards, 159, 163–4; issues of public concern, 155–9, 172–9; risk communication on, 158, 163, 173, 175–9. See also genetically modified organisms (GMOs)
bioweapons, 325–7
Blackburn, George, 330–1
Blakemore, Colin, 9
blastocysts, 313
boll weevil 171
Bolton, Dan, 109
bovine somatotropin: see RBST
bovine spongiform encephalopathy: see BSE
Braley, Silas, 110
Brassica napas, 164. See also canola
Brassica rapa (B. campestris), 161–2. See also canola
breast-feeding, and PCBS, 186, 190–1, 199, 201–3, 207–8, 215

breast implants: history, 103–4
Briggs, Robert, 299
Bristol-Meyers Squibb: breast implants, 100, 120
British Petroleum, 290–1
Brody, Jane, 96
Broughton Island, 201–2, 204, 207
BSE (mad cow disease), 4, 32, 213, 216; and Agriculture and Agri-Food; Alberta inspections, 249; and animal feed, 248–9, 250, 258–9; animal-health risk, 251; annual incidence rates, 237–8; British response, 3–5, 6–16, 22–5; in Canada, 217, 229, 231–2; Canadian response, 17, 229, 231–3; and CFIA. See CFIA; compensation payments, 3; discovery, 5; in "downers," 256; economic risk, 248, 251, 259–60; E.U. response, 3, 13, 233; first (index) case, 234, 235, 250; in France, 238; human health risk, 251; hypothetical numerical prevalence, 253–4; international policy, 233; in Ireland, 237–8; in Japan, 238; luminescence immunoassay, 257; minimal versus negligible risk, 253–4, 260; "one cow and you're out," 233, 234, 243; in Portugal, 237; precautionary principle, 238; science versus policy, 245–8, 254–5, 257, 260–1; second case, 235, 252; surveillance for, 233, 246, 247–8, 253, 254–8; testing, 248, 249, 253, 255, 257–8; trans-

mission from cow to calf, 14; in U.K., 231, 237; U.S. response, 16–18. See also beef
BST: international studies, 124–6. See also RBST
Bt gene, 135, 324
Btt, 167, 170. See also Cry-3 genes
bubble baby syndrome, 312
Bureau of Veterinary Drugs (BVD), and RBST, 125–6, 140
Bush, George W., 289–90, 293
Byrd-Hagel Resolution, 293

calcium ion channels, 330
Calman, Sir Kenneth, 241, 245
Canadian Coalition for Responsible Government, 291
Canada Emissions Outlook (CEO), 277, 280–1
Canadian Cattlemen's Association (CCA), 395n69
Canadian Food Inspection Agency (CFIA). See CFIA
Canadian Manufacturers and Exporters, 274, 276, 278
Cancer Prevention Coalition (Chicago), 123
cannabinoid receptors (CB1s), 330–1
canola: and gene escape, 155, 160–6; transgenic varieties, 160–3; as weed, 165
carbon dioxide concentrations, 284
carbonomics, 278
Carson, Rachel, 56
Caulfield, Tim, 333, 337
cells: division of, 299; germline, 329; sex, 329; somatic nuclear cell

transplantation, 313; stem. *See* stem cells

Cellucci, Paul, 290

Centers for Disease Control, U.S. (CDC), 18, 49, 79, 89, 81, 91, 92–3

CFCS, 284

CFIA (Canadian Food Inspection Agency), 230, 232–3, 234, 238, 239, 240, 250, 256, 260

chloracne, 44, 46, 50, 56, 76, 183, 194

Chrétien, Jean, 271

chromosomes, 319–20

chronic wasting disease, 230

chymosin, 130, 135

CJD (Creutzfeld-Jakob Disease): causes of infection, 4, 9; media coverage, 8, 9, 10, 16, 18–19; new-variant, 230; occurrence rates, 4; recommendations for prevention, 12; transmission, 4, 9, 15, 230; victims, 7–8, 11–12, 16

Clarke, Graham, 21

climate change, 262; and Canada, 285–6, 295; consensus science and, 264, 293–4; costs of, 268, 273; economics of, 268, 273, 279–80, 294; emissions reductions and, 269–70, 292 (*see also* emissions reductions); GHGs and, 266; and industrialized West, 285–6; and Kyoto Protocol. *See* Kyoto Protocol; made-in-Canada approach, 286–9; national expert assessment, 265–6, 293, 294; Pascal's wager and, 267–8, 273; policy, 262, 294–5; time lags in response, 284–5

Climate Change Plan for Canada, 271–2, 279, 282

climate system: global, 268–9; stability versus instability of, 269

Clinton, Bill, 93, 94, 217

cloning, 313, 338: adult DNA, 313; of animals, 298–9; of humans, 299–300, 337, 338; mammalian, 298, 338; by nuclear transfer, 299–300; of sheep, 299; therapeutic, 313, 318, 333, 336t, 337

Cohen, Robert, 144–5

Collinge, John, 15, 20

Colorado Potato Beetle (CPB), 166, 168–9, 171

communication theory: encoding/decoding, 119; "hypodermic needle" model, 228; "magic seven" theory, 229

Comrie, Peter, 248

consensus science, 264, 265

corn: Bt, 324; hybrid varieties, 322

cotton, Bt-engineered, 171

Council of Canadians (COC), and RBST, 123–4, 139, 142, 143

Courtney, Diane, 41

Crick, Francis, 302

crops: genetically modified (GM), 308, 321; genetically uniform, 322; non-hybrid varieties, 322; pollen from, 232–4; seeds from. *See* seeds

Curry, David, 7

Crudwell, Lord Lucas, 8

Cry-3 gene, 167, 169–70

CWD (chronic wasting disease), 230

D'Aliesio, Renata, 238–9

daminozide. *See* Alar

Daubert v. Merrell Dow Pharmaceuticals Inc., 102

Dealler, Stephen, 13

Delta and Pine Land Company, 322

developing countries: emissions reductions in, 286; Kyoto Protocol and, 289–90, 293; seed buying in, 323–4

Dibb, Sue, 10

dioxins, 32, 214, 215, 216, 242n2; allowable daily intake, 50–1; animal study results, 50, 51–2; cause of virulence, 45; definition, 45; Environmental Protection Agency, 48, 51, 53, 54, 56, 58, 59, 60, 68, 246n49; and Environment Canada, 245n48; hormone mimicking, 43, 54, 55, 71; industrial incidents, 46, 47; "mega-ugly," 41, 42, 214; as pesticides, 56, 66; risks to wildlife, 54, 55, 73; sources of creation, 42, 45, 75; toxic effects on humans, 52–3, 54; "virtual elimination," 214, 247, 272n6, 269n55

diseases: cures for, 298; gene therapy, 311; genetic testing for, 307; pre-symptomatic treatments, 36

DNA: and chronological age, 200; crime scene testing for, 329; databases, 303, 307; flow of heredity information from, 304–5; identification of responders, 344t; microarray analysis, 305; sequencing, 302–3; shuffling, 314, 322

Doherr, Marcus, 249

Dolly (cloned sheep), 299, 300, 313

Donnelly, Aldyen, 275t

dopamine, 330–1
Dorrell, Stephen, 9, 12, 22–5
Dow Chemical Company, 44, 323
Dow Corning Corp. and silicone breast implants, 99–120; bankruptcy declaration, 99, 100, 120, 251n4; class-action litigation, 100, 120, 213; "dog study," 110–12, 113; "expert testimony" issue, 102; failure to communicate risks to patients, 105, 107–8, 114–16, 118; failure to conduct extensive risk research, 104–5, 116–17; fraud charges, 99; internal memos, 109; leakage or bleeding of implants, 105, 106–7, 109; media response, 102, 111; revision of decisions, 102–3; risk communication and management, analysis of, 100–1, 108–9, 114–18; victim settlements against 99–100, 252n5; warnings issued to surgeons, 105–6, 107. See also silicone breast implants
Downie, Jocelyn, 333, 337
Doyle, Michael, 92
Drexhage, John, 272, 280
drugs: adverse reactions to, 304; designer, 329–30; individualized, 306; hallucinogenic, 330
DuPont, 323
Durant, John, 154

E. (Escherichia) coli O157: cause of meat contamination, 80–1; causes of infection, 78, 82, 98; and FDA, 79, 81, 87; H7 food poisoning, 78, 79, 216; and Health Canada, 78, 79, 83; incidence rates, 78, 79, 85, 95–6; media coverage, 82–3, 84–5, 87, 88–9, 91, 93, 94–5; outbreaks, 78, 82, 84; percentage of meat contaminated, 81; person-to-person transmission, 82; in salami, 91–2; and U.S. Centers for Disease Control and Prevention (CDC), 79, 81, 92–3; and U.S. Department of Agriculture (USDA), 83–4, 85, 89, 92; and U.S. National Research Council, 84; victims, 77, 89, 93, 94, 96
Eli/Lilly: and RBST, 127, 138, 140, 143, 147
embryonic defects: gene therapy, 327–8, 334t
emissions: and carbon dioxide concentrations, 284; business-as-usual scenario, 280–1; intensity targets, 287; taxes on, 295
emissions reduction, 269–70; benefits from, 282; and climate change, 292; costs of, 273, 279–82, 285; in developing world, 286; economic instruments, 295; global coordination, 285–6, 287; in industrializing countries, 285–6; rate of, 284; targets, 280–1; technology transfer and, 286, 287; in U.S., 290
emissions trading, 271, 272, 281–2, 290: cap and trade scheme, 288–9; domestic, 289, 295; and environmental policy, 288; as flexible mechanism, 288; international, 287–8; as transfer of wealth, 287
endocrine disruptors, 61, 74, 215, 244n28. See also dioxins
endocytosis, 329
environmental risks, control of, 315
eosinophilia-myalgia syndrome (EMS), 174–5
Epstein, Samuel, 123, 124, 146
erythropoetin (Epo), 290
Espy, Mike, 87, 88, 89, 90
ETC group, 321–2
eugenics, 307–8
Evans, Brian, 258

Fagan, John, 174
feline spongiform encephalopathy, 6, 7, 230
Fifth Estate, 139, 140, 143, 150
Fischler, Franz, 15
Food and Water (Vermont), 123
food crops. See crops
food irradiation, 96
Foodmaker Inc., 86, 94, 96
food poisoning: costs, 79; incidence rates, 79; symptoms, 80, 89
foot and mouth disease, 259
Forbes, Dean, 77
Foreman, Carol Tucker, 91
Foundation on Economic Trends, 131, 132
Francis, Diane, 277
Franco, Don, 20
Frankenstein, 297–8

Gardener, W., 320–1
Gelsinger, Jesse, 311–12

Genbank, 303
gene enhancement, 309–10, 320–1, 335t; benefits, 332; social effects, 333; subversive uses, 329–32
Genentech Inc., 130, 134
genes, 302; allele frequencies, 321; alterations, 321; daughter, 314; defective, 311; epistatic interactions, 312; pleiotropic expression, 312; recombinase, 322; repressor, 322; splicing, 308; terminator, 321–2; toxin, 322
gene therapy, 296, 307–8, 310–13; benefits, 332, 335t; Biologics and Genetic Therapies Directorate (BGTD) and, 312; in Canada, 312; and CB1 receptors, 330; disease cures and, 311; forensic uses, 329; gene enhancement versus, 309; germline, 311, 332; Health Canada and, 312; health versus procreation in, 320; opiate receptors and, 330; PGD and, 327–8; and population growth, 331; pre-symptomatic, 334t; and recombination events, 328–9; and research granting agencies, 312; risks, 318, 335t; social effects, 328, 333; somatic, 311; subversive uses, 329–32; transformative nature, 319; in U.S., 311, 312
genetically engineered crops, 32–3, 133, 308, 321. See also crops
genetically modified organisms (GMOs), 154,

308–9; U.S. guidelines, 153
genetically modified plants (GMPs), 180
genetic engineering, 308, 340
genetics: benefits/risks array, 335–6t; defined, 302; extrinsic risks, 318, 331–2, 333; informed debate on, 338; intersection with other technologies, 331–2; intrinsic risks, 318, 332–3; precautionary approach, 338; public policy, 338; research, 298; transformative nature, 319
genetic screening, 332, 334t
genetic testing, 306, 307
genomes: defined, 302; engineering of, 301, 316–17; minimally necessary, 319
genomics: benefits/risks, 334t, 339; bioweapons and, 325–7; and concept of risk, 301–2; defined, 302; extrinsic risks, 307, 331–2, 333; intersection with other technologies, 331–2; intrinsic risks, 307, 332–3; policies, 338; risks, 318, 334t, 339; social effects, 301, 339
germline: cells, 329; engineering, 310, 333; gene therapy, 332
Gilbert, Walter, 302
Glickman, Dan, 94
g proteins, 330
greenhouse gases (GHGs), 266, 269, 291; climate forcing by, 292; economic costs of reductions, 293; emission reductions, 270–1, 283,

292 (see also emissions reductions); emission stabilization, 283
Greenpeace: and agricultural biotechnology, 224; and dioxins, 32, 42, 59–64, 66, 68, 69–70; and PCBs, 187
Groenewegen, Paul, 144–5
Grogan, Heidi, 17
growth hormones, 296
Gummer, John, 7, 9
Gurdon, John, 299
GURTS (Genetic Use Restriction Technologies), 322: human, 331; and population growth, 331; public backlash against, 324. See also T-GURTS; V-GURTS

hamburgers, minimum cooking temperatures, 81, 83, 86
Hansen, James, 284
harmful substances, exposure to, 262–3
Harvard Center for Risk Analysis (HCRA), 233, 253
Hazard Analysis Critical Control Points (HACCP), 20, 22, 83–4, 90, 91, 92, 94
Health Action Network, 143
Health Canada, BSE and, 232–3
health risks: control of, 315, 316
hemolytic uremic syndrome (HUS), 80
Hertzman, Clyde, 41
Hickman, Roy, 67
Hogg, Douglas, 10
Hollis vs. Dow Corning Corp., 118–20
Hopkins 1991, 99, 108, 109, 111, 113

Human Genome Project, 303, 319
hybrids: corn varieties, 322; crops, 322; fitness of, 320; human-animal, 307; inviable; 320; plant varieties, 298; sterile, 320

IGF-1 (insulin-like growth factor-1), 123, 125, 143, 145; and FDA, 145–6, 148; in mice/rats, 296, 309–10; and NAFTA, 149; and special interest groups, 143–4. See also RBST
industrialization, and climate change, 266–7
Intergovernmental Panel on Climate Change (IPCC), 264, 265, 271, 316
International Convention on Biological and Toxic Weapons, 405n50
Inuit: food supply contamination by PCBs, 198–209; and media reports, 215, 224
in vitro fertilization (IVF), 327

Jaccard, Mark, 280
Jack-in-the-Box restaurant, 77, 79, 81, 85–96
Jensen, Sören, 183
Johnson, Julius, 44
Jones, Gwilym, 10

Kalter, Robert, 134
Kamei, Yoshiyuki, 248
Karmali, Mohammed, 80
Kawano, Yutaka, 248
Kenora, Ontario, 184–5, 188, 191
Kerry, John, 293
Kessler, David, 20, 106, 111–12
"Kessler package," 111–12, 115
Kihm, Ulrich, 246

King, Thomas, 299
Kinner, Brianne, 94
Klein, Ralph, 235–6, 246, 247, 252, 257
kuru, 4
Kyoto Protocol, 262, 263, 264, 270; Alberta and, 236, 291; Bonn Accord, 271, 281; cap and trade mechanism, 289; Clean Development Mechanism, 271; climate change and. See climate change; Conference of the Parties (COP), 270–1, 281; costs of ratification, 273–9; and developing countries, 289–90, 293; and E.U., 292; and emissions reductions. See emissions reductions; flexibility mechanisms, 271, 281; and global coordination, 287; made-in-Canada approach versus, 289; Marrakesh Accord, 271, 281, 282; ratification of, 263, 264, 271, 273, 285, 291; Russia and, 281, 282; U.S. and, 281, 289–90

labelling, of genetically engineered food, 176–7, 221
Lacey, Richard, 13, 16
Laird, Melvin, 44
Land 'O Lakes Dairy, 127–8
Lang, Michelle, 238–9
Lang, Tim, 13
Lappe, Marc, 110
Large Final Emitters Group (LFEG), 272, 282
Laval University Hospital Community Health Department, 202–3
"learned intermediary" rule, 117–19
Lederberg, Joshua, 326

Life-Pharma companies, 323
L-tryptophan, 174
Lu Guangxiu, 337
Lyman, Howard, 16, 19

McBean, Gordon, 266
McBride, Brian, 144–5
McCain-Lieberman bill (U.S.), 292
McDonald's, 78, 81, 86, 136
McKitrick, Ross, 275
Maclean, David, 6, 7
Macmillan Bloedel, 60
MacRae, Rod, 141
mad cow disease. See BSE, CJD
Major, John, 10, 15
Major, Justice J.C., 119
Marleau, Diane, 124, 148
Marsden, James, 90, 92
Martin, Don, 250
Maxam, Allan, 302
Mayo Clinic, 101, 103
meat inspection and testing, 87, 89–90, 91
media: agenda-setting, 235–6; and anxiety, role of, 230; and believability, 229; on BSE, 236, 238–9, 245–6, 250; exemplars, effectiveness of, 229–30; and health issues, 233; narrow-casting, 229; propaganda analysis, 228; and public education, 230–3; and science information, 227, 230–3, 245–6
media analysis, 227, 228, 234; electronic data bases, 235; history of, 228–30; indexes, 235; manual searches, 235; quantitative data analysis, 235
"mega-reg," 92, 93
Mendel, Gregor, 302
Meselson, Matthew, 58

messenger RNA (mRNA),
350
milk, cultural value, 220
molecular genetic engi-
neering. *See* RBST
Monsanto Canada, 213,
170–1; allegations of
bribery over RBST, 144;
and RBST, 127, 138–9,
140, 142, 143, 150–1
Monsanto Chemical, 190
Monsanto Corp., 220–1;
and GM crops, 322,
323; New Leaf potato,
135; and RBST, 126,
130, 134, 139, 143;
and sterile seeds, 324;
and terminator gene
patent, 321
mousepox, 327
Mullholland, Ross, 44
Murphy, Michael, 274
muscle-wasting diseases,
296, 310

nanotechnology, 328,
335t
National Academy of
Sciences (NAS), 294
National Breast Implant
Task Force, 106
National Center for Bio-
technology Informa-
tion (NCBI), 404n24
National Climate Change
Process, 279
National Research
Council, 241
Nelkin, Dorothy, 151
Nole, Michael, 77, 89
Novartis, 324
nuclear power: controls
over weapons, 320–1;
risks, 242; U.S. Nuclear
Regulatory Commis-
sion, 242; waste, 35, 37,
217
nuclear transfer, 299–300
nucleotide bases, 302
Nugent, Robert, 86
Nunavik, health studies,
200, 203

Nunavimmiut (northern
Quebec), health
studies, 200–1, 203
NVCJD disease, 11–12, 15,
212. *See also* CJD

obesity, 330–1
occupational risks, 316
Odwalla Inc., 78, 96–7
offal: processing, 5, 13;
use as feed supplement,
7, 13, 16, 17–20, 22
OIE (l'Office interna-
tional des épizooties),
237, 252, 260
opiate receptors, 329–30
ornithine transcarboxy-
lase deficiency (OTCD),
311
ozone thinning, 284

Packer, Richard, 13
Parker, Allen, 143
Pascal's wager, 267–8, 273
PCBs (Polychlorinated
biphenyls), 32, 45, 46,
47, 182–209, 215, 216;
carcinogenic potential,
193, 195; chemical
composition, analysis,
188–9; contamination
levels, 190–1, 269n54;
disposal, 184, 193,
196–8, 269n55,
270n64, n65; early
concerns over, 183;
human body burdens,
190, 206; impact on
aboriginal peoples,
198–209; incineration
units, 192, 196–8;
inventory estimates,
190; Kenora spill, 184–
5, 188, 191; media
coverage, 193–4, 205,
208–9, 265n15–18;
properties, 183–4, 190;
regulation, 186, 191–3,
197–8; risk informa-
tion vacuum, 186, 193–
6, 204–9; St-Basile-le-
Grand fire, 185–6, 192,

193; toxicity, 183, 189,
267n22; uses, 182–3;
264n2, 268n50
Pembina Institute, 277,
287, 290
pesticides, 56, 84, 217
Peterson, Bob, 265, 275,
277
Pharmacia, 321
pharmacogenics, 303–4,
334t
pharmacogenomics, 338
plants, reproduction of,
298. *See also* crops
"platform of life," 319
pluripotency, 313–14
PNTs (plants with novel
traits), regulation, 155
Polly (transgenic sheep),
299
polymerase chain reac-
tion, 90
potatoes: Bt-engineered,
167–71, 176; New Leaf,
168, 170
preimplantation genetic
diagnostics (PGD),
327–8
prenatal diagnostics,
334t
Prionics AG, 257
prions, 5–6, 13–14, 20,
230–1, 232, 258
proteins, heredity infor-
mation and, 304–5
proteomics, 303, 306,
334t
Prusiner, Stanley, 5, 230,
258
public relations, 228
pulp mills, 60, 72
Pure Food Campaign,
132–3
PVC (polyvinyl chloride),
61, 69–70

QRA. See risk assessment:
quantitative

*Rachel's Environment and
Health Weekly*, 145–6
racial profiling, 307

rBGH (recombinant bovine growth hormone). *See* rBST

rBST (recombinant bovine somatotropin), 123–52, 220–1; and breast cancer, 140; consumer studies, 127; and Dairy Farmers of Canada, 136; economic issue, 131, 135; and FDA, 125–6, 132, 136, 137, 217; and Health Canada, 125, 126, 137–9, 147, 148; herd management, 150; and mad cow disease, 140, 141; mastitis, 132, 141; media coverage (Canada), 134–52; media coverage (U.S.), 123, 125, 130–4, 144–6, 149–62; moratorium, Canada, 124, 126, 136– 8, 143, 149; moratorium, U.S., 137; National Dairy Council (Canada), 123–4, 136, 142, 148; as non-tariff trade barrier, 149–50; and PCBS, 143; Toronto Food Policy Council, 143; and U.S. Dairy Coalition, 146; and U.S. Department of Agriculture, 217; and U.S. International Dairy Foods Assn (IDFA), 133; and U.S. National Institutes of Health, 126; and U.S. National Milk Board, 133, 148; and U.S. Office of Technology Assessment, 150. *See also* IGFI-1, BST, Monsanto Canada, Monsanto Corp.

refugia, 169–71

Reno, Janet, 90

rice-oil disease, 46, 47

Rifkin, Jeremy, 17, 131–2, 135, 146

risk: of action versus inaction, 267–8; agenda setting, 42; amplification, 33; battles over, 316; catastrophic, 243; classification, 241, 243, 245; concept of, and genomics, 301–2; and consensus science, 264; distribution of, 316; domains, 317; and domination over nature, 301; estimates, 212; negligible, 232, 233–4, 241, 242; negligible versus low, 230, 232–3; occupational, 316; order of magnitude difference, 243; outcomes and, 301; probability versus consequence, 240; ranking of, 243; reduction, 216; scenarios, 268, 294; sensitive, 339; and uncertainties, 301; voluntary versus involuntary, 29

risk assessment: characterizing hazards, 218, 315; and consequences, 241–3; "expert" versus "public," 26–30, 34, 35–6, 124, 265–6; as forecasting, 262–3; formula, 240, 243; frequency versus consequences, 241, 243–4; low-probability, high-consequence, 242, 243; qualitative/quantitative, 301; quantitative, 28, 35, 240; and science, 246; zero, 241

risk communication, 26–40; defined, 33–4; diagnostic for failures, 27, 38–9; government responsibility, 215–16, 218, 223–4, 229–30, 232, 245; industry, 217–19; and the Internet, 220, 224; and lifestyle choices, 27–9; and lobbying, 219; and media, 31, 39, 151–2; as public engagement, 331, 338; and public panic, 229–30; regulatory agencies, 215–16; relation to risk management, 224–5, 234–5; research, 34–6; and science, 150; three phases, 35–8, 211–12; trust, 212, 213, 214; wording of, 230

risk control: and "no-risk" messages, 223; precautionary, 332; and public education, 222– 3; role of science, 214, 220–3; step-wise procedure, 315; versus risk elimination, 216

risk controversy: analysis methodology, 124

risk factors: and adverse outcomes, 315–16, 317; communication of, 331; intrinsic versus extrinsic, 318; risk-taking behaviour, 317; for technologies, 318

risk information vacuum, 31–4, 214–15, 226; costs, 213; and dioxins, .42; and public policy, 31

risk management: international collaboration, 315; and language, 26–30, 234; precautionary mode, 315, 332, 340; purpose of, 315; and science, 35, 264; and social consensus, 29, 30, 37; and technological innovations, 314–15; and trust, 30, 36–8

risk perception: and media, 227, 228–9, 233–5

Ritter, Len, 140

RNA (ribonucleic acid), 304–5
Roth, William, 94
Roulet, Nigel, 266
Rowe, Verald K., 44
Royal Society of Canada, 294
Royal Society (U.K.), 294
Rural Advancement Foundation International (RAFI), 321–2

Safe, Stephen, 52, 194
Safe Food Coalition, 91
St-Basile-le-Grand, Quebec, 185–6, 192, 193
Sanger, Frederick, 302
Schulz, Karl, 46
science writing, 230–3; relation to research funding, 231–3
scientific method, 264–5
scrapie, 4, 230
seeds: antibiotics and, 322, 323; sterile, 321–2, 324–5; suicide, 325; terminator genes and, 321–2
Seveso, 49–50, 53, 57
sex cells, 329
Shalala, Donna, 20
sheep: anthrax tests on, 325–6; cloning, 299
Shelley, Mary, 297–8, 340
silicone breast implants, 32, 215, 255n43; Canadian legal suits, 100, 118; connective-tissue disease, 252n10, n19; fibrous capsule formations, 106–7; immune system diseases, 100–5, 107–8, 110–12, 113, 114–15, 120, 253n21; Mayo Clinic Studies, 101–2, 103; moratoriums (FDA), 99, 112, 255n43; moratoriums, Health Canada, 112; physiological problems,

107; rupturing, 106, 254n28, n29; and U.S. FDA, 102, 103–4, 106–7, 111–12, 115; warnings to surgeons, 253n26, 30. See also Dow Corning Corp. and silicone breast implants
Sinclair, Upton, 95
SNPs (single nucleotide polymorphisms), 304, 309, 312, 334t
Society of Environmental Toxicology and Chemistry (SETAC), 265
somatic nuclear cell transplantation, 313
Soulsby, Lord of Swaffam Prior, 13
Spemann, Hans, 298–9
Spock, Benjamin, 129
spongiform encephalopathies, 14, 214. See also BSE, CJD, scrapie, feline spongiform encephalopathy
Steltenpohl, Greg, 97
stem cell research: 313–14, 336t, 337, 338; embryonic, 314; risk factors, 318
Stern lawsuit 1984, 99, 104, 109–11, 113, 117, 251n1
stigmatization, 42
sulphur dioxide, 288
Suzuki Foundation, 277
Swan Hills, Alberta, 192
Sweeney, Lee, 296, 310
Swerdlow, David, 91
Syngenta, 323, 324
synthetic pathogens, 314

Tabuns, Peter, 137
Taylor, Michael, 90–1
technological innovations: in Canada versus U.S., 290; convergence of, 336t, 338; cycle of, 297; extrinsic versus intrinsic risk factors, 318

telomeres, 200
terminator patents, 324
T-GURTS, 322–3
Third Assessment Report (TAR), 264
3-M Company (Minnesota Mining and Manufacturing): breast implants, 100, 120
Times Beach, Missouri, 48, 49, 56–7, 217
Tipton, E. Linwood, 133
tobacco, 316, 317
tobacco-related fatalities, 28
tomatoes, genetically engineered, 128; Flavr Savr tomato, 176
Tomlinson, Sir Bernard, 9
Toronto Board of Health, and rBST, 138
Toronto Food Policy Council, 138, 141
Tour de France (1998), 309
transcript profiling, 305
transcriptomics, 303, 304–5
transcriptosomes, 305, 334t
transgenics, 308
transmissible spongiform encephalopathies (TSEs), 230
Tschirley, Fred, 44
2,4,5-trichlorophenol (2,4,5-T), 44–6, 48, 56, 58, 67, 243n6. See also dioxins

Vanclief, Lyle, 235–6, 246, 247–8
Ventner, Craig, 319
verotoxin, 78
verotoxogenic E. coli (VTECH), 78–82, 84, 90, 94, 96–8. See also E. coli 0157:H7
V-GURTS, 322, 323
Vons Inc., 86

Watson, James, 302
Watson, Robert, 271

Weaver, Andrew, 266
Weber, Gary, 19
Weissmann, Charles, 6, 15
Westaway, David, 394n65
Weyant, John, 279
Wigle, Randall, 282
Willadsen, Steen, 299
Williams, Roger, 303
Willis, Norman, 21
Wilmut, Ian, 299

Winfrey, Oprah, 18
Winter Olympic Games
  (Innsbruck, 1964),
  309
World Wildlife Fund, 277

X-Files, 144
x-linked severe combined
  immunodeficiency
  disease (x-scid), 312

xenotransplantation, 308,
  318, 336t

Yusho rice-oil incident,
  46–8, 183. See also rice-
  oil disease

Zeneca, 324
Zerr, Inga, 14
Ziman, John, 265